McGraw Hill

TEAS
REVIEW

McGraw Hill

TEAS REVIEW

Fourth Edition

Wendy Hanks

New York Chicago San Francisco Athens London Madrid
Mexico City Milan New Delhi Singapore Sydney Toronto

1 2 3 4 5 6 7 8 9   LHS   28 27 26 25 24 23

ISBN   978-1-265-67359-8
MHID   1-265-67359-4

e-ISBN   978-1-265-67738-1
e-MHID   1-265-67738-7

TEAS is a trademark of Assessment Technologies Institute™ LLC, which was not involved in the production of, and does not endorse, this product.

McGraw Hill products are available at special quantity discounts for use as premiums and sales promotions, or for use in corporate training programs. To contact a representative, please visit the Contact Us pages at www.mhprofessional.com.

McGraw Hill is committed to making our products accessible to all learners. To learn more about the available support and accommodations we offer, please contact us at accessibility@mheducation.com. We also participate in the Access Text Network (www.accesstext.org), and ATN members may submit requests through ATN.

Contents

McGraw Hill

TEAS REVIEW

Introduction

If you're applying to health science school and you've picked up a copy of this book, chances are you're already familiar with the ATI Test of Essential Academic Skills (TEAS) and have decided you'd like help with reviewing what's on the test before taking the exam. This book focuses on just that: content review and review questions. Inside, you'll see content review regarding the major topics on all four subjects tested on the ATI TEAS, hundreds of review questions to help reinforce your skills, and a full-length practice test.

Before we begin, let's take a look at the subjects you'll encounter on the TEAS. We'll also make some recommendations regarding how to use this book for optimal results.

TEAS OVERVIEW

The Test of Essential Academic Skills is a test administered to health science school candidates to test exactly what the name implies: essential academic skills. These are fundamental skills that are considered to be required for success in health science school. The skills tested fall into four subject categories: Reading, Mathematics, Science, and English and Language Usage. You will see them on the TEAS in that order. The TEAS test has four sections, as described in the table below:

Subject	Number of Questions	Time Allowed
Reading	45	55 minutes
Mathematics	38	57 minutes
Science	50	60 minutes
English and Language Usage	37	37 minutes
Total	170	209 minutes

Of the 170 questions on the test, 20 questions are experimental test items that are not scored. There are six experimental questions on the Reading section, four on the Mathematics section, six on the Science section, and four on the English and Language Usage section. These questions are scattered throughout the section and you will not know which questions are experimental. The Reading section of the test covers three main areas: main ideas and supporting information, passage organization, and synthesis of information. Main idea questions test your understanding of what you read when reviewing various forms of written communication (such as academic passages, articles, advertisements, and e-mails) and graphic sources (such as maps, labels, diagrams, and other resources). Passage organization questions test your understanding of structure, purpose, and meaning. Synthesis questions test your ability to evaluate, compare, and contrast.

The Mathematics section of the test covers four subjects: numbers and operations, algebraic applications, data interpretation, and measurement. Numbers and operations questions test your ability to perform basic math and to solve problems involving fractions, ratios, proportions, and percentages. Algebraic applications questions test your ability to solve problems involving an unknown quantity. Data interpretation questions require you to answer questions based on information obtained from graphs and charts. Measurement questions require you to measure various dimensions and to convert measurements from one form to another.

The Science section of the test covers four main areas: human anatomy and physiology, biology, chemistry, and scientific reasoning. Anatomy and physiology questions test your knowledge of specific body systems. Biology questions test your knowledge of macromolecules, cells, DNA and RNA, and genetics. Chemistry questions test your understanding of the periodic table, the properties and states of matter, and chemical reactions. Scientific reasoning questions test your understanding of the scientific method and principles underlying scientific inquiry.

Finally, the English and Language Usage section of the test covers three subcategories. The first assesses your knowledge of the rules of spelling, capitalization, and punctuation. The second subcategory tests your understanding of grammar and the process of composition. The third English subcategory tests your ability to determine the meanings of words based on their context and your knowledge of roots, prefixes, and suffixes.

QUESTION FORMATS

The majority of the TEAS exam is made up of multiple-choice questions, which almost everyone has experienced at one point or another. About 15% of the questions on the test are in technology-enhanced formats, which may take some getting used to. Here is what to expect:

Multi-select: Multi-select questions look very similar to multiple-choice questions, but you will select *more* than one answer choice. You must select all of the correct answers (and no incorrect answers) to receive credit on these questions—there is no partial credit.

Here is an example:

Which of the following are functions of connective tissue? Select all that apply.

- protect organs
- remove toxins from the blood
- store fat
- transport nutrients
- control the level of white blood cells

For this question, you would select three of the five choices:

- protect organs
- store fat
- transport nutrients

Fill in the blank: This is a question type that is familiar to most people. On these questions, you will be asked a question and no answer choices will be provided. You will simply type the correct answer in a box on the screen. Expect to see several of these questions in the mathematics section. Always read the question carefully because you may be required to round a number to a particular decimal place or enter your answer in some other specific manner.

Here is an example:

How many cups are in four gallons?

To answer this question, you have to click with your mouse in the box and type in your answer. In this case, you would enter the number 64 since there are 64 cups in four gallons.

Ordering: Ordering questions ask you to put a series of items or steps in the correct order. You will be presented with several items or steps in boxes on the left side of your screen, and you will use the computer mouse to select one of the boxes and drag it into the correct position in an empty box on the right. You can move the items around as much as you like until you have all the items in the proper order, and then you will submit your response. If any item is out of order, the question is scored as incorrect—there is no partial credit. If you use a computer, you are probably familiar with the concept of "dragging" and "dropping." These questions use that skill.

Here is an example:

Put the steps of the scientific method (shown on the left below) into the correct order in the box on the right.

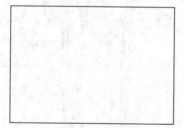

| gather data |
| draw conclusions |
| define a question |
| make predictions |
| analyze data |

For this question, you will select one of the item boxes on the left and drag it into the empty box on the right. Then select another item on the left and drag it into the box on the right, either above or below the first one you put there. Continue this process until all the items on the left are in the correct order on the right. The completed box should look like this:

| define a question |
| make predictions |
| gather data |
| analyze data |
| draw conclusions |

For ordering questions in this book, you can just write the items or steps in the correct order.

Hot spot: Hot spot items require you to indicate points on a drawing, chart, table, or graph by clicking with your mouse on the correct points. Hot spot items may have two to five clickable areas.

Here is an example:

Click on the diagram below to identify the sacrum.

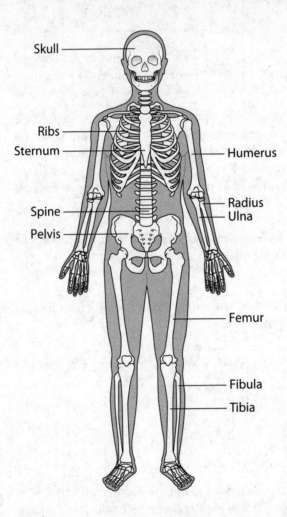

To answer this question, you have to click with your mouse on the correct point on the diagram. In this case, you would click on the bone at the base of the spine in the middle of the pelvis. For hot spot questions in this book, you can circle the spot you wish to indicate with your pen or pencil.

HOW TO USE THIS BOOK

The content review presented in this book does not include every possible topic that might be tested on the TEAS. Instead it presents a review of important topics you are likely to see on the test, and it explains different question types you may encounter.

Sometimes understanding what a question is asking for can be key to identifying the correct answer. In the Reading sections, for instance, you'll see some questions that ask about details from the passage and other questions that ask you to draw conclusions based on information given in the passage. The answer to a detail question will *always* be given right in the passage, and the answer to a conclusions question will *never* be stated directly. Just knowing what to expect on these different question types can help you choose the correct answer.

While understanding the question types is important, there's no substitute for learning the content actually covered on the exam. This book is chock-full of relevant content, but how you choose to learn that content will depend on where the gaps in your knowledge lie—and the time you have to prepare.

If you feel fairly confident about certain sections of the test, you can focus your study on just those topics or sections that you feel are your weak areas. This approach works best if you have limited time to study as well. However, if you'd like to brush up on the content of the test as a whole, you can review each chapter of the book in its entirety. This "whole book" approach requires time and will work best if you have ample time in your study schedule to prepare for the test. It also has another distinct advantage: in addition to helping you improve your weak areas, it can help you strengthen the areas that are your strong suits. This way, you can pick up more points in the areas that you're already successful in to help boost your score.

TEST INFORMATION AND REGISTRATION

The TEAS is administered by ATI Nursing Education. To register for the test or to obtain more information, contact ATI at:

ATI Nursing Education

11161 Overbrook Road

Leawood, KS 66211

(800) 667-7531

www.atitesting.com/teas

comments@atitesting.com

For further practice on this exam we recommend *McGraw Hill Education: 5 TEAS Practice Tests.*

TEST-TAKING TIPS

Use Process of Elimination

The majority of the questions on the TEAS are multiple-choice questions with four answer choices. That means the correct answer is right in front of you. All you have to do is pick it out from among three incorrect choices. For most questions, even if you do not know the answer, you will be able to rule out one or two of the wrong answers. Use the process of elimination to help you make an educated guess. The more answers you rule out, the easier it is to make the right choice. Guessing well is a skill that comes with practice, so incorporate it into your preparation program.

Answer Every Question

There is no penalty for choosing a wrong answer. Therefore, if you do not know the answer to a question, you have nothing to lose by guessing. Make sure that you answer every question. If you see that you are running out of time, make sure to enter an answer for the questions that you have not tackled. With luck, you may be able to pick up a few extra points, even if your guesses are totally random. By the way, if you **are** randomly guessing, it is statistically slightly better to always choose the same answer choice on a multiple-choice question; for example, if you are running out of time with three questions left, choose Choice D on all three of them. No letter is better than another—just choose the same one each time.

Answer Easy Questions First, Then Go Back and Do Hard Ones

Keep in mind that each section of the TEAS has a specific time limit. You cannot go back to a section after you have completed it, but within each of the four sections, you can skip hard questions and do the easier ones first. After you've picked up all those easy points, you can go back and do the harder questions. There are three reasons why you should do this:

1. Every question counts the same. Spend your time answering the easier questions, where you are sure to pick up points. Work on harder ones after that until you finish or run out of time.

2. Later in the test, you might come to a question or a set of answer choices that jogs your memory and helps you go back and answer a question you skipped.

3. Answering easier questions first builds your confidence. It will help you get into a good rhythm. When you go back to a question you skipped, you may find that it is not as hard as you first thought.

Read Each Question and Answer Choice Carefully

Often, when the test-makers are designing questions, they will use distractor answers that use familiar words or phrases. If you are moving quickly or not totally paying attention, you might be tempted to pick one of these choices. A question might ask you which answer choice is NOT true, and if you are going too quickly, you might pick a choice that is true. That's why it is also a good practice to reread the question before you finalize your answer choice. If possible, answer the question in your own words before you even look at the answer choices. Pay attention to the wording of fill-in-the-blank questions. They may require a specific unit or decimal place for the answer, so read carefully.

Trust Your Instincts

Have you ever struggled to choose between two answers, picked one, changed your mind and changed your answer, and then found out that the correct answer was the one you chose the first time?! It usually is better to trust your instincts and stay with your first answer. If you overthink the question, you are likely to get it wrong.

Watch the Clock, but Don't Panic

While you practice for each section of the TEAS, work on your pacing. Since there are so many questions to answer in a short time period, you are not going to have a lot of time to spare. Check yourself at 10- or 15-minute intervals using your watch or timer to make sure that you are on track to answer all of the questions within the time allowed. Don't spend too much time on any one question. If you find yourself stuck for more than a minute, move on and come back to it at the end. If you pace yourself and keep track of your progress, you should have enough time to complete each section of the exam. If you do find yourself running out of time, do not panic. There is no guessing penalty, so enter answers to all the remaining questions. If you are able to make educated guesses, you will probably be able to improve your score. However, even random guesses may help you pick up a few points.

If You Have Extra Time, Check Your Work

If you have time left over at the end of a section, go back and check your work. If you flagged any questions because you were not sure about your answer, go back and try to answer them now. Maybe you will have remembered something that will help you. Resist the urge to second-guess too many of your answers, however, because this may lead you to change an already correct answer to a wrong one. Remember to trust your instincts!

ON THE DAY OF THE ACTUAL EXAM

What to Expect on Test Day

- The staff at the testing center will check you in (bring your photo ID!), take you to the testing room, and direct you to a seat.
- The test proctor will give you scratch paper to use during the test. You cannot use the scratch paper before the exam or during the break, and you must return the scratch paper to the proctor at the end of your test session.
- You will have access to a four-function calculator to use on the test. Computer-based exams have a built-in, on-screen calculator. If you are taking a paper exam, the testing center will provide you with a calculator. You may not bring your own calculator.
- After the Mathematics session, you may take a 10-minute break that does not count against your total testing time. During the break, you may not access any personal items. If you need to leave your seat at any time other than during the break, raise your hand and let the proctor know. The timer for the exam section you are working on will not stop and you cannot make up lost time, so only do this in an emergency.
- The proctors in the room are monitoring testers for odd or disruptive behavior. Do not be disruptive to other testers and do not attempt to engage in any misconduct. If you do, you will be asked to leave the testing center and your exam will not be scored.
- If you have a technical issue with your computer during the exam, raise your hand and let the proctor know.
- Any testing room complaints should be reported to the proctor before you leave the room on exam day.

What to Bring on Test Day

- **Photo ID:** A driver's license, passport, or green card. **You will not be admitted to the test if you do not have your ID or if your ID does not meet the following requirements**: government-issued, current photograph, examinee signature, and permanent address. A credit card photo, temporary license, or student ID does not meet these criteria.
- **Your ATI log-in information:** If you are taking the online version of the ATI TEAS Exam, you will need to have created a student account at www.atitesting.com prior to test day (you will most likely have done this to register for the exam) and have your log-in information with you. The testing center cannot look up this information for you.
- **Pencils:** Two sharpened No. 2 pencils with attached erasers. No other writing instruments are allowed.
- **Anything required by your school:** Please refer to the confirmation e-mail you received following your ATI TEAS registration. Some schools require additional items be brought to the exam.

What NOT to Bring on Test Day

Leave these items at home or in your car. They are not allowed in the testing room.

- **Extra clothing or accessories:** Do not bring a jacket, coat, hat, and so on. There may not be anywhere to store these items, so do not wear anything you might take off. Discretionary allowances are made for religious apparel and all apparel is subject to inspection by the proctor.
- **Personal items:** Do not bring a purse, computer bag, backpack, or sunglasses. All you should have with you is your ID, pencils, and possibly your car keys.
- **Electronics:** Do not bring a phone, a calculator, or even a digital watch. For real.
- **Food or drink:** Do not bring a snack. Food or drink is only permitted as a documented, medically necessary item.

Finally, Stay Calm

You are as prepared as you are ever going to be, so be calm. There is no point in panicking. Focus your energy on being careful in answering questions and marking your answer choices.

If you see a question that is particularly difficult, do not panic. Take a nice, slow breath and remember that 20 of the 170 questions do not count and tell yourself that the question you are looking at may not count. Even if it does count, telling yourself that it doesn't and remaining calm gives you a better chance of answering it correctly!

PART I

READING

TEAS Reading questions test two different types of comprehension: paragraph and passage comprehension, and informational source comprehension. Paragraph and passage comprehension questions are accompanied by a single paragraph or an entire passage. These questions test your ability to understand the text that you have read. Informational source comprehension questions often include figures, such as maps or graphs, and excerpts from other resources, such as outlines, directions, or ingredient lists.

The questions that you'll see on the TEAS can be grouped into different question types, depending on the issues they address. They range in scope from overarching, big-picture questions to questions that test more in-depth detail.

CHAPTER 1

Text Structures and Writing Styles

Identifying text structures and writing styles questions may ask about the type of writing that a passage represents, the author's rhetorical intent in writing a passage, and the type of text structure reflected in a passage.

TYPES OF WRITING

Passages may represent four different **types of writing:** technical, narrative, persuasive, and expository.

- **Technical writing** conveys complex or difficult subject matter in a specific manner with great accuracy.
- **Narrative writing** conveys a series of events.
- **Persuasive writing** attempts to convince the reader of a particular point of view.
- **Expository writing** describes a topic and may even review its features in detail.

The questions that accompany the following two passages ask you to identify the types of writing reflected in the passage:

Maslow's hierarchy postulates that human beings must have certain basic needs met before they can realize their potential by mastering more sophisticated and complex abilities. For example, people must be confident that they have reliable sources of food, clothing, and shelter before they can start to focus on needs such as being loved. This belief system serves as the foundation for early education programs like Head Start.

> The above passage is reflective of which of the following types of writing?
>
> A) Narrative
> B) Persuasive
> C) Technical
> D) Expository

The correct answer is **D**. This passage is an example of expository writing, which describes a subject and explains its features. Choice A is incorrect because narrative writing tells a story or relates a series of events. Choice B is incorrect because persuasive writing attempts to persuade the reader to accept a particular point of view or take a certain action. Choice C is incorrect because technical writing explains highly complex topics in an accurate and often formally structured manner.

Let's look at another example.

Dear Dean Jeffries,

I am writing to oppose the imposition of an administrative fee for the use of the main student parking lot located at 765 Liberty Street on the west campus. This administrative fee would be detrimental for students and for the university. The student parking lot is currently used by students who live off-campus and must park their cars in order to attend school. Since on-campus housing is highly limited and there is no public transportation located close to campus, most students must live off-campus and must drive or share rides with others, thus necessitating parking when they come to school. The main parking lot is the most convenient to campus buildings, so it attracts the greatest amount of traffic. Imposing a fee for the use of this lot would pose a financial hardship for many off-campus students, who are already paying higher rental fees for apartments outside the campus housing system.

The fee would also have a negative impact on the university, if imposed as proposed. The fee is higher than parking fees found at any other local college or university. Students who have to incur substantial costs for parking might tend to drive less to school, missing more classes and performing less well. This could affect the university's reputation, since poorly performing students are less likely to attract top faculty to the teaching staff. Students might also choose to transfer to other schools where on-campus housing is more widely available, thus avoiding parking costs altogether and increasing enrollment at local competitor colleges. This could further negatively affect the university's standing among top programs in the area. In sum, the parking fee is a poor idea and would not serve the interests of university students or the school.

Sincerely,

Rolinda Wallach

The above letter is reflective of which of the following types of writing?

A) Expository
B) Persuasive
C) Narrative
D) Technical

The correct answer is **B**. The author's intent is to persuade. Choice A is incorrect because the author does not simply give information; she also requests a change in behavior. Choice C is incorrect because the author does not relay a story or describe a series of events. Choice D is incorrect because the writing addresses a parking issue and is not technical in nature.

RHETORICAL INTENT

Closely related to the four types of writing is the concept of rhetorical intent. An author's **rhetorical intent** may be to inform, to persuade, to entertain, or to express feelings.

- **Informational writing** is designed to give the reader information about a particular topic.
- **Persuasive writing** attempts to convince the reader to accept a perspective or to take a certain action.
- **Entertainment writing** is designed to provide entertainment.
- **Expressive writing** serves the purpose of conveying the author's feelings or bringing up certain feelings in the reader.

The questions that accompany the following two passages ask you to identify the author's rhetorical intent:

Maslow's hierarchy postulates that human beings must have certain basic needs met before they can realize their potential by mastering more sophisticated and complex abilities. For example, people must be confident that they have reliable sources of food, clothing, and shelter before they can start to focus on needs such as being loved. This belief system serves as the foundation for early education programs like Head Start.

Which of the following is the author's intent in the passage?

A) To inform
B) To entertain
C) To persuade
D) To express feelings

The correct answer is **A**. The author's intent is to inform. Choice B is incorrect because the author does not attempt to engage the reader in an entertaining or captivating manner. Choice C is incorrect because the author does not make an argument and attempt to convince the reader to believe a particular idea or take a certain action. Choice D is incorrect because the author does not attempt to express feelings or bring out emotions in the reader; instead, the passage is written from an objective, neutral perspective.

Now consider this example:

To All Restaurant Staff:

It has come to my attention that some employees have been using the kitchen's silver serving platters to serve large parties when the porcelain serving platters are all in use. This causes a problem with serving some of our VIP guests, who may arrive unexpectedly or with short notice. Please refrain from using the silver serving platters unless they have been specifically designated to serve a reserved party. The list of reservations can be found on the back bulletin board for any given night; silver service will be marked next to a reservation with a circled S.

Additional porcelain serving platters are currently on order to ensure that we have adequate servingware to accommodate all of our guests.

Thank you for helping us to serve our VIP patrons with the level of professionalism they have come to know and expect.

George Gario,

Proprietor

Which of the following is the author's intent in the memo?

A) To entertain
B) To describe
C) To persuade
D) To express feelings

The correct answer is **C**. The author's intent is to persuade. Choice A is incorrect because the author does not attempt to engage the reader in an entertaining or captivating manner. Choice B is incorrect because the author does not simply give information without also requesting a change in behavior. Choice D is incorrect because while the author does hope to appeal to the reader's feelings, he does this only for the purpose of moving the reader to action.

TEXT STRUCTURE

Along with reflecting four different types of writing and four rhetorical intentions, TEAS Reading passages may reflect five **types of text structure**: sequence, problem-solution, comparison-contrast, cause-effect, and description.

- **Sequence text structures** convey ideas in order or describe steps in a process.
- **Problem-solution text structures** present a problem and provide a solution to solve that problem.
- **Comparison-contrast text structures** discuss the similarities and differences between two or more elements.
- **Cause-effect text structures** explain an outcome as the result of a particular cause, or they show how one factor leads to a certain outcome.
- **Description text structures** merely describe topics or events in a general way.

The following examples ask you to identify the text structures in each passage.

Athletes are extremely aware of how physical motion and its properties can affect the human body as well as the outcomes of competitions. Figure skating, for example, involves concentric motion for spins. Skaters learn how to use their arms to bring in their centers of gravity. In the same way that runners adopt a certain leg stance or swimmers use their arms to move quickly through the water, skaters also use their knowledge of physics to improve their skating.

Which of the following text structures is used in the last sentence of the above passage?

A) Comparison-contrast
B) Cause-effect
C) Sequence
D) Problem-solution

The correct answer is **A**. Comparison-contrast text structures highlight similarities and differences between or among entities. Choice B is incorrect because a cause-effect text structure focuses on how one factor or variable produces a specific outcome. Choice C is incorrect because a sequence text structure describes steps in a process or presents information in chronological form. Choice D is incorrect because a problem-solution text structure presents a problem and then provides a solution to that problem.

Consider this next passage:

In the animal kingdom, many symbiotic relationships exist between two species that take actions known to be mutually beneficial for both parties. In the water, clownfish have such a relationship with sea anemones. The fish are one of the only species that can swim unharmed in the anemone's waving tentacles, as typically the tentacles would sting any animal that swam near it. However, the clownfish is immune to the sting of the tentacles and is therefore protected by them; in return, its presence helps the anemone stay clean, avoid attack by parasites, and remain free from infection.

Which of the following text structures is used to organize the above passage?

A) Description
B) Sequence
C) Comparison-contrast
D) Problem-solution

The correct answer is **A**. In this passage, the clownfish and sea anemone's relationship is described. Choice B is incorrect because a sequence text structure describes steps in a process or presents information in chronological form. Choice C is incorrect because comparison-contrast text structures highlight similarities and differences between or among entities. Choice D is incorrect because a problem-solution text structure presents a problem and then provides a solution to that problem.

Let's look at one final example related to text structure:

Arguably, the most well-known Siamese cat is the seal point. The dark brown ears, face, and tail are famous markers of this popular breed of cat. Many cats that appear in popular culture, including the mischievous Siamese cats in Disney animated films, are patterned after this type of Siamese. However, cat aficionados are well aware that other types of Siamese cats also exist. Two of these include the blue point and the snowshoe. Snowshoe Siamese are characterized by the white markings on their paws along with the dark "boots": these markings earn them their name and make the cats look as though they have been walking in the snow. Blue point Siamese cats do not have dark brown "points"; rather, their ears, paws, tails, and noses are characterized by bluish patches on their fur. Some Siamese cats are even hairless. They exhibit the darker pigment on their noses, tails, ears, and paws similar to their fur-covered counterparts of the same breed. However, hairless Siamese cats exhibit these "points" on their skin instead of their fur. This type of Siamese is rather rare and not very well known. Despite the contrasts between the external appearances of these varying types of Siamese, all Siamese cats are known for being vocal, loyal, and rather mischievous.

Which of the following text structures is used to organize the above passage?

A) Sequence
B) Cause-effect
C) Comparison-contrast
D) Problem-solution

The correct answer is **C**. In the passage, the author compares different types of Siamese cats. Choice A is incorrect because a passage with a sequence text structure describes steps in a process or presents information in chronological form. Choice B is incorrect because a cause-effect text structure focuses on how one factor or variable produces a specific outcome. Choice D is incorrect because a problem-solution text structure presents a problem and then provides a solution to that problem.

REVIEW QUESTIONS

Saltwater fish and freshwater fish are related, but their natural environments prove rather distinctive. In terms of being kept as pets, freshwater fish require less maintenance. They live in water that can be adapted from tap water, and they can be kept in many different types of containers in addition to aquariums. Saltwater fish, on the other hand, require a specific type of salt-infused water. Careful watch of the pH balance of the water must also be maintained.

The next two questions are based on this passage.

1. The author's description of saltwater and freshwater fish is reflective of which of the following types of text structures?

A) Sequence
B) Problem-solution
C) Cause-effect
D) Comparison-contrast

2. The above passage is reflective of which of the following types of writing?

A) Technical
B) Expository
C) Narrative
D) Persuasive

To All Department Supervisors:

The Acme Records Retrieval System will be undergoing scheduled maintenance this Friday, from 4:00 P.M. to midnight. Please inform all department personnel of the system outage so that researchers can make alternative arrangements to access necessary data.

An archived copy of the Core Business Records Database will be accessible in the Web Services department office from 4:00 P.M. to 8:00 P.M. on Friday. However, this database contains only core records data and is limited in its scope.

Please direct any questions to Marcus Sampson, Web Services Maintenance Officer, at (617) 555-0004.

The next two questions are based on this memo.

3. Which of the following is the author's intent in the memo?

A) To entertain
B) To express feelings
C) To persuade
D) To inform

4. Put the following elements of the organizational structure of the memo in order from first (1) to last (3).

_____ proposal of a solution
_____ caveat to the solution
_____ description of a problem

The acoustics of various performance venues emerge as the result of careful planning and extensive decision making. Sound travels differently when it moves through air, and the objects it encounters in a particular environment strongly impact the way that listeners hear the sound.

Venues that are designed primarily to house symphony orchestra performances require vastly different acoustic designs than do venues that cater to more intimate performances. Engineers must take into account a wide variety of variables during the design process, including vibration, sound, ultrasound, and infrasound.

A sound wave consists of a fundamental, followed by a series of sequential overtones. The way that listeners perceive these sound waves is impacted by the material used in the listening environment, the physical layout of the environment, the position of the stage relative to the audience's seating, and even the height of the ceiling. Many acoustic engineers also must take into consideration the manner in which transducers impact listening. Transducers include loudspeakers, microphones, and sonar projectors. The addition of these tools to an acoustic environment can strongly influence and transform how audience members in different locations in the room perceive any sound being transmitted.

The next two questions are based on this passage.

5. Which of the following text structures is used to organize the above passage?

A) Description
B) Sequence
C) Problem-solution
D) Comparison-contrast

6. Which of the following is the author's intent in the passage?

A) To persuade
B) To entertain
C) To inform
D) To express feelings

Aficionados of classical music frequently appreciate the characteristics of jazz, and some laypersons think the two genres are somewhat similar. However, jazz musicians are noted for their improvisational abilities, whereas classically trained musicians are often very reliant upon printed music. Although musicians in both genres must be very well versed in scales and various musical keys, jazz musicians must possess impeccable knowledge of this material in order to be able to perform and fulfill the requirements of their chosen genre.

The next two questions are based on this passage.

7. The above passage is reflective of which of the following types of writing?

A) Narrative
B) Expository
C) Technical
D) Persuasive

8. Which of the following text structures is used to organize the above passage?

   A) Comparison-contrast
   B) Description
   C) Sequence
   D) Problem-solution

9. When artists achieve commercial successes, their emotional mindsets can be influenced by this experience. Claude Monet was one such example of this phenomenon. Monet's innovative style earned him considerable fame and public acclaim. In addition, he was extremely prolific as an artist because of his industrious work ethic. As a result, he was successful at his craft, and his paintings reflect a more contemplative and calm perspective than those of artists whose life experiences were fraught with poverty and struggle.

   Which of the following is the author's intent in the passage?

   A) To persuade
   B) To entertain
   C) To inform
   D) To express feelings

As one of the most prolific female poets in nineteenth-century America, today Emily Dickinson is a household name. However, during her lifetime, she lived as a recluse and wrote most of her poetry from the solitude of her bedroom. She presents a unique perspective from this time period, when few women wrote about the themes she discusses. For this reason, critics are frequently interested in her perspective as a female author even beyond the contributions she made as an American nineteenth-century writer.

The next two questions are based on this passage.

10. Which of the following text structures is used to organize the last two lines of the above passage?

    A) Problem-solution
    B) Cause-effect
    C) Description
    D) Comparison-contrast

11. Which of the following is the author's intent in the passage?

    A) To persuade
    B) To entertain
    C) To express feelings
    D) To inform

Literary scholars have often speculated as to the personal characteristics of William Shakespeare. The Bard is known to many as the greatest writer the English language has ever known, but we have very few examples of his handwriting or even his own name written out in his hand. Some academics have gone so far as to speculate that Shakespeare was a pseudonym for an aristocrat. However, the majority of scholars have dismissed this proposal, and they concentrate instead on Shakespeare's thoughtful insights and dexterous construction of language.

The next two questions are based on this passage.

12. Which of the following text structures is used to organize the above passage?

    A) Cause-effect
    B) Sequence
    C) Description
    D) Comparison-contrast

13. The above passage is reflective of which of the following types of writing?

    A) Narrative
    B) Expository
    C) Technical
    D) Persuasive

14. The physician William Harvey was the first who discovered and demonstrated the true mechanism of the heart's action. No one before his time conceived that the movement of the blood was entirely due to the mechanical action of the heart as a pump. There were all sorts of speculations about the matter, but nobody had formed this conception. Harvey is as clear as possible about it. He says the movement of the blood is entirely due to the contractions of the walls of the heart—that it is the propelling apparatus—and all recent investigation tends to show that he was perfectly right.

    Which of the following is the author's intent in the passage?

    A) To inform
    B) To entertain
    C) To express feelings
    D) To persuade

15. To All Restaurant Staff:

    It has come to my attention that some employees have been using the kitchen's silver serving platters to serve large parties when the porcelain serving platters are all in use. This causes a problem with serving some of our VIP guests, who may arrive unexpectedly or with short notice. Please refrain from using the silver serving platters unless they have been specifically designated to serve a reserved party. The list of reservations can be found on the back bulletin board for any given night; silver service will be marked next to a reservation with a circled S.

Additional porcelain serving platters are currently on order to ensure that we have adequate servingware to accommodate all of our guests.

Thank you for helping us to serve our VIP patrons with the level of professionalism they have come to know and expect.

George Gario,

Proprietor

Which of the following text structures is used to organize the above memo?

A) Description
B) Sequence
C) Comparison-contrast
D) Problem-solution

ANSWER KEY

1. D
2. B
3. D
4. 2, 3, 1
5. A

6. C
7. B
8. A
9. A
10. B

11. D
12. C
13. B
14. A
15. D

ANSWERS AND EXPLANATIONS

1. (D) In the passage, the author compares and contrasts the environmental needs of freshwater and saltwater fish. Choice A is incorrect because a sequence text structure describes steps in a process or presents information in chronological form. Choice B is incorrect because a problem-solution text structure presents a problem and then provides a solution to that problem. Choice C is incorrect because a cause-effect text structure focuses on how one factor or variable produces a specific outcome.

2. (B) This passage is an example of expository writing, which describes a subject and explains its features. Choice A is incorrect because technical writing explains highly complex topics in an accurate and often formally structured manner. Choice C is incorrect because narrative writing tells a story or relates a series of events. Choice D is incorrect because persuasive writing attempts to convince the reader to accept a particular position or take a certain action.

3. (D) This memo offers details regarding a database shutdown, so the author's intent is to inform. Choice A is incorrect because the author does not attempt to engage the reader in an entertaining or captivating manner. Choice B is incorrect because the author does not attempt to express feelings or bring out emotions in the reader; instead, the memo is written from an objective, neutral perspective. Choice C is incorrect because the author does not make an argument and attempt to convince the reader to accept a particular position or take a certain action.

4. (2, 3, 1) The memo begins by describing a problem (system outage), then proposes a solution (a copy is available), and finally adds a caveat to the solution (limited scope).

5. (A) In this passage, the author describes acoustics. Choice B is incorrect because a sequence text structure describes steps in a process or presents information in chronological form. Choice C is incorrect because a problem-solution text structure presents a problem and then provides a solution to that problem. Choice D is incorrect because a comparison-contrast text structure focuses on highlighting the similarities and differences between or among entities.

6. (C) The author's intent in this passage is to inform. Choice A is incorrect because the author does not make an argument and attempt to convince the reader to accept a particular position or take a certain action. Choice B is incorrect because the author does not attempt to engage the reader in an entertaining or captivating manner. Choice D is incorrect because the author does not attempt to express feelings or bring out emotions in the reader.

7. (B) This passage is an example of expository writing, which describes a subject and explains its features. Choice A is incorrect because narrative writing tells a story or relates a series of events. Choice C is incorrect because technical writing explains highly complex topics in an accurate and often formally structured manner. Choice D is incorrect because persuasive writing attempts to persuade the reader to accept a particular position or take a certain action.

8. (A) In the passage, the author compares and contrasts jazz and classical musicians. Choice B is incorrect because a passage with a description text structure simply provides information about an entity. Choice C is incorrect because a sequence text structure describes steps in a process or presents information in chronological form. Choice D is incorrect because a problem-solution text structure presents a problem and then provides a solution to that problem.

9. (A) The author makes an argument in this passage by presenting a central claim and providing evidence to support that claim. In doing so, he or she attempts to convince the reader to accept a particular position, namely that *when artists achieve commercial successes, their emotional mindsets can be influenced by this experience*. Choice B is incorrect because the author does not attempt to engage the reader in an entertaining or captivating manner. Choice C is incorrect because the author is not simply offering information to describe a phenomenon; the description that is provided is given to support the author's point. Choice D is incorrect because the author does not attempt to express feelings or evoke emotions in the reader; instead, the passage is written from an objective, neutral perspective.

10. (B) In the last two lines of this passage, the author shows a cause-effect relationship between two factors. First, the author notes that Dickinson's perspective is unique; *for this reason*, the author explains, critics are often more interested in her point of view as a female author. Choice A is incorrect because a problem-solution text structure presents a problem and then provides a solution to that problem. Choice C is incorrect because description text structures merely present information about a subject. Choice D is incorrect because comparison-contrast text structures highlight similarities and differences between or among entities.

11. (D) The author's intent is to inform. Choice A is incorrect because the author does not make an argument and attempt to convince the reader to believe a particular point of view or take a certain action. The author instead presents facts about Dickinson's life and work and the interests of the scholars who study her. Choice B is incorrect because the author does not attempt to engage the reader in an entertaining or captivating manner. Choice C is incorrect because the author does not attempt to express feelings or bring out emotions in the reader; instead, the passage is written from an objective, neutral perspective.

12. (C) In the passage, the author uses a descriptive text structure to present information about Shakespeare. Choice A is incorrect because cause-effect text structures focus on how one factor or variable produces a specific outcome. Choice B is incorrect because a sequence text structure describes steps in a process or presents information in chronological form. Choice D is incorrect because a comparison-contrast text structure focuses on highlighting the similarities and differences between or among entities.

13. (B) This passage is an example of expository writing, which describes a subject and explains its features. Choice A is incorrect because narrative writing tells a story or relates a series of events. Choice C is incorrect because technical writing explains highly complex topics in an accurate and often formally structured manner. Choice D is incorrect because persuasive writing attempts to persuade the reader to accept a particular position or take a certain action.

14. (A) The author's intent here is to inform. Choice B is incorrect because the author does not attempt to engage the reader in an entertaining or captivating manner. Choice C is incorrect because the author does not attempt to express feelings or bring out emotions in the reader; instead, the passage is written from an objective, neutral perspective. Choice D is incorrect because the author does not make an argument and attempt to convince the reader to accept a particular position or take a certain action.

15. (D) In the passage, the author presents a problem; he also presents solutions. Choice A is incorrect because a description text structure simply provides information about a subject. Choice B is incorrect because a sequence text structure describes steps in a process or presents information in chronological form. Choice C is incorrect because a comparison-contrast text structure focuses on highlighting the similarities and differences between or among entities.

CHAPTER 2

Topic

Topic questions may reflect one of two types. The first type asks the test taker to differentiate between the topic, theme, main idea, and supporting details in a Reading passage. The **topic** of a passage is the general subject matter addressed in the passage. A passage regarding key battles of the Civil War might address the topic of history (very general), military conflict (more specific), or Civil War battles (very specific).

Here is an example of a topic question:

Imagine living in the year 1800. The railroads then were very scarce. Gas lights were not yet invented, and electric lights were not even dreamed of. Even kerosene wasn't used at that point. This was the world into which Samuel Morse, the inventor of the telegraph, was born.

Samuel Morse was born in Charlestown, Massachusetts, shortly before the turn of the century, in 1791. When he was seven years old, he was sent to boarding school at Phillips Academy, Andover. While he was there, his father wrote him letters, giving him good advice. He told him about George Washington and about a British statesman named Lord Chesterfield, who was able to achieve many of his goals. Lord Chesterfield was asked once how he managed to find time for all of his pursuits, and he replied that he only ever did one thing at a time, and that he "never put off anything until tomorrow that could be done today."

Morse worked hard at school and began to think and act for himself at quite a young age. His biggest accomplishment was in painting, and he established himself as a successful painter after graduating from college at Yale. But he also had an interest in science and inventions. He was passionate about the idea of discovering a way for people to send messages to each other in short periods of time.

In the early 1800s, it took a long time to receive news of any sort, even important news. Whole countries had to wait weeks to hear word of the outcomes of faraway wars. The mail was carried by stagecoach. In emergency situations, such as when ships were lost at sea, there was no way to send requests for help. Electricity had been discovered, but little application had been made of it up until that point. This was about to change when Morse set his mind to his invention.

On October 1, 1832, Morse was sailing to America from a trip overseas on a ship called the *Sully*. He became preoccupied with the thought of inventing a machine that would later become the telegraph. Morse thought about the telegraph night and day. As he sat upon the deck of the ship after dinner one night, he took out a little notebook and began to create a plan.

If a message could be sent ten miles without dropping, he wrote, "I could make it go around the globe." He said this over and over again during the years after his trip.

One morning at the breakfast table, Morse showed his plan to some of the other *Sully* passengers. Five years later, when the model of the telegraph was built, it was exactly like the one shown that morning to the passengers on the *Sully*.

Once he arrived in America, Morse worked for twelve long years to get people to notice his invention. Though some supported the idea of the telegraph, many people scoffed at it. Morse persisted, and eventually a bill was passed by Congress in 1842. It authorized the funds needed to build the first trial telegraph line.

After two years, the telegraph line was complete. Morse and his colleagues tested it in May 1844. The device worked, and the telegraph became a huge success. Morse's persistence had finally paid off.

> Which of the following describes the word *telegraph* as it relates to the passage?
>
> A) Main idea
> B) Topic
> C) Supporting detail
> D) Purpose

The correct answer is **B**. The word *telegraph* is the topic of the passage, because that is the passage's central focus.

Let's consider a second example:

Historically, the study of creativity has concentrated on persons known for their innovation. Early creativity studies focused on creative "geniuses," such as Einstein, Mozart, or Shakespeare. This type of creativity is known as "Big C" creativity. However, as research on creativity progressed, a corresponding interest in how people could be creative in smaller ways—on an everyday basis—emerged in the discipline. Scholars began to investigate how ordinary tasks, such as cleaning, driving particular familiar routes, and completing work and schoolwork, could be conducted in innovative ways. This focus of creativity research has been labeled "little c" creativity.

> Is *creative geniuses* a topic, main idea, supporting detail, or purpose of the above passage? Write your answer in the blank: _____

The correct answer is "supporting detail." *Creative geniuses* is a supporting detail of this passage. The topic of the passage is the study of creativity, and the main idea is that the study of creativity addresses both "Big C" and "little c" types of creativity.

Now consider this passage:

The current tests for measuring IQ, or an individual's intelligence quotient, were developed during the early and mid-twentieth century. Their use was popularized by Terman, who designed specific tests for use in the U.S. Army. Some psychologists today assert that the traditional system of measuring IQ should remain the sole method of assessing intelligence. Historically, the test has been constructed based on the assumption that there exists one general intelligence factor that impacts an individual's intellectual capacity.

The validity of this assumption has been challenged by other psychologists. In particular, Howard Gardner has emphasized that a unified conception of intelligence based on a single factor remains highly limited and unnecessarily constraining. Gardner has postulated an alternative theory concerning the existence of multiple intelligences. He posits that individuals can possess intelligence in particular areas, including linguistic intelligence, spiritual intelligence, spatial intelligence, intrapersonal intelligence, interpersonal intelligence, musical intelligence, mathematical intelligence, and kinesthetic intelligence, among others. Gardner asserts that individuals can be extremely intelligent and exhibit talent in one area, while failing to demonstrate the same level of prowess in another area. His theory has been discussed widely, although efforts to obtain empirical evidence to support his ideas remain in progress.

> Which of the following describes the phrase *IQ measurement* as it relates to the passage?
>
> A) Main idea
> B) Topic
> C) Supporting detail
> D) Purpose

The correct answer is **B**. The phrase *IQ measurement* reflects the topic of this passage. This phrase is too broad to be a supporting detail of the passage.

The second type of Topic question asks the test taker to identify the topic sentence or summary sentence of a paragraph or passage. **Topic sentences** are introductory sentences that encapsulate the main idea to be developed in that paragraph or passage. **Summary sentences** are concluding sentences that restate the main idea of the paragraph or passage. They may also draw a conclusion based on information given in the paragraph or passage.

Normally we might think of topic sentences and summary sentences as applying only to text at the paragraph level. The topic sentence of a full passage would be referred to as its thesis statement, and the summary sentence of a full passage would be referred to as its conclusion. On the TEAS, however, the term *topic sentence* is sometimes used to refer to a sentence at either the paragraph level or the level of the full passage. The term *summary sentence* is also used to refer to the concluding sentence for a single paragraph or the conclusion of a full passage. Consider this passage.

CPR, an acronym that stands for cardiopulmonary resuscitation, is a widely utilized method of attempting to save someone's life. It is especially applicable to scenarios in which a patient's heart has stopped beating. Frequently, it is also used in cases where a person is in danger of drowning.

Almost all approaches to CPR suggest that a person begin resuscitation efforts with chest compressions. To perform a chest compression, the individual places both hands flat on the patient's chest and then begins pushing down carefully but firmly, most likely at equal intervals. The compressions should be counted, so that the individual can keep track of how many compressions have been administered. The unofficial recommendation of how many chest compressions to provide is around 100 per minute.

There are many resources through which potential lifesavers can acquire training and even certification so that they can more effectively administer this lifesaving technique to a potential patient. However, the American Heart Association stresses that even if someone has not received any type of formal training, attempting to help a person who needs to be resuscitated is far better than offering no help. This is why 911 operators sometimes request that bystanders at the scene of an emergency administer CPR. The operators may even coach the bystanders verbally, over the phone. These approaches have been shown to be effective in many cases.

If a bystander at an emergency scene has received CPR training—even if the training occurred a long time ago—the bystander should attempt further techniques in addition to chest compressions, especially if the patient has been underwater. The lifesaver should start first by checking the patient's airway. He or she might also administer mouth-to-mouth rescue breathing. However, lifesavers should only perform these additional techniques if they are confident of their skills and remember their training. Otherwise, any potential lifesaver should just administer chest compressions.

Some important items to remember in administering CPR are as follows. First, the lifesaver should always check whether the patient is conscious or not. Verbal interaction or communication can be a key way of determining if a person is conscious. If the emergency is related to drowning, the lifesaver should start chest compressions. These should be conducted for about a minute or so, before the lifesaver calls 911. However, if one person can perform the compressions and there is another person available who can call 911, then these steps should happen simultaneously.

For persons who are trained in CPR, one of the best ways to remember the order in which steps should be administered is to recall the memory cue CAB. This cue stands for Circulation, Airway, Breathing. The goal of CPR is to help an unresponsive person to start breathing on his or her own. First, use chest compressions to restore circulation. This is the C of CAB. Second, check the patient's airway for possible blockages. The A in CAB stands for airway. Finally, administer rescue breathing. This is, of course, the B of CAB.

Which of the following sentences is the topic sentence for paragraph two?

A) Almost all approaches to CPR suggest that a person begin resuscitation efforts with chest compressions.

B) The unofficial recommendation of how many chest compressions to provide is around 100 per minute.

C) The compressions should be counted, so that the individual can keep track of how many compressions have been administered.

D) To perform a chest compression, the individual places both hands flat on the patient's chest and then begins pushing down carefully but firmly, most likely at equal intervals.

The correct answer is **A**. Paragraph two focuses on how to give chest compressions. Choice A reflects the topic sentence, as this sentence comes first in the paragraph and describes the idea to be developed. Choices B, C, and D reflect supporting details of the paragraph.

Let's look at another example:

Christopher Columbus was particularly influenced by the maps of the ancient geographer Ptolemy. Ptolemy argued that the world was round, which went against the belief of the day that the world was flat. Columbus sided with Ptolemy on this question and set out to prove that it was so.

At the time it was widely held that sailing west from Europe would lead to certain death. Believing that the world was round, Columbus thought that one who sailed west would wind up in the east. Other scientists of the day rejected this idea, so Columbus wrote to a respected Italian scholar, Paolo Toscanelli, to ask for his opinion on the matter.

Toscanelli supported the idea of Columbus's trip and sent word back to Columbus in 1474. After receiving Toscanelli's encouragement, Columbus focused all of his thoughts and plans on traveling westward. To make the journey, he would require the help of a generous financial backer, so he went to seek the aid of the king of Portugal. Columbus asked the king for ships and sailors to make the journey. In return, he promised to bring back wealth and to help to convert natives living on the lands to the Church. Portugal refused, and Columbus approached Italy unsuccessfully as well. He went to Spain next.

Queen Isabella of Spain agreed to support the journey. It took some time for Columbus to convince her, but he did succeed, and she paid for the trip. Part of what led the queen to believe in Columbus was the way that he focused on his goal for such a long time with great intent. He spent the best years of his life working toward his dream, remaining persistent and determined. Legend has it that even during his first voyage, members of his crew became frightened and uncertain, wanting to return home, but Columbus pressed on. The eventual discovery of the Americas was the reward for his commitment.

More than 500 years later, the geography of the world is often taken for granted, but Columbus was an early visionary whose results proved at least some of his theories correct.

> Which of the following sentences is the summary sentence for the entire passage?
>
> A) Christopher Columbus was particularly influenced by the maps of the ancient geographer Ptolemy.
> B) More than 500 years later, the geography of the world is often taken for granted, but Columbus was an early visionary whose results proved at least some of his theories correct.
> C) Part of what led the queen to believe in Columbus was the way that he focused on his goal for such a long time with great intent.
> D) Legend has it that even during his first voyage, members of his crew became frightened and uncertain, wanting to return home, but Columbus pressed on.

The correct answer is **B**. The passage continually emphasizes how Columbus worked to prove his belief that the world was round. His commitment to his vision enabled him to win the backing of Queen Isabella and eventually discover America. The statement in choice C summarizes how the persistence of Columbus impressed Queen Isabella. This statement highlights an important theme of the passage, *persistence*, rather than summarizing the entire passage.

REVIEW QUESTIONS

Saltwater fish and freshwater fish are related, but their natural environments prove rather distinctive. In terms of being kept as pets, freshwater fish require less maintenance. They live in water that can be adapted from tap water, and they can be kept in many different types of containers in addition to aquariums. Saltwater fish, on the other hand, require a specific type of salt-infused water. Careful watch of the pH balance of the water must also be maintained.

> 1. Which of the following describes the phrase *fresh versus saltwater fish* as it relates to the passage?
>
> A) Main idea
> B) Topic
> C) Supporting detail
> D) Theme

Laurel Hill Botanic Gardens is pleased to announce the installation of the sculpture series by Laurel Hill artist-in-residence, Darryl C. Grant. The installation features mixed-media sculptures emphasizing the floral designs prominent in Mr. Grant's paintings, many of which are also on exhibit in the Michael and Frieda Sachs Viewing Room.

The sculpture exhibit will open at 10:00 A.M. on Thursday, June 5. The Botanic Gardens' art curator, Jessalyn Jones, will present an overview of the sculptures and lead a guided tour of the installation. The opening ceremony will end with refreshments served in the Nature Observatory from 2:00–3:00 P.M.

This is a members-only event. All Botanic Gardens members and their guests are invited to attend. Tickets are $50.00 per person and can be purchased at the registration desk beginning Monday, May 5.

The next two questions are based on this passage.

2. Is *floral designs* a topic, main idea, supporting detail, or theme of the above announcement?

    A) Theme
    B) Topic
    C) Supporting detail
    D) Main idea

3. Underline the topic sentence that describes the purpose of the announcement.

To Whom It May Concern,

I am writing to request a refund of the charge made to my credit card for the purchase of a water filter on Friday, September 18. The filter was the wrong type for my filtration system, so I had to return it. I returned the filter to the store on Saturday, September 19, and the customer service clerk had me complete the paperwork to refund my charges for the purchase. However, the credit never appeared on my credit card account. Please reverse the charges in the amount shown on the credit receipt attached to this e-mail.

Thank you for your assistance.

Claire Glendheim

The next two questions are based on this passage.

4. Which of the following sentences is a summary sentence for the e-mail above?

    A) I am writing to request a refund of the charge made to my credit card for the purchase of a water filter on Friday, September 18.
    B) The filter was the wrong type for my filtration system, so I had to return it.
    C) However, the credit never appeared on my credit card account.
    D) Please reverse the charges in the amount shown on the credit receipt attached to this e-mail.

5. Which of the following describes the phrase *credit card refund request* as it relates to the above e-mail?

A) Topic
B) Theme
C) Supporting detail
D) Main idea

6. Jan,

Arthur from Human Resources let me know that you were requesting recommendations for interns who might fill the open position in the Graphics department. I would highly recommend Alex Hastings, who has worked with me this summer on several book designs. His work is consistently top quality. He has not only the experience we are looking for, but also the motivation and drive to excel. Alex will be graduating this fall and would be an ideal candidate to fill the position.

If I can provide you with any additional information, just let me know.

Henry

Is *intern recommendation* a topic, main idea, supporting detail, or theme of the above passage?

A) Main idea
B) Topic
C) Supporting detail
D) Theme

Historically, the study of creativity has concentrated on persons known for their innovation. Early creativity studies focused on creative "geniuses," such as Einstein, Mozart, or Shakespeare. This type of creativity is known as "Big C" creativity. However, as research on creativity progressed, a corresponding interest in how people could be creative in smaller ways—on an everyday basis—emerged in the discipline. Scholars began to investigate how ordinary tasks, such as cleaning, driving particular familiar routes, and completing work and schoolwork, could be conducted in innovative ways. This focus of creativity research has been labeled "little c" creativity.

The next two questions are based on this passage.

7. Is *types of creativity* a topic, main idea, supporting detail, or theme of the above passage?

A) Supporting detail
B) Theme
C) Main idea
D) Topic

8. Which of the following describes the phrase *driving particular familiar routes* as it relates to the above passage?

A) Main idea
B) Theme
C) Topic
D) Supporting detail

The way that scientists have envisioned the makeup of the universe has shifted and transformed as the centuries have passed. Prior to the work of Copernicus, people believed that the earth was at the center of the universe. The idea that the earth revolved around the sun was initially taken as heresy. The progression and gradual acceptance of these originally controversial ideas paved the way for the acceptance of later discoveries by Newton and Einstein. Their theories have revolutionized the ways in which science itself is conducted today.

9. Which of the following sentences is the topic sentence for the entire passage?

A) The way that scientists have envisioned the makeup of the universe has shifted and transformed as the centuries have passed.
B) Prior to the work of Copernicus, people believed that the earth was at the center of the universe.
C) The progression and gradual acceptance of these originally controversial ideas paved the way for the acceptance of later discoveries by Newton and Einstein.
D) Their theories have revolutionized the ways in which science itself is conducted today.

The best method of treating individuals facing psychological difficulties is a blend of cognitive-behavioral therapy and medication. This approach not only serves to address the patient's potential chemical imbalances, but it also emancipates the patient by allowing him or her some autonomy in dealing with the issues associated with a possible malaise.

Cognitive-behavioral therapy requires the patient to examine his or her own behavior and to make moderations in a rational and well-thought-out manner. If a person's chemical makeup is preventing him or her from being able to carry out such a responsibility, then medication can help alleviate specific symptoms to allow the patient to deal with the underlying emotional and psychological issues in an effective manner. Nevertheless, psychologists have wide-ranging opinions on how to help these patients cope with challenges such as depression or anxiety.

Some trained professionals assert that medication alone can best serve psychological patients. Other psychologists believe that the utilization of Freud's psychoanalytic approach represents the best method for assisting persons with these emotional symptoms. Some counselors believe that each person's set of individual circumstances should be considered. Other counselors depend on the characteristics of behaviorism to modify the patients' behavior so that their behavioral patterns become more effective. Overall, however, many professionals agree that the combination of cognitive-behavioral therapy and medication will ultimately best serve the patient.

The next two questions are based on this passage.

10. Which of the following sentences is the summary sentence for the passage?

A) The best method of treating individuals facing psychological difficulties is a blend of cognitive-behavioral therapy and medication.

B) Some counselors believe that each person's set of individual circumstances should be considered.

C) Overall, however, many professionals agree that the combination of cognitive-behavioral therapy and medication will ultimately best serve the patient.

D) Nevertheless, psychologists have wide-ranging opinions on how to help these patients cope with challenges such as depression or anxiety.

11. Is *cognitive-behavioral therapy versus medication* a topic, main idea, supporting detail, or theme of the above passage?

A) Main idea
B) Topic
C) Supporting detail
D) Theme

12. One of the most important gymnastic exercises in the original Montessori school approach is that of the "line." For this exercise, a line is drawn in chalk or paint on the floor. Instead of one line, there may also be two lines drawn. The children are taught to walk on these lines like tightrope walkers, placing their feet one in front of the other.

To keep their balance, the children must make efforts similar to those of real tightrope walkers, except that they have no danger of falling, since the lines are drawn only on the floor. The teacher herself performs the exercise first, showing clearly how she places her feet, and the children imitate her without her even needing to speak. At first it is only certain children who follow her, and when she has shown them how to walk the line, she leaves, letting the exercise develop on its own.

The children for the most part continue to walk, following with great care the movement they have seen, and making efforts to keep their balance so they don't fall. Gradually the other children come closer and watch and try the exercise. In a short time, the entire line is covered with children balancing themselves and continuing to walk around, watching their feet attentively.

Music may be used at this point. It should be a very simple march, without an obvious rhythm. It should simply accompany and support the efforts of the children.

When children learn to master their balance in this way, Dr. Montessori believed, they can bring the act of walking to a remarkable standard of perfection.

Is *the line* a topic, main idea, supporting detail, or theme of the above passage?

A) Supporting detail
B) Main idea
C) Topic
D) Theme

ANSWER KEY

1. B
2. C
3. All Botanic Gardens members and their guests are invited to attend.
4. D
5. A
6. B
7. D
8. D
9. A
10. C
11. B
12. C

ANSWERS AND EXPLANATIONS

1. (B) *Fresh versus saltwater fish* is the general topic of this passage.

2. (C) *Floral designs* is a supporting detail of this announcement. The announcement mentions in the first paragraph that the installation features sculptures emphasizing the floral designs prominent in Mr. Grant's paintings.

3. (All Botanic Gardens members and their guests are invited to attend.) This is the topic sentence of the entire announcement, because it introduces the main idea developed in the announcement. This announcement's purpose is to invite members of the Botanic Gardens to an event. The topic sentence is unusually positioned in that it appears in the middle of the announcement rather than at the beginning.

4. (D) Choice D provides a summary sentence for the ideas addressed in the entire e-mail. Here, the author restates her main reason for the writing the e-mail: to have her credit card charges reversed. Choice A is the topic statement of the e-mail, while choices B and C are supporting details.

5. (A) The topic of this passage is a credit card refund request. The main idea of this e-mail might be stated as follows: "The author returned a water filtration system and is placing a second request for a credit card refund."

6. (B) The phrase *intern recommendation* is the specific topic of this passage. Two possible supporting details of the e-mail could be *motivation* and *extensive experience,* both of which describe the intern's qualifications.

7. (D) *Types of creativity* is the general topic of this passage, because it is what the passage is about.

8. (D) The phrase *driving particular familiar routes* is a supporting detail of the passage. This detail is mentioned as an example of an everyday task.

9. (A) Choice A is the topic sentence of the entire article, because it introduces the main idea developed in the article. Choice B is a supporting detail for the topic sentence. Choice C is another supporting detail.

10. (C) Choice C provides a summary sentence for the passage, while choice A is the topic sentence.

11. (B) *Cognitive-behavioral therapy versus medication* is the topic of this passage.

12. (C) *The line* is the general topic of this passage because it is what the passage is about.

CHAPTER 3

Main Idea

Main idea questions test understanding of the overall content of a passage or selection. They ask about the general point or "big picture" idea. They are commonly phrased "What is the passage mainly about?" or "Which of the following best reflects the main idea of the passage?"

When answering main idea questions, keep in mind the following:

> The answer to a main idea question must not be too broad or too specific. It must be just right to capture the "big picture" of the passage.

Consider this example:

Public highways are used constantly with little thought of how important they are to the everyday life of a community. It is understandable that most people think about their local public highway only when it affects their own activities. People usually don't focus on highway improvements unless the subject is brought to their attention by increased taxes or advertising.

Highway improvements are an important issue, however. It is important for the economies of most communities to keep highways in good repair. Products purchased in one location are often manufactured in other locations, and safe highways are required to transport the products to their final destination. Good transportation facilities contribute greatly to community prosperity.

The type and amount of the highway improvement needed in any area depend on the traffic in that area. In low-population areas, the amount of traffic on local roads is likely to be small, and highways will not require as much work. But as an area develops, the use of public highways increases, and maintenance demands increase. In small towns, residents are also more able to adapt to the condition of the roads. A road shutdown does not have the same impact on business as it would in busy areas. In large districts with many activities, however, roads must be usable year-round in order for business progress to continue.

In planning improvements of highway systems, several different types of traffic may be encountered. These range from business traffic to agricultural shipping to residential transportation. Improvement activities must meet the requirements of all classes of traffic, with the most important provided for first. Those improvements of lesser importance can be performed as soon as finances permit.

Which title best conveys the main idea of the passage?

A) Highways: How They Contribute to Economic Growth
B) Highways: Their History and Development
C) Highways: What Can Be Done About Traffic
D) Highways: Why Improvement Is Important

The correct answer is **D**. Most of the article focuses on why improvement is an important issue for those who use highways. Therefore, choice D best captures the main idea of the passage. The passage mentions the economic role of the highways, but that is not the main idea, so choice A can be eliminated. There is little attention to history in the passage, and the passage does not focus on traffic control as an issue in itself, so choices B and C are also incorrect.

Some main idea questions ask you to identify what a passage is "mainly about," as in the example below. This passage concerns the town of Stratford-upon-Avon, where Shakespeare was born.

The English town of Stratford-upon-Avon is visited yearly by tourists wanting to view the birthplace of William Shakespeare. William's father, John Shakespeare, bought the family home on Henley Street, and it is here that William is believed to have been born in 1564. Shakespeare's birth home remained in his family until the early 1800s, and it is now a public museum.

Shakespeare attended school at the King Edward VI Grammar School, which occupied the first floor of a building known as the Guildhall. It was in this Guildhall that Shakespeare first experienced theater, when he saw a theatrical performance given by a group of traveling actors. The Royal Shakespeare Company still performs in the town at the Royal Shakespeare and Swan Theaters.

Close to the Guildhall is the site of a house known as New Place, which was bought by Shakespeare himself. Here Shakespeare lived during the later part of his life, until his death in 1616. Although he spent most of his career in London, with trips back to Stratford, he moved permanently to New Place in the last years of his life and is believed to have written some of his later works there. Only the foundations of the New Place house now remain.

In the town of Shottery, one mile from Stratford, is the cottage where Shakespeare's wife, Anne Hathaway, was born. The Hathaway cottage, now also a museum, is actually a large, thatch-roofed farmhouse with sprawling gardens where Shakespeare is believed to have developed his relationship with Anne. They married in 1582 and had three children.

What is this passage mainly about?

A) The importance of Stratford-upon-Avon for theatrical performances
B) The importance of Stratford-upon-Avon in Shakespeare's plays
C) The importance of Stratford-upon-Avon in Shakespeare's life
D) The importance of Stratford-upon-Avon in English history

The correct answer is **C**. This passage focuses on Shakespeare's relationship to Stratford-upon-Avon throughout his life. It does not mention whether the town appeared in his plays, although there is a short statement that he wrote some of his plays there. The passage does deal with theatrical performances and history, but those are broad topics and not the main idea.

Main idea questions may sometimes ask you to identify which statement from the passage best reflects the "big picture" of the passage. Here, we are looking for the sentence that comes closest to describing the main idea, without being too broad or too specific.

One of the most important gymnastic exercises in the original Montessori school approach is that of the "line." For this exercise, a line is drawn in chalk or paint on the floor. Instead of one line, there may also be two lines drawn. The children are taught to walk on these lines like tightrope walkers, placing their feet one in front of the other.

To keep their balance, the children must make efforts similar to those of real tightrope walkers, except that they have no danger of falling, since the lines are drawn only on the floor. The teacher herself performs the exercise first, showing clearly how she places her feet, and the children imitate her without her even needing to speak. At first it is only certain children who follow her, and when she has shown them how to walk the line, she leaves, letting the exercise develop on its own.

The children for the most part continue to walk, following with great care the movement they have seen, and making efforts to keep their balance so they don't fall. Gradually the other children come closer and watch and try the exercise. In a short time, the entire line is covered with children balancing themselves and continuing to walk around, watching their feet attentively.

Music may be used at this point. It should be a very simple march, without an obvious rhythm. It should simply accompany and support the efforts of the children.

When children learn to master their balance in this way, Dr. Montessori believed, they can bring the act of walking to a remarkable standard of perfection.

Which of the following sentences best reflects the main idea of the entire passage?

A) Instead of one line, there may also be two lines drawn.
B) Music may be used at this point.
C) One of the most important gymnastic exercises in the original Montessori school approach is that of the "line."
D) The children for the most part continue to walk, following with great care the movement they have seen, and making efforts to keep their balance so they don't fall.

The correct answer is **C**. Choice C best reflects the main idea of the entire passage, because it introduces the "big picture" concept developed in the passage. The entire passage talks about the Montessori exercise of the "line." Choices A, B, and D reflect details from the passage; they are too narrow to be the main idea.

Let's look at two more examples:

Percy Bysshe Shelley was one of the second-generation Romantic poets. Along with John Keats and Lord Byron, Shelley was considered one of the most masterful poets of his generation.

Shelley was born in England in 1792, as a member of the aristocracy. He was educated at two prestigious English schools, Eton College and Oxford University. Shelley believed that poets were visionaries who could serve as societal leaders because of the creative power of their imaginations. The second generation of Romantic poets, in particular, believed that poets were going to help change the world. Shelley's generation believed that through the imagination, anything was possible. They believed that they could use the creative power of the mind to change the government and even change the world. Shelley's poems reflect this belief. He was a truly idealistic thinker, and he claimed that poets were the "unacknowledged legislators of the world." The poet's creative vision could let him or her see things that other people could not.

Shelley's ideas were heavily influenced by the politics of his time. He grew up at a time when governments were under transformation. In fact, he came of age in the shadow of the French Revolution. This period was very violent, and since France was so close to England, Shelley was acutely aware of the violence that was occurring there. That may have led him to concentrate even more on his belief that artists were able to change the world and improve living conditions.

Shelley's poem "Mont Blanc" focuses on the Romantic notion of the sublime. The Romantic poets believed that when people interacted with nature, it sometimes caused them to be in a state of wonder—or it caused them to be awestruck. For example, when a person gazed at a mountain, the huge size of the mountain could cause the person to become speechless with wonder. This was the effect that the sublime quality of nature could have on a viewer.

In "Mont Blanc," Shelley describes the mountain in a way that attempts to explain its effects on the viewer's mind. According to Shelley, the mountain itself causes the viewer's thoughts to enter a kind of strange trance, and to be affected in a way that resembles how a poet or an artist feels whenever he or she is caught in the midst of a creative inspiration. In the poem, Shelley draws a comparison between the effect of the mountain on the viewer and the power that the imagination has over the artist's mind.

What is the passage mainly about?

A) It focuses on the history of the French Revolution.
B) It discusses English poetry that addresses nature.
C) It covers Shelley's ideas about the imagination.
D) It deals generally with the artist's role in society.

The correct answer is **C**. The passage is mainly about how Shelley explores the role of the creative imagination and what it means for a poet. Choice A is incorrect because the discussion about the French Revolution is only a reference to the historical background in which Shelley lived; choice A is therefore too narrow to reflect the main idea. Although the passage does discuss English poetry that addresses nature, the main focus of the passage concerns Shelley's views on how poets could use the power of imagination to help change the world. The passage describes what Shelley thought about the imagination specifically, so choice D can be eliminated, as it is too broad to capture the main idea.

Now try this passage:

CPR, an acronym that stands for cardiopulmonary resuscitation, is a widely utilized method of attempting to save someone's life. It is especially applicable to scenarios in which a patient's heart has stopped beating. Frequently, it is also used in cases where a person is in danger of drowning.

Almost all approaches to CPR suggest that a person begin resuscitation efforts with chest compressions. To perform a chest compression, the individual places both hands flat on the patient's chest and then begins pushing down carefully but firmly, most likely at equal intervals. The compressions should be counted, so that the individual can keep track of how many compressions have been administered. The unofficial recommendation of how many chest compressions to provide is around 100 per minute.

There are many resources through which potential lifesavers can acquire training and even certification so that they can more effectively administer this life-saving technique to a potential patient. However, the American Heart Association stresses that even if someone has not received any type of formal training, attempting to help a person who needs to be resuscitated is far better than offering no help. This is why 911 operators sometimes request that bystanders at the scene of an emergency administer CPR. The operators may even coach the bystanders verbally, over the phone. These approaches have been shown to be effective in many cases.

If a bystander at an emergency scene has received CPR training—even if the training occurred a long time ago—the bystander should attempt further techniques in addition to chest compressions, especially if the patient has been underwater. The lifesaver should start first by checking the patient's airway. He or she might also administer mouth-to-mouth rescue breathing. However, lifesavers should only perform these additional techniques if they are confident of their skills and remember their training. Otherwise, any potential lifesaver should just administer chest compressions.

Some important items to remember in administering CPR are as follows. First, the lifesaver should always check whether the patient is conscious or not. Verbal interaction or communication can be a key way of determining if a person is conscious. If the emergency is related to drowning, the lifesaver should start chest compressions. These should be conducted for about a minute or so before the lifesaver calls 911. However, if one person can perform the compressions, and there is another person available who can call 911, then these steps should happen simultaneously.

For persons who are trained in CPR, one of the best ways to remember the order in which steps should be administered is to recall the memory cue CAB. This cue stands for Circulation, Airway, Breathing. The goal of CPR is to help an unresponsive person to start breathing on his or her own. First, use chest compressions to restore circulation. This is the C of CAB. Second, check the patient's airway for possible blockages. The A in CAB stands for airway. Finally, administer rescue breathing. This is, of course, the B of CAB.

What is the passage mainly about?

A) It focuses on how to administer CPR techniques.
B) It focuses on several ways to save people in danger.
C) It covers various ways that people can learn about CPR.
D) It presents a review of how people can use CPR daily.

The correct answer is **A**. The passage is mainly about how to administer CPR techniques. Choice B is incorrect because the passage focuses more on CPR than on lifesaving approaches in general. The passage discusses how to use CPR and not how to learn about it, per se, so choice C can be eliminated.

REVIEW QUESTIONS

1. Literary scholars have frequently compared the characteristics of poetry written by the first and second generation of Romantic poets. Poets such as William Wordsworth established the foundations of the exaltation of the imagination that later influenced writers such as John Keats and Percy Bysshe Shelley. The first generation of poets was attempting to advocate for the importance of artistry and creativity. The second generation of poets built on this foundation and went even further in their speculations about what creativity could achieve, especially perhaps in a political sense. However, the second generation was also negatively impacted by their observation of the French Revolution, and this experience tempered their idealism.

Which of the following best states the main idea of the passage?

A) To describe the distinctions between the first and second generation Romantic poets
B) To explain the influence of William Wordsworth as a poet
C) To illustrate the importance of Percy Bysshe Shelley as a poet
D) To discuss the political viewpoints of the British Romantic poets

2. The acoustics of various performance venues emerge as the result of careful planning and extensive decision making. Sound travels differently when it moves through air, and the objects it encounters in a particular environment strongly impact the way that listeners hear the sound. Venues that are designed primarily to house symphony orchestra performances require vastly different acoustic designs than do venues that cater to more intimate performances. Engineers must take

into account a wide variety of variables during the design process, including vibration, sound, ultrasound, and infrasound.

A sound wave consists of a fundamental, followed by a series of sequential overtones. The way that listeners perceive these sound waves is impacted by the material used in the listening environment, the physical layout of the environment, the position of the stage relative to the audience's seating, and even the height of the ceiling. Many acoustic engineers also must take into consideration the manner in which transducers impact listening. Transducers include loudspeakers, microphones, and sonar projectors. The addition of these tools to an acoustic environment can strongly influence and transform how audience members in different locations in the room perceive any sound being transmitted.

Which of the following best states the main idea of the passage?

A) Sound is a multifaceted and complex phenomenon impacted by numerous factors.
B) Acoustic engineers need to acquire an advanced degree to become qualified.
C) Acoustic engineering is a sophisticated science that requires complex decision making.
D) Multiple acoustic engineers should work on a single project to combine their expertise.

3. Michelangelo was arguably the most talented and prolific artist to emerge from the Italian Renaissance. Not only did he spend three years on his back lying on a scaffold to create the famous paintings adorning the Sistine Chapel, but he also created a sculpture of the Biblical hero David that has been emulated for centuries. Michelangelo himself reflected that he simply took a block of marble and removed all the pieces that did not belong to the David statue. Michelangelo is considered a consummate artist because he created works in so many different media, including painting and sculpture.

The passage is primarily concerned with which of the following?

A) Justifying the value of Michelangelo's art
B) Explaining why Michelangelo could create in multiple media
C) Analyzing the humility of great artists from the Renaissance
D) Arguing that Michelangelo's accomplishments are some of the greatest of his time

4. The current tests for measuring IQ, or an individual's intelligence quotient, were developed during the early and mid-twentieth century. Their use was popularized by Terman, who designed specific tests for use in the U.S. Army. Some psychologists today assert that the traditional system of measuring IQ should remain the sole method of assessing intelligence. Historically, the test has been constructed based on the assumption that there exists one general intelligence factor that impacts an individual's intellectual capacity.

The validity of this assumption has been challenged by other psychologists. In particular, Howard Gardner has emphasized that a unified conception of intelligence based on a single factor remains highly limited and unnecessarily constraining. Gardner has postulated an alternative theory concerning the existence of multiple intelligences. He posits that individuals can possess intelligence in particular areas, including linguistic intelligence, spiritual intelligence, spatial intelligence, intrapersonal intelligence, interpersonal intelligence, musical intelligence, mathematical intelligence, and kinesthetic intelligence, among others. Gardner asserts that individuals can be extremely intelligent and exhibit talent in one area, while failing to demonstrate the same level of prowess in another area. His theory has been discussed widely, although efforts to obtain empirical evidence to support his ideas remain in progress.

Which of the following best states the main idea of the passage?

A) Traditional IQ tests are faulty and should be eliminated.
B) Howard Gardner's theory of IQ measurement focuses on multiple intelligences.
C) Both traditional IQ tests and Gardner's assessments should be used to measure intelligence.
D) Gardner's IQ test focuses predominantly on linguistic intelligence.

5. To All Department Supervisors:

The Acme Records Retrieval System will be undergoing scheduled maintenance this Friday, from 4:00 P.M. until midnight. Please inform all department personnel of the system outage, so that researchers can make alternative arrangements to access necessary data.

An archived copy of the Core Business Records Database will be accessible in the Web Services department office from 4:00 P.M. until 8:00 P.M. on Friday. However, this database contains only core records data and is limited in its scope.

Please direct any questions to Marcus Sampson, Web Services Maintenance Officer, at (617) 555-0004.

What is the memo mainly about?

A) It notifies employees of maintenance on the Records Retrieval System.
B) It notifies employees regarding who to contact in the Web Services office.
C) It describes the scope of the company's Core Business Records Database.
D) It explains the public availability of the Core Business Records Database.

6. The Beatles influenced the genre of rock and roll just as Beethoven expanded the genre of the symphony. John Lennon, Paul McCartney, George Harrison, and Ringo Starr expanded the public's understanding of their musical genre and reclassified it as an anthem for rebellion. Their music transformed into the hippies' theme songs of the sixties. Beethoven similarly altered the public's understanding of the symphony. His addition of a chorus in the last movement of the Ninth Symphony attests to this feat.

What is the passage mainly about?

A) It compares the effects that the Beatles and Beethoven had on their genres.
B) It explains how the Beatles helped reclassify rock and roll as a genre.
C) It contrasts the music styles of the Beatles with those of Beethoven.
D) It describes how the music of the Beatles became the hippies' theme songs.

7. In the animal kingdom, many symbiotic relationships exist between two species that take actions known to be mutually beneficial for both parties. In the water, clownfish have such a relationship with sea anemones. The fish are one of the only species that can swim unharmed in the anemone's waving tentacles, as typically the tentacles would sting any animal that swam near it. However, the clownfish is immune to the sting of the tentacles and is therefore protected by them; in return, its presence helps the anemone stay clean, avoid attack by parasites, and remain free from infection.

Which of the following best states the main idea of the passage?

A) Clownfish are one of the only species that can swim unharmed near sea anemones.
B) Clownfish and sea anemones have a mutually beneficial symbiotic relationship.
C) Sea anemones are able to protect clownfish and offer them a safe place to reside.
D) Clownfish typically help sea anemones to stay clean and avoid being attacked.

8. To Whom It May Concern,

I am writing to request a refund of the charge made to my credit card for the purchase of a water filter on Friday, September 18. The filter was the wrong type for my filtration system, so I had to return it. I returned the filter to the store on Saturday, September 19, and the customer service clerk had me complete the paperwork to refund my charges for the purchase. However, the credit never appeared on my credit card account. Please reverse the charges in the amount shown on the credit receipt attached to this e-mail.

Thank you for your assistance.

Claire Glendheim

The e-mail is primarily concerned with which of the following?

A) Explaining the reason for a return
B) Reporting a product failure
C) Complaining about poor service
D) Requesting a refund

9. Historically, the study of creativity has concentrated on persons known for their innovation. Early creativity studies focused on creative "geniuses," such as Einstein, Mozart, or Shakespeare. This type of creativity is known as "Big C" creativity. However, as research on creativity progressed, a corresponding interest in how people could be creative in smaller ways—on an everyday basis—emerged in the discipline. Scholars began to investigate how ordinary tasks, such as cleaning, driving particular familiar routes, and completing work and schoolwork, could be conducted in innovative ways. This focus of creativity research has been labeled "little c" creativity.

Which sentence best describes the main idea of this passage?

A) Creativity occurs not just in large ways, but through small, everyday actions.
B) The study of creativity has historically concentrated on innovative persons.
C) The study of creativity addresses both "Big C" and "little c" types of creativity.
D) Driving familiar routes to a destination can be considered an example of creativity.

10. Laurel Hill Botanic Gardens is pleased to announce the installation of the sculpture series by Laurel Hill artist-in-residence, Darryl C. Grant. The installation features mixed-media sculptures emphasizing the floral designs prominent in Mr. Grant's paintings, many of which are also on exhibit in the Michael and Frieda Sachs Viewing Room.

The sculpture exhibit will open at 10:00 A.M. on Thursday, June 5. The Botanic Gardens' art curator, Jessalyn Jones, will present an overview of the sculptures and lead a guided tour of the installation. The opening ceremony will end with refreshments served in the Nature Observatory from 2:00–3:00 P.M.

This is a members-only event. All Botanic Gardens members and their guests are invited to attend. Tickets are $50.00 per person and can be purchased at the registration desk beginning Monday, May 5.

What is the memo mainly about?

A) It invites Botanic Gardens members to a sculpture installation.
B) It explains the history of floral sculptures at the Botanic Gardens.
C) It describes details regarding the work of sculptor Darryl C. Grant.
D) It explains the role of the art curator in presenting the exhibit.

ANSWER KEY

1. A	**5.** A	**9.** C
2. C	**6.** A	**10.** A
3. D	**7.** B	
4. B	**8.** D	

ANSWERS AND EXPLANATIONS

1. (A) The passage describes the distinctions between the first and second generations of British Romantic poets. Choice D is incorrect because the poets' political sensibilities are included as an example of a factor that impacted their perspectives.

2. (C) The passage emphasizes the fact that performance venues have excellent acoustics as the result of extensive planning and careful decision making. Choice A is incorrect because this statement is too broad.

3. (D) The first sentence emphasizes Michelangelo's status as a master artist, and the passage describes his most well-known art works. Choice A is incorrect because the passage is more of an advocacy for Michelangelo rather than a defense of the value of his art.

4. (B) The passage describes Gardner's theory and indicates that it focuses on the idea of multiple intelligences. Choice C is incorrect because the passage does not address this topic directly.

5. (A) This memo is designed mainly to notify Acme employees of maintenance on the Records Retrieval System. Choices B, C, and D are mentioned in the memo, but they are details of the memo as opposed to the main idea.

6. (A) The focus of the passage is conveyed in the first sentence, which states that "the Beatles influenced the genre of rock and roll just as Beethoven expanded the genre of the symphony." The passage mainly compares the effects that the Beatles and Beethoven had on their respective genres. Choice B is a detail mentioned in the passage, and choice C can be eliminated because the passage does not contrast the styles of the artists but instead compares their impact.

7. (B) The main idea of the passage is that clownfish and sea anemones have a mutually beneficial symbiotic relationship. Choices A, C, and D all represent supporting details of the passage, not the main idea.

8. (D) The e-mail is primarily concerned with requesting a refund. The first sentence of the e-mail clarifies the reason for the author's message. The author does explain why she returned the product, as choice A indicates, but this is a supporting detail of the e-mail, not its main focus.

9. (C) The main idea of the passage is that the study of creativity addresses both "Big C" and "little c" types of creativity. The passage focuses mainly on the study of creativity, not on defining what creativity is, so choice A can be eliminated. Choice B presents a supporting detail of the passage.

10. (A) The memo mainly invites Botanic Gardens members to a sculpture installation. Choice B is incorrect, because the memo does not discuss the history of floral sculptures. Choices C and D convey details mentioned in the passage, not the main idea.

CHAPTER 4

Identifying Purpose

Identifying purpose questions test your understanding of the purpose of a passage or part of a passage. The answer choices for purpose questions usually start with the word "to." A question might ask, for example, "Why does the author mention X?" The answer choices would all give reasons for why the particular detail might have been mentioned.

The example below asks about a specific detail, whereas the example that follows it asks about the entire passage.

Percy Bysshe Shelley was one of the second-generation Romantic poets. Along with John Keats and Lord Byron, Shelley was considered one of the most masterful poets of his generation.

Shelley was born in England in 1792, as a member of the aristocracy. He was educated at two prestigious English schools, Eton College and Oxford University. Shelley believed that poets were visionaries who could serve as societal leaders because of the creative power of their imaginations. The second generation of Romantic poets, in particular, believed that poets were going to help change the world. Shelley's generation believed that through the imagination, anything was possible. They believed that they could use the creative power of the mind to change the government and even change the world. Shelley's poems reflect this belief. He was a truly idealistic thinker, and he claimed that poets were the "unacknowledged legislators of the world." The poet's creative vision could let him or her see things that other people could not.

Shelley's ideas were heavily influenced by the politics of his time. He grew up at a time when governments were under transformation. In fact, he came of age in the shadow of the French Revolution. This war was very violent, and since France was so close to England, Shelley was acutely aware of the violence that was occurring there. That may have led him to concentrate even more on his belief that artists were able to change the world and improve living conditions.

Shelley's poem "Mont Blanc" focuses on the Romantic notion of the sublime. The Romantic poets believed that when people interacted with nature, it sometimes caused them to be in a state of wonder—or it caused them to be awestruck. For example, when a person gazed at a mountain, the huge size of the mountain could cause the person to become speechless with wonder. This was the effect that the sublime quality of nature could have on a viewer.

In "Mont Blanc," Shelley describes the mountain in a way that attempts to explain its effects on the viewer's mind. According to Shelley, the mountain itself causes the viewer's thoughts to enter a kind of strange trance, and to be affected in a way that resembles how a poet or an artist feels whenever he or she is caught in the midst of a creative inspiration. In the poem, Shelley draws a comparison between the effect of the mountain on the viewer and the power that the imagination has over the artist's mind.

Why does the author mention the English schools of Eton College and Oxford University?

A) To give a description of Shelley's background
B) To present a critique of Shelley's education
C) To explain why Shelley disappointed his father
D) To describe why Shelley disliked aristocrats

The correct answer is **A**. The author mentions the English schools of Eton College and Oxford University to give a description of Shelley's background. Only wealthy students, such as those in the aristocracy, usually went to these schools.

The next passage is an example of a question that asks about the author's purpose in the full passage.

The current tests for measuring IQ, or an individual's intelligence quotient, were developed during the early and mid-twentieth century. Their use was popularized by Terman, who designed specific tests for use in the U.S. Army. Some psychologists today assert that the traditional system of measuring IQ should remain the sole method of assessing intelligence. Historically, the test has been constructed based on the assumption that there exists one general intelligence factor that impacts an individual's intellectual capacity.

The validity of this assumption has been challenged by other psychologists. In particular, Howard Gardner has emphasized that a unified conception of intelligence based on a single factor remains highly limited and unnecessarily constraining. Gardner has postulated an alternative theory concerning the existence of multiple intelligences. He posits that individuals can possess intelligence in particular areas, including linguistic intelligence, spiritual intelligence, spatial intelligence, intrapersonal intelligence, interpersonal intelligence, musical intelligence, mathematical intelligence, and kinesthetic intelligence, among others. Gardner asserts that individuals can be extremely intelligent and exhibit talent in one area, while failing to demonstrate the same level of prowess in another area. His theory has been discussed widely, although efforts to obtain empirical evidence to support his ideas remain in progress.

What statement best describes the author's purpose in this passage?

A) The author is trying to prove that Gardner's theory is superior to the traditional method of measuring IQ.
B) The author believes that the traditional method of measuring IQ remains the best.
C) The author is comparing Gardner's theory to the traditional method of measuring IQ.
D) The author is demonstrating why IQ cannot be measured scientifically.

The correct answer is **C**. In this passage the author is comparing Gardner's theory to the traditional method of measuring IQ, but he does not favor either approach. Choices A and B can therefore be ruled out. Although the author points out that Gardner's theory has not been proven with empirical evidence, the passage does not state that IQ can never be measured with such evidence, so choice D is incorrect.

Additional examples of purpose questions are given below. In each of these, the correct answer explains the *reason* an author mentions a particular element in the passage.

Literary scholars have frequently compared the characteristics of poetry written by both the first and second generation of Romantic poets. Poets such as William Wordsworth established the foundations of the exaltation of the imagination that later influenced writers such as John Keats and Percy Bysshe Shelley. The first generation of poets was attempting to advocate for the importance of artistry and creativity. The second generation of poets built on this foundation and went even further in their speculations about what creativity could achieve, especially perhaps in a political sense. However, the second generation was also negatively impacted by their observation of the French Revolution, and this experience tempered their idealism.

The author mentions that the second generation was negatively impacted by their observations of the French Revolution most likely to accomplish which of the following?

A) To make the assertion that the second generation was cynical and bitter
B) To posit that the second generation purposely differentiated themselves from the first
C) To explain why the second generation was less idealistic than the first
D) To support the claim that they were not as prolific as the first generation

The correct answer is **C**. The author mentions how the second generation's observation of the French Revolution negatively impacted their perspectives in order to explain why the second generation was less idealistic than the first. Choice B is incorrect because the second generation's intention was not to differentiate themselves from their predecessors.

Let's look at another example.

As one of the most prolific female poets in nineteenth-century America, today Emily Dickinson is a household name. However, during her lifetime, she lived as a recluse and wrote most of her poetry from the solitude of her bedroom. She presents a unique perspective from this time period, when few women wrote about the themes she discusses. For this reason, critics are frequently interested in her perspective as a female author even beyond the contributions she made as an American nineteenth-century writer.

The author mentions the dual classification of Emily Dickinson most likely to demonstrate which of the following?

A) As an author, Dickinson can be classified by either focus or genre, but not both.

B) As an author, Dickinson can fit into more than one general classification.

C) Writers should be classified according to their personal practices.

D) Writers should be classified according to how much writing they do.

The correct answer is **B**. The passage mentions that some literary scholars are more interested in Dickinson's perspective as a female author than they are in her contributions as a nineteenth-century writer. This discussion reveals that Dickinson has been and can be classified in more than one manner.

Now consider this passage.

The best method of treating individuals facing psychological difficulties is a blend of cognitive-behavioral therapy and medication. This approach not only serves to address the patient's potential chemical imbalances, but it also emancipates the patient by allowing him or her some autonomy in dealing with the issues associated with a possible malaise.

Cognitive-behavioral therapy requires the patient to examine his or her own behavior and to make moderations in a rational and well-thought-out manner. If a person's chemical makeup is preventing him or her from being able to carry out such a responsibility, then medication can help alleviate specific symptoms to allow the patient to deal with the underlying emotional and psychological issues in an effective manner. Nevertheless, psychologists have wide-ranging opinions on how to help these patients cope with challenges such as depression or anxiety.

Some trained professionals assert that medication alone can best serve psychological patients. Other psychologists believe that the utilization of Freud's psychoanalytic approach represents the best method for assisting persons with these emotional symptoms. Some counselors believe that each person's set of individual circumstances should be considered. Other counselors depend on the characteristics of behaviorism to modify the patients' behavior so that their behavioral patterns become more effective. Overall, however, many professionals agree that the combination of cognitive-behavioral therapy and medication will ultimately best serve the patient.

The author notes that "cognitive-behavioral therapy requires the patient to examine his or her own behavior" primarily for which of the following reasons?

A) To advocate for the superiority of this therapeutic approach

B) To emphasize the negative aspects of this therapeutic approach

C) To describe a positive characteristic of this treatment strategy

D) To explain why this option is an inferior treatment method

The correct answer is **C**. The sentence is explaining a positive characteristic of this type of therapeutic approach. The next sentence describes how this course of treatment corresponds well with medication as adjunct treatment if necessary to alleviate specific symptoms. Choice A is incorrect because the sentence's primary function is to describe a beneficial aspect of this approach, not to advocate for its superiority.

REVIEW QUESTIONS

1. Christopher Columbus was particularly influenced by the maps of the ancient geographer Ptolemy. Ptolemy argued that the world was round, which went against the belief of the day that the world was flat. Columbus sided with Ptolemy on this question and set out to prove that it was so.

   At the time it was widely held that sailing west from Europe would lead to certain death. Believing that the world was round, Columbus thought that one who sailed west would wind up in the east. Other scientists of the day rejected this idea, so Columbus wrote to a respected Italian scholar, Paolo Toscanelli, to ask for his opinion on the matter.

   Toscanelli supported the idea of Columbus's trip and sent word back to Columbus in 1474. After receiving Toscanelli's encouragement, Columbus focused all of his thoughts and plans on traveling westward. To make the journey, he would require the help of a generous financial backer, so he went to seek the aid of the king of Portugal. Columbus asked the king for ships and sailors to make the journey. In return, he promised to bring back wealth and to help to convert natives living on the lands to the Church. Portugal refused, and Columbus approached Italy unsuccessfully as well. He went to Spain next.

   Queen Isabella of Spain agreed to support the journey. It took some time for Columbus to convince her, but he did succeed, and she paid for the trip. Part of what led the queen to believe in Columbus was the way that he focused on his goal for such a long time with great intent. He spent the best years of his life working toward his dream, remaining persistent and determined. Legend has it that even during his first voyage, members of his crew became frightened and uncertain, wanting to return home, but Columbus pressed on. The eventual discovery of the Americas was the reward for his commitment.

   More than 500 years later, the geography of the world is often taken for granted, but Columbus was an early visionary whose results proved at least some of his theories correct.

   What is the author's purpose in writing this passage?

   A) To compare and contrast the theories of Ptolemy and Columbus
   B) To dispute the claim that Columbus discovered the Americas
   C) To offer the reader glimpses into the regrets of Columbus
   D) To argue that Columbus was a persistent and committed explorer

2. The English town of Stratford-upon-Avon is visited yearly by tourists wanting to view the birthplace of William Shakespeare. William's father, John Shakespeare, bought the family home on Henley Street, and it is here that William is believed to have been born in 1564. Shakespeare's birth home remained in his family until the early 1800s, and it is now a public museum.

Shakespeare attended school at the King Edward VI Grammar School, which occupied the first floor of a building known as the Guildhall. It was in this Guildhall that Shakespeare first experienced theater, when he saw a theatrical performance given by a group of traveling actors. The Royal Shakespeare Company still performs in the town at the Royal Shakespeare and Swan Theaters.

Close to the Guildhall is the site of a house known as New Place, which was bought by Shakespeare himself. Here Shakespeare lived during the later part of his life, until his death in 1616. Although he spent most of his career in London, with trips back to Stratford, he moved permanently to New Place in the last years of his life and is believed to have written some of his later works there. Only the foundations of the New Place house now remain.

In the town of Shottery, one mile from Stratford, is the cottage where Shakespeare's wife, Anne Hathaway, was born. The Hathaway cottage, now also a museum, is actually a large, thatch-roofed farmhouse with sprawling gardens where Shakespeare is believed to have developed his relationship with Anne. They married in 1582 and had three children.

Why does the author mention William Shakespeare's wife in a passage about Stratford-upon-Avon?

A) Because Shakespeare's wife's parents favored the town
B) Because Anne Hathaway was an important founder of the town
C) Because William Shakespeare preferred Shottery to Stratford
D) Because Hathaway was born nearby, and her cottage is now a local museum

3. One of the most important gymnastic exercises in the original Montessori school approach is that of the "line." For this exercise, a line is drawn in chalk or paint on the floor. Instead of one line, there may also be two lines drawn. The children are taught to walk on these lines like tightrope walkers, placing their feet one in front of the other.

To keep their balance, the children must make efforts similar to those of real tightrope walkers, except that they have no danger of falling, since the lines are drawn only on the floor. The teacher herself performs the exercise first, showing clearly how she places her feet, and the children imitate her without her even needing to speak. At first it is only certain children who follow her, and when she has shown them how to walk the line, she leaves, letting the exercise develop on its own.

The children for the most part continue to walk, following with great care the movement they have seen, and making efforts to keep their balance so they don't fall. Gradually the other children come closer and watch and try the exercise. In a short time, the entire line is covered with children balancing themselves and continuing to walk around, watching their feet attentively.

Music may be used at this point. It should be a very simple march, without an obvious rhythm. It should simply accompany and support the efforts of the children.

When children learn to master their balance in this way, Dr. Montessori believed, they can bring the act of walking to a remarkable standard of perfection.

For what reason does the author focus all five paragraphs on *walking the line?*

A) The main idea of the passage is to explain the importance of this exercise.
B) Walking the line is the most important aspect of a Montessori education.
C) The concept is a difficult one to grasp and needs extensive explanation.
D) The passage's genre is nonfiction, so it includes detailed instructions.

4. Public highways are used constantly with little thought of how important they are to the everyday life of a community. It is understandable that most people think about their local public highway only when it affects their own activities. People usually don't focus on highway improvements unless the subject is brought to their attention by increased taxes or advertising.

Highway improvements are an important issue, however. It is important for the economies of most communities to keep highways in good repair. Products purchased in one location are often manufactured in other locations, and safe highways are required to transport the products to their final destination. Good transportation facilities contribute greatly to community prosperity.

The type and amount of the highway improvement needed in any area depends on the traffic in that area. In low-population areas, the amount of traffic on local roads is likely to be small, and highways will not require as much work. But as an area develops, the use of public highways increases, and maintenance demands increase. In small towns, residents are also more able to adapt to the condition of the roads. A road shutdown does not have the same impact on business as it would in busy areas. In large districts with many activities, however, roads must be usable year-round in order for business progress to continue.

In planning improvements of highway systems, several different types of traffic may be encountered. These range from business traffic to agricultural shipping to residential transportation. Improvement activities must meet the requirements of all classes of traffic, with the most important provided for first. Those improvements of lesser importance can be performed as soon as finances permit.

What is the author's purpose in writing this passage?

A) To advise city planners about how to build and maintain highways
B) To prove that areas with low populations do not need highways
C) To highlight the necessity of highway improvements in daily life
D) To provide an objective view of how rural highways function

5. Personality is the combination of traits that make up an individual's sense of self. Traits can range from descriptors of behavior, such as "calm" or "emotional," to modes of experiencing the world, such as "thinking" or "sensing." One Swiss theorist named Carl Jung influenced the development of the Myers-Briggs personalities (sixteen total), a system that is now well known. These sixteen personalities consist of some combination of four dimensions: introversion–extroversion, sensing–intuiting, thinking–feeling, and judging–perceiving.

What is the author's primary purpose in writing this passage?

A) To share a biography about a famous theorist
B) To provide additional details about a topic
C) To introduce and define a particular topic
D) To argue that a topic is of prominent importance

6. Imagine living in the year 1800. The railroads then were very scarce. Gas lights were not yet invented, and electric lights were not even dreamed of. Even kerosene wasn't used at that point. This was the world into which Samuel Morse, the inventor of the telegraph, was born.

Samuel Morse was born in Charlestown, Massachusetts, shortly before the turn of the century, in 1791. When he was seven years old, he was sent to boarding school at Phillips Academy, Andover. While he was there, his father wrote him letters, giving him good advice. He told him about George Washington and about a British statesman named Lord Chesterfield, who was able to achieve many of his goals. Lord Chesterfield was asked once how he managed to find time for all of his pursuits, and he replied that he only ever did one thing at a time, and that he "never put off anything until tomorrow that could be done today."

Morse worked hard at school and began to think and act for himself at quite a young age. His biggest accomplishment was in painting, and he established himself as a successful painter after graduating from college at Yale. But he also had an interest in science and inventions. He was passionate about the idea of discovering a way for people to send messages to each other in short periods of time.

In the early 1800s, it took a long time to receive news of any sort, even important news. Whole countries had to wait weeks to hear word of the outcomes of faraway wars. The mail was carried by stagecoach. In emergency situations, such as when ships were lost at sea, there was no way to send requests for help. Electricity had been discovered, but little application had been made of it up until that point. This was about to change when Morse set his mind to his invention.

On October 1, 1832, Morse was sailing to America from a trip overseas on a ship called the *Sully*. He became preoccupied with the thought of inventing a machine that would later become the telegraph. Morse thought about the telegraph night and day. As he sat upon the deck of the ship after dinner one night, he took out a little notebook and began to create a plan.

If a message could be sent ten miles without dropping, he wrote, "I could make it go around the globe." He said this over and over again during the years after his trip.

One morning at the breakfast table, Morse showed his plan to some of the other *Sully* passengers. Five years later, when the model of the telegraph was built, it was exactly like the one shown that morning to the passengers on the *Sully*.

Once he arrived in America, Morse worked for twelve long years to get people to notice his invention. Though some supported the idea of the telegraph, many people scoffed at it. Morse persisted, and eventually a bill was passed by Congress in 1842. It authorized the funds needed to build the first trial telegraph line.

After two years, the telegraph line was complete. Morse and his colleagues tested it in May 1844. The device worked, and the telegraph became a huge success. Morse's persistence had finally paid off.

Why do the first few paragraphs sketch a biography of Morse's early life?

A) Because the main idea of the passage is the early life of Samuel Morse

B) Because the passage is written in narrative form, with events presented chronologically

C) Because it was when Morse was young that he invented the telegraph

D) Because the author wants to demonstrate that Morse's discovery was random

7. Percy Bysshe Shelley was one of the second-generation Romantic poets. Along with John Keats and Lord Byron, Shelley was considered one of the most masterful poets of his generation.

Shelley was born in England in 1792, as a member of the aristocracy. He was educated at two prestigious English schools, Eton College and

Oxford University. Shelley believed that poets were visionaries who could serve as societal leaders because of the creative power of their imaginations. The second generation of Romantic poets, in particular, believed that poets were going to help change the world. Shelley's generation believed that through the imagination, anything was possible. They believed that they could use the creative power of the mind to change the government and even change the world. Shelley's poems reflect this belief. He was a truly idealistic thinker, and he claimed that poets were the "unacknowledged legislators of the world." The poet's creative vision could let him or her see things that other people could not.

Shelley's ideas were heavily influenced by the politics of his time. He grew up at a time when governments were under transformation. In fact, he came of age in the shadow of the French Revolution. This war was very violent, and since France was so close to England, Shelley was acutely aware of the violence that was occurring there. That may have led him to concentrate even more on his belief that artists were able to change the world and improve living conditions.

Shelley's poem "Mont Blanc" focuses on the Romantic notion of the sublime. The Romantic poets believed that when people interacted with nature, it sometimes caused them to be in a state of wonder—or it caused them to be awestruck. For example, when a person gazed at a mountain, the huge size of the mountain could cause the person to become speechless with wonder. This was the effect that the sublime quality of nature could have on a viewer.

In "Mont Blanc," Shelley describes the mountain in a way that attempts to explain its effects on the viewer's mind. According to Shelley, the mountain itself causes the viewer's thoughts to enter a kind of strange trance, and to be affected in a way that resembles how a poet or an artist feels whenever he or she is caught in the midst of a creative inspiration. In the poem, Shelley draws a comparison between the effect of the mountain on the viewer and the power that the imagination has over the artist's mind.

Why does the author mention the French Revolution?

A) To explain a historical event that affected Shelley's beliefs
B) To show why Shelley included violence in his poems
C) To illustrate how Shelley achieved a poetic effect
D) To describe why Shelley disliked the French so strongly

8. The Beatles influenced the genre of rock and roll just as Beethoven expanded the genre of the symphony. John Lennon, Paul McCartney, George Harrison, and Ringo Starr expanded the public's understanding of their musical genre and reclassified it as an anthem for rebellion. Their music transformed into the hippies' theme songs of the sixties. Beethoven similarly altered the public's understanding of the symphony. His addition of a chorus in the last movement of the Ninth Symphony attests to this feat.

Which of the following reflects the primary purpose of the passage?

A) To describe the Beatles' contribution to rock music
B) To explain Beethoven's influence on the Beatles
C) To describe how the Beatles and Beethoven affected their genres
D) To delineate the terms of the Beatles' musical genius

9. Athletes are extremely aware of how physical motion and its properties can affect the human body as well as the outcomes of competitions. Figure skating, for example, involves concentric motion for spins. Skaters learn how to use their arms to bring in their centers of gravity. In the same way that runners adopt a certain leg stance or swimmers use their arms to move quickly through the water, skaters also use their knowledge of physics to improve their skating.

Why does the passage mention concentric motion?

A) To suggest that a certain leg stance can impact a skater's motion
B) To differentiate it from paracentric motion, which skiers use
C) To show how skaters use their knowledge of physical motion
D) To suggest that skaters have a better sense of physical motion than other athletes

10. Bees are <u>a natural part of the pollination cycle</u> of plants. Many plants require the assistance of bees in order to transfer their pollen so that flowers can be produced. Bees travel from flower to flower, and minuscule grains of pollen attach to the bees' legs. The pollen travels much more efficiently via bees than it might if it had to rely on the wind, for example. In this manner, bees assist in the natural pollination cycle <u>through the action of gathering nectar from flowers</u>. Bees are a critical component of this process; without them, <u>plants would face much greater challenges</u> in their reproduction.

Circle the underlined phrase in the passage that explains the primary action through which bees contribute to the pollination process.

Arguably, the most well-known Siamese cat is the seal point. The dark brown ears, face, and tail are famous markers of this popular breed of cat. Many cats that appear in popular culture, including the mischievous Siamese cats in Disney animated films, are patterned after this type of Siamese. However, cat aficionados are well aware that other types of Siamese cats also exist. Two of these include the blue point and the snowshoe. Snowshoe Siamese are characterized by the white markings on their paws along with the dark "boots": these markings earn them their name and make the cats look as though they have been walking in the snow. Blue point Siamese cats do not have dark brown "points"; rather, their ears, paws, tails, and noses are characterized by bluish patches on their fur. Some Siamese cats are even hairless. They exhibit the darker pigment on their noses, tails, ears, and paws, similar to their fur-covered counterparts of the same breed. However, hairless Siamese cats exhibit these "points" on their skin instead of their fur. This type of

Siamese is rather rare and not very well known. Despite the contrasts between the external appearances of these varying types of Siamese, all Siamese cats are known for being vocal, loyal, and rather mischievous.

The next three questions are based on this passage.

11. Which of the following best states the purpose of the passage?

   A) To assert that the seal point is the most well-known type of Siamese cat
   B) To provide a physical description of different types of Siamese cats
   C) To propose that snowshoe Siamese tend to live in colder environments
   D) To indicate that all Siamese cats in popular culture have seal point markings

12. The author mentions the Siamese cats in Disney animated films for which of the following reasons?

   A) To support the idea that seal points appear frequently in popular culture
   B) To provide a contrast between how seal points and blue points are presented
   C) To explain how Siamese cats are construed as being mischievous
   D) To explain how seal point Siamese are typically portrayed in popular culture

13. The author notes that "all Siamese cats are known for being vocal, loyal, and mischievous" in order to accomplish which of the following?

   A) To provide a contrast between blue point and snowshoe Siamese
   B) To make a generalization about all cats of this breed
   C) To indicate that the different types have distinct personalities
   D) To explain differences among the three types of Siamese cats

14. Aficionados of classical music frequently appreciate the characteristics of jazz, and some laypersons think the two genres are somewhat similar. However, jazz musicians are noted for their improvisational abilities, whereas classically trained musicians are often very reliant upon printed music. Although musicians in both genres must be very well versed in scales and various musical keys, jazz musicians must possess impeccable knowledge of this material in order to be able to perform and fulfill the requirements of their chosen genre.

   The author of the passage mentions jazz players' improvisational abilities in order to do which of the following?

   A) To demonstrate their classical music skills
   B) To differentiate them from classical players
   C) To provide evidence of the merits of their performance
   D) To explain how they receive their training

15. The acoustics of various performance venues emerge as the result of careful planning and extensive decision making. Sound travels differently when it moves through air, and the objects it encounters in a particular environment strongly impact the way that listeners hear the sound. Venues that are designed primarily to house symphony orchestra performances require vastly different acoustic designs than do venues that cater to more intimate performances. Engineers must take into account a wide variety of variables during the design process, including vibration, sound, ultrasound, and infrasound.

A sound wave consists of a fundamental, followed by a series of sequential overtones. The way that listeners perceive these sound waves is impacted by the material used in the listening environment, the physical layout of the environment, the position of the stage relative to the audience's seating, and even the height of the ceiling. Many acoustic engineers also must take into consideration the manner in which transducers impact listening. Transducers include loudspeakers, microphones, and sonar projectors. The addition of these tools to an acoustic environment can strongly influence and transform how audience members in different locations in the room perceive any sound being transmitted.

Which of the following most likely reflects the primary purpose of the passage?

A) To indicate that a new type of material should be used to improve acoustics in performance venues
B) To indicate that unexpected elements can impact the way people hear sounds
C) To illustrate how the purpose for which a performance hall is intended impacts its acoustic design
D) To explain some of the factors that acoustic engineers consider in designing performance venues

ANSWER KEY

1. D	**7.** A	**11.** B
2. D	**8.** C	**12.** A
3. A	**9.** C	**13.** B
4. C	**10.** through the action	**14.** B
5. C	of gathering nectar	**15.** D
6. B	from flowers	

ANSWERS AND EXPLANATIONS

1. (D) Ptolemy is only briefly mentioned in the passage's first paragraph and is not contrasted theory-wise with Columbus; hence, choice A is incorrect. Choice B is incorrect because nowhere does the author suggest that Columbus did not discover the Americas. Finally, this passage does not concern the regrets of Columbus, but rather his discovery of the Americas, indicating that choice C is incorrect.

2. (D) Choices A, B, and C are incorrect because their content is neither mentioned nor suggested in the passage. Since the passage is about the town of Stratford-upon-Avon, it is appropriate to mention important buildings located nearby, which indicates that choice D is the correct answer.

3. (A) All paragraphs in a nonfiction passage should focus on or support the main idea of the covered subject, in this case *walking the line*. Choice B can be eliminated because of its absolute phrase *the most important*, which is not true; instead, walking the line is *one of the most important gymnastic exercises*.

4. (C) This passage is directed to a general audience as indicated by its first sentence, so choice A is incorrect. The first sentence of paragraph two makes the statement that highway improvements are an important issue, which is an opinion that gives away the author's purpose for writing this passage. Choice D is concerned with explaining highway function, which is not the author's purpose. Choice C is correct.

5. (C) The passage begins by defining the term to be discussed: *personality*. Such definitions are generally provided at the introduction of a new topic, as choice C states. Choice A is incorrect because while the passage mentions a theorist, Carl Jung, his life is not the topic of focus, as would be the case in a biography. Choice D is also incorrect because the passage offers no opinions about the subject matter.

6. (B) The main idea of the passage is the invention of the telegraph, not the early life of Samuel Morse, so choice A is incorrect. Choice C is also incorrect because the information in the passage leads the reader to conclude that Morse was over 40 years old when the telegraph was invented. Finally, the author demonstrates that Morse was a deep thinker and a hard worker from an early age, which would make choice D incorrect; given these qualities, his invention could not have been random. This passage is a narrative that flows chronologically, with earlier events appearing before later ones, making choice B correct.

7. (A) The author mentions the French Revolution to explain a historical event that affected Shelley's beliefs. The violence of this war affected Shelley and his contemporaries, possibly leading Shelley to strengthen his belief that artists could change the world. Choice C is incorrect, because the author does not talk about Shelley's poetic effects in relation to the French Revolution.

8. (C) The passage explains how the Beatles' compositional style challenged and expanded the genre of rock and roll. The passage uses Beethoven as an example of a musician who accomplished a similar feat in his genre.

9. (C) The passage mentions concentric motion to explain how skaters use their knowledge of physical motion when performing spins. Choice A is incorrect because it is not related to the passage's discussion of concentric motion.

10. (through the action of gathering nectar from flowers) The passage describes how bees gather nectar in order to illustrate the primary action that bees take in their role in the pollination process.

11. (B) The passage provides a physical description of different types of Siamese cats. Choices A and D are incorrect because the seal point is only one type of Siamese cat discussed in the passage.

12. (A) The passage uses the Disney animated cats as examples of how seal points frequently appear in the popular media. Choice D is incorrect because the passage does not explain how seal points are portrayed. Other than describing them as *mischievous*, it merely states that they appear often.

13. (B) The author ends the passage by listing characteristics common to all Siamese cats. The sentence focuses on all Siamese, so choices A, C, and D are incorrect.

14. (B) The passage mentions jazz players' improvisational abilities to differentiate them from classical players. This ability is the primary distinction that provides a contrast between jazz musicians and the abilities of their classical counterparts.

15. (D) The passage mainly explains factors that acoustic engineers have to consider to achieve their desired results in a performance venue. Choice B is incorrect because the passage focuses more on the design factors that must be considered by acoustic engineers.

CHAPTER 5

Identifying Details

Identifying details questions ask about specific facts from the passage. They often start with the phrase "According to the author." They typically ask "how" and "what" questions. In a sense, detail questions are the opposite of main idea questions. They ask about smaller issues raised in the passage rather than "big picture" ideas. When answering detail questions, keep in mind the following:

> The answer to a detail question is always given directly in the passage.

Some detail questions may ask you to identify the correct order of events given in the passage, as in this example.

Imagine living in the year 1800. The railroads then were very scarce. Gas lights were not yet invented, and electric lights were not even dreamed of. Even kerosene wasn't used at that point. This was the world into which Samuel Morse, the inventor of the telegraph, was born.

Samuel Morse was born in Charlestown, Massachusetts, shortly before the turn of the century, in 1791. When he was seven years old, he was sent to boarding school at Phillips Academy, Andover. While he was there, his father wrote him letters, giving him good advice. He told him about George Washington and about a British statesman named Lord Chesterfield, who was able to achieve many of his goals. Lord Chesterfield was asked once how he managed to find time for all of his pursuits, and he replied that he only ever did one thing at a time, and that he "never put off anything until tomorrow that could be done today."

Morse worked hard at school and began to think and act for himself at quite a young age. His biggest accomplishment was in painting, and he established himself as a successful painter after graduating from college at Yale. But he also had an interest in science and inventions. He was passionate about the idea of discovering a way for people to send messages to each other in short periods of time.

In the early 1800s, it took a long time to receive news of any sort, even important news. Whole countries had to wait weeks to hear word of the outcomes of faraway wars. The mail was carried by stagecoach. In emergency situations, such as when ships were lost at sea, there was no way to send requests for help. Electricity had been discovered, but little application had been made of it up until that point. This was about to change when Morse set his mind to his invention.

On October 1, 1832, Morse was sailing to America from a trip overseas on a ship called the *Sully*. He became preoccupied with the thought of inventing a machine that would later become the telegraph. Morse thought about the telegraph night and day. As he sat upon the deck of the ship after dinner one night, he took out a little notebook and began to create a plan.

If a message could be sent ten miles without dropping, he wrote, "I could make it go around the globe." He said this over and over again during the years after his trip.

One morning at the breakfast table, Morse showed his plan to some of the other *Sully* passengers. Five years later, when the model of the telegraph was built, it was exactly like the one shown that morning to the passengers on the *Sully*.

Once he arrived in America, Morse worked for twelve long years to get people to notice his invention. Though some supported the idea of the telegraph, many people scoffed at it. Morse persisted, and eventually a bill was passed by Congress in 1842. It authorized the funds needed to build the first trial telegraph line.

After two years, the telegraph line was complete. Morse and his colleagues tested it in May 1844. The device worked, and the telegraph became a huge success. Morse's persistence had finally paid off.

Put the events below into chronological order (1 = first / 3 = last).

_____ Morse returns to America aboard the *Sully*.
_____ Morse attends Yale.
_____ Morse becomes a painter.

The correct order is 3, 1, 2. Paragraph three states that Morse became a painter after graduating from Yale, and paragraph five describes Morse as sailing to America aboard the *Sully* after that. The passage states that Morse was returning to America from a trip overseas.

As the question in the following example shows, some detail questions may ask you to identify a statement that paraphrases, or restates, information given in the passage.

Literary scholars have often speculated as to the personal characteristics of William Shakespeare. The Bard is known to many as the greatest writer the English language has ever known, but we have very few examples of his handwriting or even his own name written out in his hand. Some academics have gone so far as to speculate that Shakespeare was a pseudonym for an aristocrat. However, the majority of scholars have dismissed this proposal, and they concentrate instead on Shakespeare's thoughtful insights and dexterous construction of language.

Which sentence below best restates, or paraphrases, the third sentence of the passage?

A) Some scholars are convinced that Shakespeare was the name of an aristocratic family that fell from grace.

B) Some scholars think that Shakespeare got most of his insights from disguising himself as an aristocrat and infiltrating wealthy circles.
C) Some scholars have speculated that aristocrats did not like Shakespeare's plays and considered his insights pseudo-intellectual.
D) Some scholars have a theory that Shakespeare's works were really written by an aristocrat who used that name as an alias.

The correct answer is **D**. The third sentence states that some scholars speculate, or have the theory, that Shakespeare was a pseudonym, or alias, used by an aristocrat who wrote his works. Choice D therefore best restates the information given in the third sentence.

In the following example the question asks about a specific detail mentioned in one part of the passage.

Austrian-born Sigmund Freud, a psychoanalytic psychologist, lived from the mid-nineteenth to the mid-twentieth century. The psychoanalytic approach refers to the school of thought that unconscious memories or desires guide our emotions and actions. In personality theory, this equates to events from childhood shaping the individual self without a person's conscious awareness. These specific childhood events continue to exert a strong influence over our lives and dominate our emotions. If you are a life-of-the-party, extroverted personality, perhaps you had a healthy upbringing; however, quiet, deep-thinker types can be just as functional. How your caregivers responded to your natural urges will determine your level of mental health, according to the psychoanalytic approach.

Freud believed that as a child, an individual's actions are driven by hidden impulses—and that repression or denial of those impulses by parents or society can lead to fixations or personality disorders. Alternatively, if the child's impulses are accepted as normative to his or her development, then a functional adult behavioral pattern should take root. Now, by no means should parents allow every impulse to dictate behavior; each of us has a "censor," which Freud referred to as the "superego." This element of the psyche is largely helpful and acts as a conscience. However, if we let the superego dominate our personality, Freud believed, it could lead to repression and inauthentic behavior.

Freud often worked with highly distressed female clients, repressed in their natural modes of expression; this is how he developed many of his theories, which some people believe are not very scientific. By today's standards, they are not, but Freud's idea that unconscious urges drive our behavior was revolutionary for his time.

According to the passage, which of the following statements best describes Freud's theory of personality?

A) Individuals are shaped by childhood experiences.
B) Individuals are shaped by a superego, or censor.
C) Healthy individuals become outgoing, while unhealthy ones become introverted.
D) Women are more likely to repress their emotions than men.

The correct answer is **A**. To answer this question, it may be helpful to reread the first paragraph of the passage. The first paragraph states that Freud's personality theory is based on how childhood events shape individuals, choice A. The paragraph also states that extroverted and introverted individuals can be equally functional, making choice B incorrect. The superego is part of Freud's theory but not the whole definition. The third paragraph states that Freud developed his theories by working with female patients who repressed their emotions, but the passage does not say whether women are more repressed than men.

The next two examples contain further explanations of detail questions that ask about specific information from each passage.

CPR, an acronym that stands for cardiopulmonary resuscitation, is a widely utilized method of attempting to save someone's life. It is especially applicable to scenarios in which a patient's heart has stopped beating. Frequently, it is also used in cases where a person is in danger of drowning.

Almost all approaches to CPR suggest that a person begin resuscitation efforts with chest compressions. To perform a chest compression, the individual places both hands flat on the patient's chest and then begins pushing down carefully but firmly, most likely at equal intervals. The compressions should be counted, so that the individual can keep track of how many compressions have been administered. The unofficial recommendation of how many chest compressions to provide is around 100 per minute.

There are many resources through which potential lifesavers can acquire training and even certification so that they can more effectively administer this lifesaving technique to a potential patient. However, the American Heart Association stresses that even if someone has not received any type of formal training, attempting to help a person who needs to be resuscitated is far better than offering no help. This is why 911 operators sometimes request that bystanders at the scene of an emergency administer CPR. The operators may even coach the bystanders verbally, over the phone. These approaches have been shown to be effective in many cases.

If a bystander at an emergency scene has received CPR training—even if the training occurred a long time ago—the bystander should attempt further techniques in addition to chest compressions, especially if the patient has been underwater. The lifesaver should start first by checking the patient's airway. He or she might also administer mouth-to-mouth rescue breathing. However, lifesavers should only perform these additional techniques if they are confident of their skills and remember their training. Otherwise, any potential lifesaver should just administer chest compressions.

Some important items to remember in administering CPR are as follows. First, the lifesaver should always check whether the patient is conscious or not. Verbal interaction or communication can be a key way of determining if a person is conscious. If the emergency is related to drowning, the lifesaver should start chest compressions. These should be conducted for about a minute or so, before the lifesaver calls 911. However, if one person can perform the compressions and there is another person available who can call 911, then these steps should happen simultaneously.

For persons who are trained in CPR, one of the best ways to remember the order in which steps should be administered is to recall the memory cue CAB. This cue stands for Circulation, Airway, Breathing. The goal of CPR is to help an unresponsive person to start breathing on his or her own. First, use chest compressions to restore circulation. This is the C of CAB. Second, check the patient's airway for possible blockages. The A in CAB stands for airway. Finally, administer rescue breathing. This is, of course, the B of CAB.

> According to the passage, what is the goal of CPR?
>
> A) To prevent a person who has lost consciousness from drowning
> B) To help an unconscious person regain consciousness
> C) To help an unresponsive person start breathing again
> D) To help an unresponsive person become mobile again

The correct answer is **C**. This detail question asks you to identify the goal of CPR, according to the passage. Paragraph six states that the goal of CPR is to help an unresponsive person start breathing on his or her own. The correct answer is stated directly in the passage, as choice C reflects.

Now consider this passage:

The English town of Stratford-upon-Avon is visited yearly by tourists wanting to view the birthplace of William Shakespeare. William's father, John Shakespeare, bought the family home on Henley Street, and it is here that William is believed to have been born in 1564. Shakespeare's birth home remained in his family until the early 1800s, and it is now a public museum.

Shakespeare attended school at the King Edward VI Grammar School, which occupied the first floor of a building known as the Guildhall. It was in this Guildhall that Shakespeare first experienced theater, when he saw a theatrical performance given by a group of traveling actors. The Royal Shakespeare Company still performs in the town at the Royal Shakespeare and Swan Theaters.

Close to the Guildhall is the site of a house known as New Place, which was bought by Shakespeare himself. Here Shakespeare lived during the later part of his life, until his death in 1616. Although he spent most of his career in London, with trips back to Stratford, he moved permanently to New Place in the last years of his life and is believed to have written some of his later works there. Only the foundations of the New Place house now remain.

In the town of Shottery, one mile from Stratford, is the cottage where Shakespeare's wife, Anne Hathaway, was born. The Hathaway cottage, now also a museum, is actually a large, thatch-roofed farmhouse with sprawling gardens where Shakespeare is believed to have developed his relationship with Anne. They married in 1582 and had three children.

What does the passage state about the importance of the Guildhall to Shakespeare?

A) Shakespeare wrote some of his most important works there.
B) The Guildhall became the first home for the Royal Shakespeare Company.
C) Shakespeare's father bought the Guildhall, and Shakespeare was born there.
D) Shakespeare first saw theater at the Guildhall when he was a student there.

The correct answer is **D**. The second paragraph tells us that Shakespeare attended school at the Guildhall and that he saw his first theater production there. The passage does not mention that the Royal Shakespeare Company found its first home at the Guildhall, so choice B is incorrect. Although Shakespeare bought a home near the Guildhall, he did not actually live there, nor did his family own the building, based on information given in the passage, so C is incorrect.

REVIEW QUESTIONS

1. Christopher Columbus was particularly influenced by the maps of the ancient geographer Ptolemy. Ptolemy argued that the world was round, which went against the belief of the day that the world was flat. Columbus sided with Ptolemy on this question and set out to prove that it was so.

At the time it was widely held that sailing west from Europe would lead to certain death. Believing that the world was round, Columbus thought that one who sailed west would wind up in the east. Other scientists of the day rejected this idea, so Columbus wrote to a respected Italian scholar, Paolo Toscanelli, to ask for his opinion on the matter.

Toscanelli supported the idea of Columbus's trip and sent word back to Columbus in 1474. After receiving Toscanelli's encouragement, Columbus focused all of his thoughts and plans on traveling westward. To make the journey, he would require the help of a generous financial backer, so he went to seek the aid of the king of Portugal. Columbus asked the king for ships and sailors to make the journey. In return, he promised to bring back wealth and to help to convert natives living on the lands to the Church. Portugal refused, and Columbus approached Italy unsuccessfully as well. He went to Spain next.

Queen Isabella of Spain agreed to support the journey. It took some time for Columbus to convince her, but he did succeed, and she paid for the trip. Part of what led the queen to believe in Columbus was the way that he focused on his goal for such a long time with great intent.

He spent the best years of his life working toward his dream, remaining persistent and determined. Legend has it that even during his first voyage, members of his crew became frightened and uncertain, wanting to return home, but Columbus pressed on. The eventual discovery of the Americas was the reward for his commitment.

More than 500 years later, the geography of the world is often taken for granted, but Columbus was an early visionary whose results proved at least some of his theories correct.

Which country was responsible for funding Columbus's voyage to the Americas? Write your answer in the blank: _____

2. The English town of Stratford-upon-Avon is visited yearly by tourists wanting to view the birthplace of William Shakespeare. William's father, John Shakespeare, bought the family home on Henley Street, and it is here that William is believed to have been born in 1564. Shakespeare's birth home remained in his family until the early 1800s, and it is now a public museum.

Shakespeare attended school at the King Edward VI Grammar School, which occupied the first floor of a building known as the Guildhall. It was in this Guildhall that Shakespeare first experienced theater, when he saw a theatrical performance given by a group of traveling actors. The Royal Shakespeare Company still performs in the town at the Royal Shakespeare and Swan Theaters.

Close to the Guildhall is the site of a house known as New Place, which was bought by Shakespeare himself. Here Shakespeare lived during the later part of his life, until his death in 1616. Although he spent most of his career in London, with trips back to Stratford, he moved permanently to New Place in the last years of his life and is believed to have written some of his later works there. Only the foundations of the New Place house now remain.

In the town of Shottery, one mile from Stratford, is the cottage where Shakespeare's wife, Anne Hathaway, was born. The Hathaway cottage, now also a museum, is actually a large, thatch-roofed farmhouse with sprawling gardens where Shakespeare is believed to have developed his relationship with Anne. They married in 1582 and had three children.

How was William Shakespeare first introduced to plays?

A) When he was a boy, the Royal Shakespeare Company visited his classroom.
B) He read many scripts at the Guildhall, where he attended school as a child.
C) He watched a traveling group of performers in the same building as the King Edward VI Grammar School.
D) His wife, Anne Hathaway, began taking him to New Place, where she performed as an actress.

3. One of the most important gymnastic exercises in the original Montessori school approach is that of the "line." For this exercise, a line is drawn in chalk or paint on the floor. Instead of one line, there may also be two lines drawn. The children are taught to walk on these lines like tightrope walkers, placing their feet one in front of the other.

To keep their balance, the children must make efforts similar to those of real tightrope walkers, except that they have no danger of falling, since the lines are drawn only on the floor. The teacher herself performs the exercise first, showing clearly how she places her feet, and the children imitate her without her even needing to speak. At first it is only certain children who follow her, and when she has shown them how to walk the line, she leaves, letting the exercise develop on its own.

The children for the most part continue to walk, following with great care the movement they have seen, and making efforts to keep their balance so they don't fall. Gradually the other children come closer and watch and try the exercise. In a short time, the entire line is covered with children balancing themselves and continuing to walk around, watching their feet attentively.

Music may be used at this point. It should be a very simple march, without an obvious rhythm. It should simply accompany and support the efforts of the children.

When children learn to master their balance in this way, Dr. Montessori believed, they can bring the act of walking to a remarkable standard of perfection.

Before the children begin to walk the line, what must they do?

A) Master their balance
B) Watch their teacher
C) Watch their feet attentively
D) Draw a line on the floor

The Myers-Briggs personality test is based on the sixteen personality types conceptualized by Carl Jung and Isabel Briggs Myers. The Myers-Briggs test was developed based on the presumption that most individuals would fall somewhere on a spectrum of the following binaries: introvert–extrovert, sensor–intuitor, thinker–feeler, and judger–perceiver. Although other personality tests measure different personality traits, the Myers-Briggs test notably bases its foundation on philosophical suppositions from Jung that are rooted in his discussion of archetypes. The test is distinctive due to its reliance on a nonempirical theoretical foundation.

The next two questions are based on this passage.

4. Which of the following statements summarizes why the Myers-Briggs test is unique?

   A) The Myers-Briggs test uses a total of 16 personality types.
   B) The Myers-Briggs test is based on the use of a set of binary traits.
   C) The Myers-Briggs test is based on empirical data rather than theory.
   D) The Myers-Briggs test is based on theory rather than empirical data.

5. Which of the following statements is true, based on the passage?

   A) Conclusions drawn from the test have no basis in reality.
   B) Conclusions drawn from the test are based on the archetypes of Carl Jung.
   C) Conclusions drawn from the test are based on neither fact nor opinion.
   D) Conclusions drawn from the test are based on historical evidence.

6. Austrian-born Sigmund Freud, a psychoanalytic psychologist, lived from the mid-nineteenth to the mid-twentieth century. The psycho-analytic approach refers to the school of thought that unconscious memories or desires guide our emotions and actions. In personality theory, this equates to events from childhood shaping the individual self without a person's conscious awareness. These specific childhood events continue to exert a strong influence over our lives and dominate our emotions. If you are a life-of-the-party, extroverted personality, perhaps you had a healthy upbringing; however, quiet, deep-thinker types can be just as functional. How your caregivers responded to your natural urges will determine your level of mental health, according to the psychoanalytic approach.

   Freud believed that as a child, an individual's actions are driven by hidden impulses—and that repression or denial of those impulses by parents or society can lead to fixations or personality disorders. Alternatively, if the child's impulses are accepted as normative to his or her development, then a functional adult behavioral pattern should take root. Now, by no means should parents allow every impulse to dictate behavior; each of us has a "censor," which Freud referred to as the "superego." This element of the psyche is largely helpful and acts as a conscience. However, if we let the superego dominate our personality, Freud believed, it could lead to repression and inauthentic behavior.

   Freud often worked with highly distressed female clients, repressed in their natural modes of expression; this is how he developed many of his theories, which some people believe are not very scientific. By today's standards, they are not, but Freud's idea that unconscious urges drive our behavior was revolutionary for his time.

Which of the following is a belief held by Sigmund Freud, according to the passage?

A) No scientific support exists for the idea that unconscious urges drive our behavior.

B) The superego serves as a censor that primarily causes repression and inauthenticity.

C) Parents should allow every impulse that a child has to dictate the child's behavior.

D) Functional adult behavior should result from accepting a child's impulses as normal.

7. The current tests for measuring IQ, or an individual's intelligence quotient, were developed during the early and mid-twentieth century. Their use was popularized by Terman, who designed specific tests for use in the U.S. Army. Some psychologists today assert that the traditional system of measuring IQ should remain the sole method of assessing intelligence. Historically, the test has been constructed based on the assumption that there exists one general intelligence factor that impacts an individual's intellectual capacity.

The validity of this assumption has been challenged by other psychologists. In particular, Howard Gardner has emphasized that a unified conception of intelligence based on a single factor remains highly limited and unnecessarily constraining. Gardner has postulated an alternative theory concerning the existence of multiple intelligences. He posits that individuals can possess intelligence in particular areas, including linguistic intelligence, spiritual intelligence, spatial intelligence, intrapersonal intelligence, interpersonal intelligence, musical intelligence, mathematical intelligence, and kinesthetic intelligence, among others. Gardner asserts that individuals can be extremely intelligent and exhibit talent in one area, while failing to demonstrate the same level of prowess in another area. His theory has been discussed widely, although efforts to obtain empirical evidence to support his ideas remain in progress.

Which of the following statements is true, based on the passage?

A) Individuals who are extremely intelligent typically demonstrate equally high levels of skills in all areas.

B) The work of Howard Gardner emphasizes a unified conception of intelligence based on a single factor.

C) The use of IQ tests was made popular by Terman, who designed specific tests for use in the U.S. Army.

D) The traditional system of measuring IQ has remained the sole method of assessing intelligence.

Percy Bysshe Shelley was one of the second-generation Romantic poets. Along with John Keats and Lord Byron, Shelley was considered one of the most masterful poets of his generation.

Shelley was born in England in 1792, as a member of the aristocracy. He was educated at two prestigious English schools, Eton College and Oxford University. Shelley believed that poets were visionaries who could serve as societal leaders because of the creative power of their imaginations. The second generation of Romantic poets, in particular, believed that poets were going to help change the world. Shelley's generation believed that through the imagination, anything was possible. They believed that they could use the creative power of the mind to change the government and even change the world. Shelley's poems reflect this belief. He was a truly idealistic thinker, and he claimed that poets were the "unacknowledged legislators of the world." The poet's creative vision could let him or her see things that other people could not.

Shelley's ideas were heavily influenced by the politics of his time. He grew up at a time when governments were under transformation. In fact, he came of age in the shadow of the French Revolution. This war was very violent, and since France was so close to England, Shelley was acutely aware of the violence that was occurring there. That may have led him to concentrate even more on his belief that artists were able to change the world and improve living conditions.

Shelley's poem "Mont Blanc" focuses on the Romantic notion of the sublime. The Romantic poets believed that when people interacted with nature, it sometimes caused them to be in a state of wonder—or it caused them to be awestruck. For example, when a person gazed at a mountain, the huge size of the mountain could cause the person to become speechless with wonder. This was the effect that the sublime quality of nature could have on a viewer.

In "Mont Blanc," Shelley describes the mountain in a way that attempts to explain its effects on the viewer's mind. According to Shelley, the mountain itself causes the viewer's thoughts to enter a kind of strange trance, and to be affected in a way that resembles how a poet or an artist feels whenever he or she is caught in the midst of a creative inspiration. In the poem, Shelley draws a comparison between the effect of the mountain on the viewer and the power that the imagination has over the artist's mind.

The next two questions are based on this passage.

8. According to the passage, how did Shelley think poets could save the world?

    A) Through the creative power of the imagination
    B) By fighting in the French Revolution
    C) By writing more about nature
    D) By speaking out against acts of violence

9. According to the passage, what effect can mountains have on a viewer?

    A) They can cause a viewer to become intimidated.
    B) They can frighten a viewer into being speechless.
    C) They can cause a viewer to become amused.
    D) They can cause a viewer to be filled with wonder.

10. CPR, an acronym that stands for cardiopulmonary resuscitation, is a widely utilized method of attempting to save someone's life. It is especially applicable to scenarios in which a patient's heart has stopped beating. Frequently, it is also used in cases where a person is in danger of drowning.

Almost all approaches to CPR suggest that a person begin resuscitation efforts with chest compressions. To perform a chest compression, the individual places both hands flat on the patient's chest and then begins pushing down carefully but firmly, most likely at equal intervals. The compressions should be counted, so that the individual can keep track of how many compressions have been administered. The unofficial recommendation of how many chest compressions to provide is around 100 per minute.

There are many resources through which potential lifesavers can acquire training and even certification so that they can more effectively administer this life-saving technique to a potential patient. However, the American Heart Association stresses that even if someone has not received any type of formal training, attempting to help a person who needs to be resuscitated is far better than offering no help. This is why 911 operators sometimes request that bystanders at the scene of an emergency administer CPR. The operators may even coach the bystanders verbally, over the phone. These approaches have been shown to be effective in many cases.

If a bystander at an emergency scene has received CPR training—even if the training occurred a long time ago—the bystander should attempt further techniques in addition to chest compressions, especially if the patient has been underwater. The lifesaver should start first by checking the patient's airway. He or she might also administer mouth-to-mouth rescue breathing. However, lifesavers should only perform these additional techniques if they are confident of their skills and remember their training. Otherwise, any potential lifesaver should just administer chest compressions.

Some important items to remember in administering CPR are as follows. First, the lifesaver should always check whether the patient is conscious or not. Verbal interaction or communication can be a key way of determining if a person is conscious. If the emergency is related to drowning, the lifesaver should start chest compressions. These should be conducted for about a minute or so, before the lifesaver calls 911. However, if one person can perform the compressions and there is another person available who can call 911, then these steps should happen simultaneously.

For persons who are trained in CPR, one of the best ways to remember the order in which steps should be administered is to recall the memory cue CAB. This cue stands for Circulation, Airway, Breathing. The goal of CPR is to help an unresponsive person to start breathing on his or her own. First, use chest compressions to restore circulation. This is the C of CAB. Second, check the patient's airway for possible blockages. The A in CAB stands for airway. Finally, administer rescue breathing. This is, of course, the B of CAB.

According to the passage, what is the best approach to using CPR for bystanders who have received CPR training? Select all that apply.

A) They should use a portable defibrillator.
B) They should refrain from using any form of CPR.
C) They should check the patient's airway.
D) They should administer rescue breathing.

11. Saltwater fish and freshwater fish are related, but their natural environments prove rather distinctive. In terms of being kept as pets, freshwater fish require less maintenance. They live in water that can be adapted from tap water, and they can be kept in many different types of containers in addition to aquariums. Saltwater fish, on the other hand, require a specific type of salt-infused water. Careful watch of the pH balance of the water must also be maintained.

According to the passage, what must people watch carefully when they have saltwater fish?

A) The type of food the fish ingest
B) The water temperature
C) The pH balance of the water
D) The type of light in the aquarium

12. Music can have a significant positive influence on individuals in many different circumstances. Persons who must spend time recuperating in the hospital are frequently soothed by the presence of soft music. Babies are trained to respond to auditory noises through the use of music. Persons going through emotional difficulties such as grief frequently listen to and create music as a means of dealing with the issues they are experiencing. Even people who simply need a short respite from the stresses of the day often use music as a calming and coping mechanism.

According to the passage, what can happen when a baby is exposed to music on a regular basis?

A) The baby can associate various sounds with different foods.
B) The baby can learn to distinguish between his or her parents' voices.
C) The baby can learn to respond to different noises.
D) The baby can learn to discriminate between the voices of siblings.

13. The acoustics of various performance venues emerge as the result of careful planning and extensive decision making. Sound travels differently when it moves through air, and the objects it encounters in a particular environment strongly impact the way that listeners hear the sound. Venues that are designed primarily to house symphony orchestra performances require vastly different acoustic designs than do venues that cater to more intimate performances. Engineers must take into account a wide variety of variables during the design process, including vibration, sound, ultrasound, and infrasound.

A sound wave consists of a fundamental, followed by a series of sequential overtones. The way that listeners perceive these sound waves is impacted by the material used in the listening environment, the physical layout of the environment, the position of the stage relative to the audience's seating, and even the height of the ceiling. Many acoustic engineers also must take into consideration the manner in which transducers impact listening. Transducers include loudspeakers, microphones, and sonar projectors. The addition of these tools to an acoustic environment can strongly influence and transform how audience members in different locations in the room perceive any sound being transmitted.

Which of the following is true regarding sound waves, according to the passage?

A) Sound waves impact the hard of hearing differently than other people.
B) Sound waves are distinctive for different musical genres.
C) Sound waves are unaffected by the physical layouts of performance venues.
D) A sound wave consists of a fundamental and a series of overtones.

14. Bees are a natural part of the pollination cycle of plants. Many plants require the assistance of bees in order to transfer their pollen so that flowers can be produced. Bees travel from flower to flower, and minuscule grains of pollen attach to the bees' legs. The pollen travels much more efficiently via bees than it might if it had to rely on the wind, for example. In this manner, bees assist in the natural pollination cycle through the action of gathering nectar from flowers. Bees are a critical component of this process; without them, plants would face much greater challenges in their reproduction.

The passage indicates which of the following about the migration of pollen via bees as opposed to migration by the wind?

A) Pollen travels much more efficiently via bees than it would by the wind.
B) Pollen can travel equally as effectively via bees or by the wind.
C) Pollen is too heavy to be transported by the wind, except during wind storms.
D) Bees are sometimes allergic to pollen, so it must be transported on the wind.

15. When artists achieve commercial successes, their emotional mindsets can be influenced by this experience. Claude Monet was one such example of this phenomenon. Monet's innovative style earned him considerable fame and public acclaim. In addition, he was extremely prolific as an artist because of his industrious work ethic. As a result, he was successful at his craft, and his paintings reflect a more contemplative and calm perspective than those of artists whose life experiences were fraught with poverty and struggle.

According to the passage, why did Monet's paintings reflect a contemplative perspective?

A) Because he did not achieve fame until after his death
B) Because he experienced artistic success during his lifetime
C) Because he became overly enthusiastic about painting
D) Because he was trying to cultivate an artistic persona

ANSWER KEY

1. Spain	**6.** D	**11.** C
2. C	**7.** C	**12.** C
3. B	**8.** A	**13.** D
4. D	**9.** D	**14.** A
5. B	**10.** C and D	**15.** B

ANSWERS AND EXPLANATIONS

1. (Spain) The passage states that Queen Isabella of Spain paid for the trip.

2. (C) Choice A is incorrect because the Royal Shakespeare Company was not yet established when William was a boy. Choice B offers information that was never stated in the passage, while choice D takes two elements of the passage, Anne Hathaway and New Place, and incorrectly links them. Choice C is, thus, correct.

3. (B) The children learn to master their balance by taking part in the activity, which requires practice; therefore, choice A is not a logical choice. Choice C occurs *after* the children have started walking the line, not before, and choice D refers to an action the teacher must take, not the children. Choice B is the correct answer.

4. (D) The author states that the test is based upon a nonempirical theoretical foundation. *Empirical data* refers to data gained by observation. Choice C is incorrect because it is the opposite of the correct answer.

5. (B) The passage states that *the Myers-Briggs test notably bases its foundation on philosophical suppositions from Jung that are rooted in his discussion of archetypes.* Choice B is therefore correct.

6. (D) Choice D is the only offered statement that Freud himself believed. Choice B misrepresents information given in the passage, and choice C is the opposite of Freud's belief, according to paragraph two.

7. (C) The statement in choice C is mentioned in the first paragraph of the passage. Choice B is the opposite of what the passage states, and choice A is incorrect as well, according to the work of Gardner described in paragraph three.

8. (A) In the beginning of the selection, the author explains that Shelley and his contemporaries believed very strongly in the power of the creative imagination. Shelley believed poets could see things that other people could not.

9. (D) The passage states that Shelley believed the size of a mountain could inspire a state of wonder in a viewer. This experience is similar to the same state of wonder a poet experiences through creative inspiration.

10. (C and D) In paragraph four of the passage, the author explains that anyone who has been trained in CPR can check the patient's airway, use chest compressions, and administer mouth-to-mouth rescue breathing to try to save the patient.

11. (C) The passage explains that saltwater aquariums require a fish owner to check the pH balance of the water carefully. Choice B is incorrect because the passage specifically describes pH balance.

12. (C) The passage suggests that babies who are exposed to music on a regular basis can learn to respond to noises. Choice A is incorrect because the passage explicitly mentions how music can foster auditory training in infants.

13. (D) The passage states that a sound wave consists of a fundamental followed by a series of sequential overtones. Choices A and B are incorrect because the passage does not mention these statements.

14. (A) The passage explains that pollen travels much more efficiently on bees' legs than it could by being blown on the wind. Choice C is incorrect because the passage never mentions the weight of pollen.

15. (B) The passage explains that when artists achieve commercial success, their emotional mindsets can be influenced by the experience. The passage mentions reasons Monet was successful and the effect this success had on his work.

CHAPTER 6

Making Inferences and Drawing Conclusions

Inference questions ask about logical deductions or implications that can be drawn from what an author says. They usually contain the phrases "What does the author imply about X?" or "What can be inferred about X?" They also contain phrases such as "most likely" and "probably." A common inference question is "Based on the passage, which of the following is most likely to be true?"

The correct answers to inference questions must be logically deduced from the information presented. When answering inference questions, therefore, it's important to remember that the correct answer will not be a detail found in the passage.

> The answer to an inference question is never given directly in the passage.

Instead, you must use logical reasoning to determine the answer. Consider this example:

Aficionados of classical music frequently appreciate the characteristics of jazz, and some laypersons think the two genres are somewhat similar. However, jazz musicians are noted for their improvisational abilities, whereas classically trained musicians are often very reliant upon printed music. Although musicians in both genres must be very well versed in scales and various musical keys, jazz musicians must possess impeccable knowledge of this material in order to be able to perform and fulfill the requirements of their chosen genre.

> Based on information given in the passage, which of the following statements is most likely to be true of jazz musicians?
>
> A) Jazz musicians must rely on printed musical scores.
> B) Jazz musicians can also play classical music if they wish.
> C) Jazz musicians do not always need printed music.
> D) Jazz musicians play better music than classical musicians.

The correct answer is **C**. The passage states that jazz musicians can improvise, whereas classical musicians rely on printed music, so we can therefore reason logically that jazz musicians do not always need printed scores. The passage does not suggest that jazz musicians can play classical music, although both types of musicians learn many of the same skills. The passage states that jazz musicians must develop excellent skills, but it does not imply that jazz is superior to classical music, so choice D is incorrect.

Here is another inference question regarding the study of Shakespeare.

Literary scholars have often speculated as to the personal characteristics of William Shakespeare. The Bard is known to many as the greatest writer the English language has ever known, but we have very few examples of his handwriting or even his own name written out in his hand. Some academics have gone so far as to speculate that Shakespeare was a pseudonym for an aristocrat. However, the majority of scholars have dismissed this proposal, and they concentrate instead on Shakespeare's thoughtful insights and dexterous construction of language.

Based on information given in the passage, how do scholars most likely learn about Shakespeare?

A) Through speculation about his personality and his true identity
B) By studying diaries, letters, and other documents written in his hand
C) By studying his plays, his poetry, and other works attributed to him
D) By studying the architecture, construction, and other physical attributes of his historical era

The correct answer is **C**. The last sentence of the passage states that most scholars focus on Shakespeare's use of insights and language, which implies that scholars learn about him through what is expressed in his works. The passage makes clear that very few documents are actually written in his hand, so choice B is incorrect. Choice D is not mentioned anywhere in the passage, so we cannot make a logical inference about it.

In this next example, concerning Michelangelo, we are asked to draw an inference based on a specific sentence in the passage.

Michelangelo was arguably the most talented and prolific artist to emerge from the Italian Renaissance. Not only did he spend three years on his back lying on a scaffold to create the famous paintings adorning the Sistine Chapel, but he also created a sculpture of the Biblical hero David that has been emulated for centuries. Michelangelo himself reflected that he simply took a block of marble and removed all the pieces that did not belong to the David statue. Michelangelo is considered a consummate artist because he created works in so many different media, including painting and sculpture.

Which of the following is implied by the third sentence of the passage?

A) Michelangelo mused that the statue of David was inside the block of marble all along, and all he had to do was free it.
B) Michelangelo created his sculpture of David by using several pieces of marble, each of which had to be dug up or removed from the quarry separately.
C) Michelangelo created a reflection of his statue of David by removing all the marble that stood between the statue and a mirrored surface.
D) Michelangelo said that he worked by trial and error, removing pieces of marble to see what happened as he sculpted his statue of David.

The correct answer is **A**. The third sentence of the passage implies that by "removing" all the marble that did not belong to the statue of David, Michelangelo was revealing something that he had envisioned within the marble all along. Choice A forms the best logical deduction that can be based on the third sentence. Choice B is outside the scope of the passage.

Drawing conclusions questions require the same deductive logic as Inference questions, except they focus specifically on overall conclusions that can be drawn from a passage or paragraph. Conclusion questions ask about the "big ideas" implied in a selection, rather than the details. They may also ask about predictions that can be made, based on the information in a passage. The question that follows asks about the third paragraph of this example specifically.

Public highways are used constantly with little thought of how important they are to the everyday life of a community. It is understandable that most people think about their local public highway only when it affects their own activities. People usually don't focus on highway improvements unless the subject is brought to their attention by increased taxes or advertising.

Highway improvements are an important issue, however. It is important for the economies of most communities to keep highways in good repair. Products purchased in one location are often manufactured in other locations, and safe highways are required to transport the products to their final destination. Good transportation facilities contribute greatly to community prosperity.

The type and amount of the highway improvement needed in any area depend on the traffic in that area. In low-population areas, the amount of traffic on local roads is likely to be small, and highways will not require as much work. But as an area develops, the use of public highways increases, and maintenance demands increase. In small towns, residents are also more able to adapt to the condition of the roads. A road shutdown does not have the same impact on business as it would in busy areas. In large districts with many activities, however, roads must be usable year-round in order for business progress to continue.

In planning improvements of highway systems, several different types of traffic may be encountered. These range from business traffic to agricultural shipping to residential transportation. Improvement activities must meet the requirements of all classes of traffic, with the most important provided for first. Those improvements of lesser importance can be performed as soon as finances permit.

What conclusion can be drawn from the third paragraph of the passage?

A) People in small towns are more adaptable than those in more developed areas.

B) People move to small towns to avoid the traffic found in developed areas.

C) Good highway maintenance is more important in developed areas than in small towns.

D) Most people do not think about highway maintenance in rural or developed areas.

The correct answer is **C**. The last sentence of the paragraph states that roads in developed areas must be usable year-round, which indicates that maintenance in those areas is more important than in small towns. Choice A is incorrect because the author does not compare the adaptability of people in small towns versus developed areas. Choice B is not suggested in the passage. Finally, the first paragraph states that most people do not usually think about highway maintenance or improvements, but this is not a topic raised in the third paragraph, so choice D is incorrect as well.

The passage below is followed by another type of drawing conclusions question—this time asking you to predict what will come next.

Austrian-born Sigmund Freud, a psychoanalytic psychologist, lived from the mid-nineteenth to the mid-twentieth century. The psychoanalytic approach refers to the school of thought that unconscious memories or desires guide our emotions and actions. In personality theory, this equates to events from childhood shaping the individual self without a person's conscious awareness. These specific childhood events continue to exert a strong influence over our lives and dominate our emotions. If you are a life-of-the-party, extroverted personality, perhaps you had a healthy upbringing; however, quiet, deep-thinker types can be just as functional. How your caregivers responded to your natural urges will determine your level of mental health, according to the psychoanalytic approach.

Freud believed that as a child, an individual's actions are driven by hidden impulses—and that repression or denial of those impulses by parents or society can lead to fixations or personality disorders. Alternatively, if the child's impulses are accepted as normative to his or her development, then a functional adult behavioral pattern should take root. Now, by no means should parents allow every impulse to dictate behavior; each of us has a "censor," which Freud referred to as the "superego." This element of the psyche is largely helpful and acts as a conscience. However, if we let the superego dominate our personality, Freud believed, it could lead to repression and inauthentic behavior.

Freud often worked with highly distressed female clients, repressed in their natural modes of expression.

What can be predicted about the next lines of the passage?

A) They will discuss Freud's theories of personality development in children.
B) They will discuss Freud's theories about dreams.
C) They will elaborate on Freud's views on the unconscious minds of women.
D) They will show how women's emotions can be studied and analyzed scientifically today.

The correct answer is **C**. The last paragraph begins to discuss Freud's work with female patients, so we should expect the next lines to continue discussing that same topic. The paragraph does not provide information to suggest that women's emotions can be studied scientifically today, so choice D is incorrect.

REVIEW QUESTIONS

1. The Beatles influenced the genre of rock and roll just as Beethoven expanded the genre of the symphony. John Lennon, Paul McCartney, George Harrison, and Ringo Starr expanded the public's understanding of their musical genre and reclassified it as an anthem for rebellion. Their music transformed into the hippies' theme songs of the sixties. Beethoven similarly altered the public's understanding of the symphony. His addition of a chorus in the last movement of the Ninth Symphony attests to this feat.

   What does the author imply about the influence that both the Beatles and Beethoven had on music?

   A) While different musically, both the Beatles and Beethoven invented radically new genres that the general public became skeptical about.
   B) The Beatles and Beethoven revolutionized the audience's perspective of their respective genres of music.
   C) Neither the Beatles nor Beethoven let societal concerns dictate the way they constructed music; as a result, their nonconformity gave birth to chaotic movements in music.
   D) Both inspired others to follow their lead to invent new genres of music.

2. Imagine living in the year 1800. The railroads then were very scarce. Gas lights were not yet invented, and electric lights were not even dreamed of. Even kerosene wasn't used at that point. This was the world into which Samuel Morse, the inventor of the telegraph, was born.

   Samuel Morse was born in Charlestown, Massachusetts, shortly before the turn of the century, in 1791. When he was seven years old, he was sent to boarding school at Phillips Academy, Andover. While he was there, his father wrote him letters, giving him good advice. He told him about George Washington and about a British statesman named Lord Chesterfield, who was able to achieve many of his goals. Lord Chesterfield was asked once how he managed to find time for all of his pursuits, and he replied that he only ever did one thing at a time, and that he "never put off anything until tomorrow that could be done today."

   Morse worked hard at school and began to think and act for himself at quite a young age. His biggest accomplishment was in painting, and he established himself as a successful painter after graduating from college at Yale. But he also had an interest in science and inventions. He was passionate about the idea of discovering a way for people to send messages to each other in short periods of time.

   In the early 1800s, it took a long time to receive news of any sort, even important news. Whole countries had to wait weeks to hear word of the outcomes of faraway wars. The mail was carried by stagecoach.

In emergency situations, such as when ships were lost at sea, there was no way to send requests for help. Electricity had been discovered, but little application had been made of it up until that point. This was about to change when Morse set his mind to his invention.

On October 1, 1832, Morse was sailing to America from a trip overseas on a ship called the *Sully*. He became preoccupied with the thought of inventing a machine that would later become the telegraph. Morse thought about the telegraph night and day. As he sat upon the deck of the ship after dinner one night, he took out a little notebook and began to create a plan.

If a message could be sent ten miles without dropping, he wrote, "I could make it go around the globe." He said this over and over again during the years after his trip.

One morning at the breakfast table, Morse showed his plan to some of the other *Sully* passengers. Five years later, when the model of the telegraph was built, it was exactly like the one shown that morning to the passengers on the *Sully*.

Once he arrived in America, Morse worked for twelve long years to get people to notice his invention. Though some supported the idea of the telegraph, many people scoffed at it. Morse persisted, and eventually a bill was passed by Congress in 1842. It authorized the funds needed to build the first trial telegraph line.

After two years, the telegraph line was complete. Morse and his colleagues tested it in May 1844. The device worked, and the telegraph became a huge success. Morse's persistence had finally paid off.

What does paragraph three imply about the character of Samuel Morse?

A) Morse was a solemn child who depended heavily on his family for support.
B) Morse had difficulty focusing on one project and so failed to find any real success early in life.
C) Morse was a well-rounded child with varied interests who exerted independence even at a young age.
D) Morse treasured independence above family; therefore, he threw himself into his projects for consolation.

One of the most important gymnastic exercises in the original Montessori school approach is that of the "line." For this exercise, a line is drawn in chalk or paint on the floor. Instead of one line, there may also be two lines drawn. The children are taught to walk on these lines like tightrope walkers, placing their feet one in front of the other.

To keep their balance, the children must make efforts similar to those of real tightrope walkers, except that they have no danger of falling, since the lines are drawn only on the floor. The teacher herself performs the exercise first, showing clearly how she places her feet, and the children imitate her without her even needing to speak. At first it is only certain children who follow her, and when she has shown them how to walk the line, she leaves, letting the exercise develop on its own.

The children for the most part continue to walk, following with great care the movement they have seen, and making efforts to keep their balance so they don't fall. Gradually the other children come closer and watch and try the exercise. In a short time, the entire line is covered with children balancing themselves and continuing to walk around, watching their feet attentively.

Music may be used at this point. It should be a very simple march, without an obvious rhythm. It should simply accompany and support the efforts of the children.

When children learn to master their balance in this way, Dr. Montessori believed, they can bring the act of walking to a remarkable standard of perfection.

The next two questions are based on this passage.

3. Based on the passage's tightrope walking example, what does the author imply about Montessori education?

    A) Dr. Montessori believed that children learned best through example and practice.
    B) Montessori schools provide unusual exercise regimens to keep children from getting bored.
    C) Dr. Montessori believed that children were incapable of learning to walk without strict instruction.
    D) Children in Montessori schools are subjected to rigorous exercise because it is believed to help children retain information.

4. Based on the passage, which of the following most likely reflects Dr. Montessori's belief about learning?

    A) Children cannot learn through experience.
    B) Not all children can learn through exercise.
    C) Children can learn only through demonstrations.
    D) Learning is less likely when fear is present.

5. Aficionados of classical music frequently appreciate the characteristics of jazz, and some laypersons think the two genres are somewhat similar. However, jazz musicians are noted for their improvisational abilities, whereas classically trained musicians are often very reliant upon printed music. Although musicians in both genres must be very well versed in scales and various musical keys, jazz musicians must possess impeccable knowledge of this material in order to be able to perform and fulfill the requirements of their chosen genre.

What does the author imply about the similarity between classical and jazz music?

A) It can be inferred that despite some opinions, classical and jazz music resemble each other quite remarkably.

B) Both genres have the same roots in folk music, so musicians from one genre can play in the other without too much trouble.

C) Despite some opinions that the classical and jazz genres are similar, musicians in the two genres have notably different skills.

D) Although the musical structures of the two are the same, jazz musicians are better at playing both kinds of music.

Christopher Columbus was particularly influenced by the maps of the ancient geographer Ptolemy. Ptolemy argued that the world was round, which went against the belief of the day that the world was flat. Columbus sided with Ptolemy on this question and set out to prove that it was so.

At the time it was widely held that sailing west from Europe would lead to certain death. Believing that the world was round, Columbus thought that one who sailed west would wind up in the east. Other scientists of the day rejected this idea, so Columbus wrote to a respected Italian scholar, Paolo Toscanelli, to ask for his opinion on the matter.

Toscanelli supported the idea of Columbus's trip and sent word back to Columbus in 1474. After receiving Toscanelli's encouragement, Columbus focused all of his thoughts and plans on traveling westward. To make the journey, he would require the help of a generous financial backer, so he went to seek the aid of the king of Portugal. Columbus asked the king for ships and sailors to make the journey. In return, he promised to bring back wealth and to help to convert natives living on the lands to the Church. Portugal refused, and Columbus approached Italy unsuccessfully as well. He went to Spain next.

Queen Isabella of Spain agreed to support the journey. It took some time for Columbus to convince her, but he did succeed, and she paid for the trip. Part of what led the queen to believe in Columbus was the way that he focused on his goal for such a long time with great intent. He spent the best years of his life working toward his dream, remaining persistent and determined. Legend has it that even during his first voyage, members of his crew became frightened and uncertain, wanting to return home, but Columbus pressed on. The eventual discovery of the Americas was the reward for his commitment.

More than 500 years later, the geography of the world is often taken for granted, but Columbus was an early visionary whose results proved at least some of his theories correct.

The next two questions are based on this passage.

6. Based on the passage, which of the following can be inferred about Queen Isabella?

    A) She wholeheartedly believed in Ptolemy's vision of the world.
    B) She was open to new ideas about the geography of the world.
    C) She was an enemy of Portugal and Italy.
    D) She believed Columbus's expedition would fail.

7. Based on the passage, what can be concluded about the king of Portugal?

    A) He lacked enough support for Columbus's vision to fund it.
    B) He agreed with Ptolemy's vision of the world.
    C) He had no financial resources to offer Columbus.
    D) He and Queen Isabella were enemies.

Public highways are used constantly with little thought of how important they are to the everyday life of a community. It is understandable that most people think about their local public highway only when it affects their own activities. People usually don't focus on highway improvements unless the subject is brought to their attention by increased taxes or advertising.

Highway improvements are an important issue, however. It is important for the economies of most communities to keep highways in good repair. Products purchased in one location are often manufactured in other locations, and safe highways are required to transport the products to their final destination. Good transportation facilities contribute greatly to community prosperity.

The type and amount of the highway improvement needed in any area depends on the traffic in that area. In low-population areas, the amount of traffic on local roads is likely to be small, and highways will not require as much work. But as an area develops, the use of public highways increases, and maintenance demands increase. In small towns, residents are also more able to adapt to the condition of the roads. A road shutdown does not have the same impact on business as it would in busy areas. In large districts with many activities, however, roads must be usable year-round in order for business progress to continue.

In planning improvements of highway systems, several different types of traffic may be encountered. These range from business traffic to agricultural shipping to residential transportation. Improvement activities must meet the requirements of all classes of traffic, with the most important provided for first. Those improvements of lesser importance can be performed as soon as finances permit.

The next two questions are based on this passage.

8. According to the passage, what can be inferred about the relationship between the lack of highway maintenance and local economies?

   A) Businesses do not consider highway systems when choosing their location.
   B) Consumers will frequent businesses despite the lack of highway maintenance.
   C) Businesses can thrive despite the lack of good highway systems.
   D) Poor roads decrease consumer traffic, which leads to a decline in business.

9. What conclusion can be drawn based on paragraph two of the passage?

   A) Public highways are important only as a means of bypassing rural areas.
   B) It costs much more to repair rural highways than city streets, so city streets are ultimately less important.
   C) Public highways play a vital role in transporting goods to and from different locations.
   D) People do not care about the upkeep of public highways because they do not understand their value.

10. Freud was the first psychologist to conceptualize the idea of the unconscious, or the proposal that people acted from motivations of which they were unaware. Freud believed that unconscious motivations were most effectively revealed through dreams, so he frequently had his patients review and analyze their dreams. Since Freud's initial proposal, psychologists have built upon his original conception.

   It can be inferred that Freud established what relationship between his theory of the unconscious and dreams?

   A) Dreams could reveal why people acted a certain way even if they were not conscious of the motives behind those actions.
   B) If people analyzed their dreams, they could learn how to motivate themselves and take action.
   C) Because dreams occurred while people were asleep, or unconscious, most people could not remember them until Freud developed his theories.
   D) Freud was the first serious scholar to study dreams and speculate on their meaning.

11. In the animal kingdom, many symbiotic relationships exist between two species that take actions known to be mutually beneficial for both parties. In the water, clownfish have such a relationship with sea anemones. The fish are one of the only species that can swim unharmed in the anemone's waving tentacles, as typically the tentacles would sting any animal that swam near it. However, the clownfish is immune to the

sting of the tentacles and is therefore protected by them; in return, its presence helps the anemone stay clean, avoid attack by parasites, and remain free from infection.

What conclusion can be drawn about the relationship between the clownfish and the sea anemone?

A) It is mutually beneficial to both creatures and allows for harmonious living.

B) It is parasitic in nature and often leads to the destruction of one of the two creatures.

C) In every pairing, one of the two creatures ends up as more of a beneficiary than the other, which leads to disharmony.

D) Separating the two would mean imminent death; therefore, the relationship is not only beneficial but also necessary.

12. Historically, the study of creativity has concentrated on persons known for innovation. Early creativity studies focused on creative "geniuses," such as Einstein, Mozart, or Shakespeare. This type of creativity is known as "Big C" creativity. However, as research on creativity progressed, a corresponding interest in how people could be creative in smaller ways—on an everyday basis—emerged in the discipline. Scholars began to investigate how ordinary tasks, such as cleaning, driving particular familiar routes, and completing work and schoolwork, could be conducted in innovative ways. This focus of creativity research has been labeled "little c" creativity.

Which of the following is the best prediction of what the author's conclusion about creativity will be?

A) It is not possible to conduct research on creativity because it is such an elusive trait.

B) Creativity is only tracked in "Big C" cases where geniuses are concerned.

C) Because creativity can now be found in even the mundane, it is no longer a subject worthy of study.

D) Creativity is multifaceted and can be found in various areas of a person's daily life.

13. The current tests for measuring IQ, or an individual's intelligence quotient, were developed during the early and mid-twentieth century. Their use was popularized by Terman, who designed specific tests for use in the U.S. Army. Some psychologists today assert that the traditional system of measuring IQ should remain the sole method of assessing intelligence. Historically, the test has been constructed based on the assumption that there exists one general intelligence factor that impacts an individual's intellectual capacity.

The validity of this assumption has been challenged by other psychologists. In particular, Howard Gardner has emphasized that a unified conception of intelligence based on a single factor remains highly limited and unnecessarily constraining. Gardner has postulated an alternative theory concerning the existence of multiple intelligences. He posits that individuals can possess intelligence in particular areas, including linguistic intelligence, spiritual intelligence, spatial intelligence, intrapersonal intelligence, interpersonal intelligence, musical intelligence, mathematical intelligence, and kinesthetic intelligence, among others.

Gardner asserts that individuals can be extremely intelligent and exhibit talent in one area, while failing to demonstrate the same level of prowess in another area. His theory has been discussed widely, although efforts to obtain empirical evidence to support his ideas remain in progress.

What conclusion can be drawn about intelligence based on Howard Gardner's findings?

A) The IQ test, while flawed, remains the most important tool we have to test intelligence.
B) Intelligence is not limited to one's ability to take a test; instead, there are multiple intelligences that a person may exhibit in any given area.
C) Intelligence is elusive and difficult to measure or determine; therefore, the IQ test has questionable meaning.
D) Intelligence can only be determined through a series of tests; therefore, students should be heavily tested in every subject area.

14. Literary scholars have frequently compared the characteristics of poetry written by both the first and second generation of Romantic poets. Poets such as William Wordsworth established the foundations of the exaltation of the imagination that later influenced writers such as John Keats and Percy Bysshe Shelley. The first generation of poets was attempting to advocate for the importance of artistry and creativity. The second generation of poets built on this foundation and went even further in their speculations about what creativity could achieve, especially perhaps in a political sense. However, the second generation was also negatively impacted by their observation of the French Revolution, and this experience tempered their idealism.

What conclusion can be drawn about the influence of the French Revolution on Romantic poets?

A) It divided the British and American Romantic poets into two very distinct movements.
B) It shifted the tone and dimmed the idealism of the Romantic movement.
C) The Revolution caused the Romantics to abandon their ideals and take up arms against tyranny.
D) It forced Romantics to cling even more to their ideals and to shun the reality of war.

15. Austrian-born Sigmund Freud, a psychoanalytic psychologist, lived from the mid-nineteenth to the mid-twentieth century. The psycho-analytic approach refers to the school of thought that unconscious memories or desires guide our emotions and actions. In personality theory, this equates to events from childhood shaping the individual self without a person's conscious awareness. These specific childhood events continue to exert a strong influence over our lives and dominate our emotions. If you are a life-of-the-party, extroverted personality, perhaps you had a healthy upbringing; however, quiet, deep-thinker types can be just as functional. How your caregivers responded to your natural urges will determine your level of mental health, according to the psychoanalytic approach.

Freud believed that as a child, an individual's actions are driven by hidden impulses—and that repression or denial of those impulses by parents or society can lead to fixations or personality disorders. Alter-natively, if the child's impulses are accepted as normative to his or her development, then a functional adult behavioral pattern should take root. Now, by no means should parents allow every impulse to dictate behavior; each of us has a "censor," which Freud referred to as the "superego." This element of the psyche is largely helpful and acts as a conscience. However, if we let the superego dominate our personality, Freud believed, it could lead to repression and inauthentic behavior.

Freud often worked with highly distressed female clients, repressed in their natural modes of expression; this is how he developed many of his theories, which some people believe are not very scientific. By today's standards, they are not, but Freud's idea that unconscious urges drive our behavior was revolutionary for his time.

Based on information given in the passage, which of the following can be concluded about the psychoanalytic approach?

A) Psychoanalysis discounts the role of desire in individuals' actions.
B) Early psychoanalytic theory guides most psychological treatments today.
C) The psychoanalytic approach is not as credible today as it was in the past.
D) The psychoanalytic approach is best used with female patients only.

ANSWER KEY

1. B	6. B	11. A
2. C	7. A	12. D
3. A	8. D	13. B
4. D	9. C	14. B
5. C	10. A	15. C

ANSWERS AND EXPLANATIONS

1. (B) The question asks you to determine what influence the respective musicians had on music. The author uses words like *expanded*, *transformed*, and *altered* to indicate the influence they had. *Revolutionize* is a synonym of these terms and best represents the intended inference. Although it may be tempting to identify the term *invented* with *revolutionize*, the second half of choice A creates an extreme that does not exist in the passage. The musicians did not create new genres; instead, they worked within their genres to expand them. In addition, the passage in no way indicates that the musicians fell out of public favor, so choice A is incorrect. The passage does not discuss societal concerns either, so choice C can be eliminated. Not only does the passage not argue that the musicians invented new genres, as discussed above, but it also does not address any inspirational effects the musicians may or may not have had on other musicians. Choice D is therefore incorrect.

2. (C) The author notes that Morse was interested in both painting and science—this implies that Morse was not pigeonholed into any one field. His interests were well rounded. The author also claims that Morse "began to think and act for himself at quite a young age," which suggests that Morse was an independent person. Since the author establishes Morse as a child who liked to think for himself, choice A can be eliminated because it suggests that Morse was dependent by nature. While the author does mention more than one interest that Morse had, Morse was able to achieve success in painting at an early age, which eliminates choice B. Regarding choice D, the author does state that Morse was independent, but there is no mention of how he might prioritize his family over his independence.

3. (A) The question asks you to identify the statement that best identifies traits of the Montessori program based on the tightrope description given in the passage. In the passage, example and practice are highlighted as methodologies used to help children learn to walk properly. Regarding choice B, although the tightrope walking exercise may be considered unusual by some, the focus of the passage is on the methodology used by Montessori, not on people's response to it. The passage also explains that the exercise helps to improve students' sense of balance, not to prevent boredom. Choice C is incorrect, because the passage never addresses any negative attitude Dr. Montessori might have had toward students, nor does it identify Montessori education with rigidity or strictness. Choice D is also incorrect because, like choices B and C, it addresses a topic that is not discussed in the passage.

4. (D) The second paragraph states that the line is drawn on the floor so that children do not have a danger of falling while walking the line. One can infer that learning is less likely when children are afraid of falling. Although this passage discusses learning through demonstration, the author does not suggest that children can learn only through demonstration. Therefore, choice C is incorrect.

5. (C) Using the word "however" after stating that "some laypersons think the two genres are somewhat similar" indicates that the author believes the opposite: they are not that similar. This eliminates choices A and B, which contend that the two genres are quite similar. Choice D is incorrect because the author does not make a judgment regarding which players may or may not be the better musicians. Instead, the focus is on the differences between the two musical genres.

6. (B) Although the passage does not state that Queen Isabella was open-minded about new ideas, it can be inferred that she was because she believed in Columbus's vision and eventually supported his expedition. Choice A is not correct because Columbus had to convince her to support his journey. If she had believed in Ptolemy's ideas wholeheartedly, she most likely would not have needed to be convinced.

7. (A) Based on the passage, we can conclude that the king lacked enough support for Columbus's vision to support it. Choices C and D are incorrect, because the passage suggests that the king had the resources to be a financial backer, and it does not discuss the king's relationship with Queen Isabella.

8. (D) This passage supports the idea that good highway systems are needed for business and local economies to thrive. If roads are in disrepair and funding for improvements is scarce, people will not be able to access the businesses along these roads. This decline in business activity is likely to negatively affect the local economy.

9. (C) The question asks you to draw a conclusion based on information presented in the second paragraph. The paragraph states that the importance of highways lies in their ability to help transfer goods from one to place to another. Choices B and D do not address the importance of highways and therefore can be eliminated.

10. (A) The first half of the second sentence states that Freud believed that dreams revealed unconscious motives. That passage does not state whether or not Freud was the first to study dreams, only that he was the first to develop a theory of the unconscious.

11. (A) The two creatures do not destroy each other, so choice B can be eliminated. The crucial component of the relationship is harmony; each of the creatures benefits equally from the other, thus eliminating choice C as well.

12. (D) The passage draws attention to the complexity of creativity and puts to rest old assumptions about how creativity should be defined. Choice D is therefore the correct answer.

13. (B) The question asks you to identify a conclusion about intelligence that could be drawn based on Gardner's findings. Gardner lists multiple areas in which people can be intelligent and believed that intelligence could manifest in a multitude of ways. Choice A does not address the traits of intelligence and instead focuses on the test, so it can be eliminated.

14. (B) The author specifically addresses a difference between first- and second-generation Romantic writers, noting that the second generation built on the foundation of the first generation but that the influence of the French Revolution served to restrain their original idealism. In this light, choice B is the logical conclusion. The other choices fail to acknowledge correctly the split between the generations and misinterpret the effect on the Romantics' idealism.

15. (C) In the first paragraph, the author states that, according to the psychoanalytic approach, events from childhood exert a strong influence on people's lives. Later in the passage, the author states that Freud's ideas are not considered scientific by today's standards. Therefore, it can be concluded that the psychoanalytic approach is not as credible today as it was in the past.

CHAPTER 7

Fact Versus Opinion

Fact versus opinion questions ask you to determine whether a portion of text is based on fact or the author's opinion. Some texts may contain a mixture of both.

These views are not necessarily based on fact or knowledge. An opinion is simply something that a person believes.

It is also important to be able to identify bias and stereotypes. **Bias** is a personal preference (like or dislike) that may interfere with a person's ability to be objective. For example, former victims of violent crime are typically excluded from serving on a jury in a case involving violent crime because they might not be able to be impartial.

A **stereotype** is an oversimplified generalization about a group, the idea that all the members of a group of people have certain characteristics. For example, the idea that senior citizens are bad drivers is a stereotype.

> Fact: Sixty-five percent of U.S. households have a pet. (This is a fact that can be verified.)
>
> Opinion: I like big dogs. (This is the author's personal opinion.)
>
> Bias: Cats and dogs both make wonderful pets, but if you want a loyal companion who is always happy to see you, get a dog. (The author clearly prefers dogs to cats.)
>
> Stereotype: Dog people are more socially outgoing. (This opinion is projected onto all dog owners.)

When examining texts, try to identify the author's point of view and potential biases. Look at the language used and whether it seems objective or biased in a certain direction. Persuasive texts will certainly show bias, but other types of texts might as well. Pay attention to the author's tone as well. **Tone** is the author's attitude about the subject. Tone can often help you identify bias.

Facts can be verified using empirical evidence, whereas **opinions** are based on the author's subjective views. Below are some examples of this question type.

Arguably, the most well-known Siamese cat is the seal point. The dark brown ears, face, and tail are famous markers of this popular breed of cat. Many cats that appear in popular culture, including the mischievous Siamese cats in Disney animated films, are patterned after this type of Siamese. However, cat aficionados are well aware that other types of Siamese cats also exist. Two of these include the blue point and the snowshoe. Snowshoe Siamese are characterized by the white markings on their paws along with the dark "boots": these markings earn them their name and make the cats look as though they have been walking in the snow. Blue point Siamese cats do not have dark brown "points"; rather, their ears, paws, tails, and noses are characterized by bluish patches on their fur. Some Siamese cats are even hairless. They exhibit the darker pigment on their noses, tails, ears, and paws, similar to their fur-covered counterparts of the same breed. However, hairless Siamese cats exhibit these "points" on their skin instead of their fur. This type of Siamese is rather rare and not very well known. Despite the contrasts between the external appearances of these varying types of Siamese, all Siamese cats are known for being vocal, loyal, and rather mischievous.

Which sentence or phrase in the passage refers mostly to traits of the Siamese cat that are stereotypes rather than facts?

A) The dark brown ears, face, and tail are famous markers of this popular breed of cat.
B) Their ears, paws, tails, and noses are characterized by bluish patches on their fur.
C) All Siamese cats are known for being vocal, loyal, and rather mischievous.
D) Snowshoe Siamese are characterized by the white markings on their paws.

The correct answer is **C**. *Loyal* and *mischievous* are traits that are matters of opinion rather than physical traits. The other phrases and sentences describe traits that are physical and can be proven through observation.

Let's consider another example:

The acoustics of various performance venues emerge as the result of careful planning and extensive decision making. Sound travels differently when it moves through air, and the objects it encounters in a particular environment strongly impact the way that listeners hear the sound. Venues that are designed primarily to house symphony orchestra performances require vastly different acoustic designs than do venues that cater to more intimate performances. Engineers must take into account a wide variety of variables during the design process, including vibration, sound, ultrasound, and infrasound.

A sound wave consists of a fundamental, followed by a series of sequential overtones. The way that listeners perceive these sound waves is impacted by the material used in the listening environment, the physical layout of the environment, the position of the stage relative to the audience's seating, and even the height of the ceiling. Many acoustic engineers also must take into consideration the manner in which transducers impact listening. Transducers include loudspeakers, microphones, and sonar projectors. The addition of these tools to an acoustic environment can strongly influence and transform how audience members in different locations in the room perceive any sound being transmitted.

The author states in paragraph two that "a sound wave consists of a fundamental, followed by a series of sequential overtones." This statement can be seen as which of the following?

A) It is a fact, because the sentence after it provides evidence and support for its veracity.
B) It is an opinion, because the author is not a scientist; he is merely a music connoisseur.
C) It is a fact, because the statement can be supported with scientific data and does not reflect the author's subjective viewpoint about sound.
D) It is an opinion, because it reveals the author's feelings about sound rather than providing an objective and empirically deduced statement.

The correct answer is **C**. While both choices A and C correctly identify this statement as a fact, only choice C gives the correct support. Choice A indicates the sentence following the one quoted in the question provides support when in fact this sentence goes on to develop another idea.

Now consider this passage:

CPR, an acronym that stands for cardiopulmonary resuscitation, is a widely utilized method of attempting to save someone's life. It is especially applicable to scenarios in which a patient's heart has stopped beating. Frequently, it is also used in cases where a person is in danger of drowning.

Almost all approaches to CPR suggest that a person begin resuscitation efforts with chest compressions. To perform a chest compression, the individual places both hands flat on the patient's chest and then begins pushing down carefully but firmly, most likely at equal intervals. The compressions should be counted, so that the individual can keep track of how many compressions have been administered. The unofficial recommendation of how many chest compressions to provide is around 100 per minute.

There are many resources through which potential lifesavers can acquire training and even certification so that they can more effectively administer this lifesaving technique to a potential patient. However, the American Heart Association stresses that even if someone has not received any type of formal training, attempting to help a person who needs to be resuscitated is far better than offering no help. This is why 911 operators sometimes request that bystanders at the scene of an emergency administer CPR. The operators may even coach the bystanders verbally, over the phone. These approaches have been shown to be effective in many cases.

If a bystander at an emergency scene has received CPR training—even if the training occurred a long time ago—the bystander should attempt further techniques in addition to chest compressions, especially if the patient has been underwater. The lifesaver should start first by checking the patient's airway. He or she might also administer mouth-to-mouth rescue breathing. However, lifesavers should only perform these additional techniques if they are confident of their skills and remember their training. Otherwise, any potential lifesaver should just administer chest compressions.

Some important items to remember in administering CPR are as follows. First, the lifesaver should always check whether the patient is conscious or not. Verbal interaction or communication can be a key way of determining if a person is conscious. If the emergency is related to drowning, the lifesaver should start chest compressions. These should be conducted for about a minute or so before the lifesaver calls 911. However, if one person can perform the compressions and there is another person available who can call 911, then these steps should happen simultaneously.

For persons who are trained in CPR, one of the best ways to remember the order in which steps should be administered is to recall the memory cue CAB. This cue stands for Circulation, Airway, Breathing. The goal of CPR is to help an unresponsive person to start breathing on his or her own. First, use chest compressions to restore circulation. This is the C of CAB. Second, check the patient's airway for possible blockages. The A in CAB stands for airway. Finally, administer rescue breathing. This is, of course, the B of CAB.

The author states that "one of the best ways to remember the order in which steps should be administered is to recall the memory cue CAB." This statement can best be described by which of the following?

A) It is a fact, because CAB is a short word and is easy to remember.
B) It is an opinion, because the author is unable to determine what is objectively "best" for all people.
C) It is a fact, because empirical research has been conducted to prove the author's statement.
D) It is an opinion, because the author introduces it with the phrase, "in my opinion."

The correct answer is **B**. While choices B and D both identify this statement correctly as an opinion, only choice B accurately indicates why. The author never states that this is an opinion, but he or she does use the subjective word *best*, which indicates opinion.

To make sure you're comfortable with fact versus opinion questions, let's look at two more examples:

Christopher Columbus was particularly influenced by the maps of the ancient geographer Ptolemy. Ptolemy argued that the world was round, which went against the belief of the day that the world was flat. Columbus sided with Ptolemy on this question and set out to prove that it was so.

At the time it was widely held that sailing west from Europe would lead to certain death. Believing that the world was round, Columbus thought that one who sailed west would wind up in the east. Other scientists of the day rejected this idea, so Columbus wrote to a respected Italian scholar, Paolo Toscanelli, to ask for his opinion on the matter.

Toscanelli supported the idea of Columbus's trip and sent word back to Columbus in 1474. After receiving Toscanelli's encouragement, Columbus focused all of his thoughts and plans on traveling westward. To make the journey, he would require the help of a generous financial backer, so he went to seek the aid of the king of Portugal. Columbus asked the king for ships and sailors to make the journey. In return, he promised to bring back wealth and to help to convert natives living on the lands to the Church. Portugal refused, and Columbus approached Italy unsuccessfully as well. He went to Spain next.

Queen Isabella of Spain agreed to support the journey. It took some time for Columbus to convince her, but he did succeed, and she paid for the trip. Part of what led the queen to believe in Columbus was the way that he focused on his goal for such a long time with great intent. He spent the best years of his life working toward his dream, remaining persistent and determined. Legend has it that even during his first voyage, members of his crew became frightened and uncertain, wanting to return home, but Columbus pressed on. The eventual discovery of the Americas was the reward for his commitment.

More than 500 years later, the geography of the world is often taken for granted, but Columbus was an early visionary whose results proved at least some of his theories correct.

> The author's statement that Columbus asked the king of Portugal "for ships and sailors to make the journey" most accurately reflects which of the following?
>
> A) It is an opinion, because the statement is based on inaccurate information.
> B) It is a fact, because it expresses a subjective belief of the author.
> C) It is a fact, because the statement can be supported with historical evidence.
> D) It is an opinion, because it is impossible to know what Columbus asked for.

The correct answer is **C**. The question of what Columbus asked for can be documented with historical evidence, making choice D incorrect and choice C the correct answer. Choice B is incorrect, because facts express objective knowledge, not subjective beliefs.

Let's consider one more example:

Literary scholars have often speculated as to the personal characteristics of William Shakespeare. The Bard is known to many as the greatest writer the English language has ever known, but we have very few examples of his handwriting or even his own name written out in his hand. Some academics have gone so far as to speculate that Shakespeare was a pseudonym for an aristocrat. However, the majority of scholars have dismissed this proposal, and they concentrate instead on Shakespeare's thoughtful insights and dexterous construction of language.

Which of the following sentences reveals a bias?

A) Literary scholars have often speculated as to the personal characteristics of William Shakespeare.

B) We have very few examples of Shakespeare's handwriting or even his own name written out in his hand.

C) Some academics have gone so far as to speculate that Shakespeare was a pseudonym for an aristocrat; however, most serious scholars have dismissed this proposal.

D) Many scholars concentrate on Shakespeare's thoughtful insights and dexterous construction of language.

The correct answer is **D**. Choice D presupposes that Shakespeare's insights are thoughtful and that his construction of language is dexterous.

REVIEW QUESTIONS

Public highways are used constantly with little thought of how important they are to the everyday life of a community. It is understandable that most people think about their local public highway only when it affects their own activities. People usually don't focus on highway improvements unless the subject is brought to their attention by increased taxes or advertising.

Highway improvements are an important issue, however. It is important for the economies of most communities to keep highways in good repair. Products purchased in one location are often manufactured in other locations, and safe highways are required to transport the products to their final destination. Good transportation facilities contribute greatly to community prosperity.

The type and amount of the highway improvement needed in any area depend on the traffic in that area. In low-population areas, the amount of traffic on local roads is likely to be small, and highways will not require as much work. But as an area develops, the use of public highways increases, and maintenance demands increase. In small towns, residents are also more able to adapt to the condition of the roads. A road shutdown does not have the same impact on business as it would in busy areas. In large districts with many activities, however, roads must be usable year-round in order for business progress to continue.

In planning improvements of highway systems, several different types of traffic may be encountered. These range from business traffic to agricultural shipping to residential transportation. Improvement activities must meet the requirements of all classes of traffic, with the most important provided for first. Those improvements of lesser importance can be performed as soon as finances permit.

The next two questions are based on this passage.

1. Read the following quotation from line 2 of the passage.

It is understandable that most people think about their local public highway only when it affects their own activities.

Which of the following statements is true concerning the quotation above?

A) This statement is an opinion, because most people probably think that it is true.

B) This statement is an opinion, because it is a viewpoint that may not be held by everyone.

C) This statement is a fact, because the claim is objective and could be proven empirically.

D) This statement is a fact, because everyone knows that people think primarily of their own interests.

2. Read the following quotation from paragraph three of the passage.

In low-population areas, the amount of traffic on local roads is likely to be small.

Which of the following statements is true regarding the quotation above?

A) This statement is a fact, because it uses a qualifier to cover any exceptions to its claim.

B) This statement is an opinion, because it is a belief that cannot be proven empirically.

C) This statement is a fact, because it has been proven through scientific experimentation.

D) This statement is an opinion, because there is evidence to support the opposite claim as well.

One of the most important gymnastic exercises in the original Montessori school approach is that of the "line." For this exercise, a line is drawn in chalk or paint on the floor. Instead of one line, there may also be two lines drawn. The children are taught to walk on these lines like tightrope walkers, placing their feet one in front of the other.

To keep their balance, the children must make efforts similar to those of real tightrope walkers, except that they have no danger of falling, since the lines are drawn only on the floor. The teacher herself performs the exercise first, showing clearly how she places her feet, and the children imitate her without her even needing to speak. At first it is only certain children who follow her, and when she has shown them how to walk the line, she leaves, letting the exercise develop on its own.

The children for the most part continue to walk, following with great care the movement they have seen, and making efforts to keep their balance so they don't fall. Gradually the other children come closer and watch and try the exercise. In a short time, the entire line is covered with children balancing themselves and continuing to walk around, watching their feet attentively.

Music may be used at this point. It should be a very simple march, without an obvious rhythm. It should simply accompany and support the efforts of the children.

When children learn to master their balance in this way, Dr. Montessori believed, they can bring the act of walking to a remarkable standard of perfection.

The next two questions are based on this passage.

3. Circle the underlined sentence or phrase from the passage that is reflective of the author stating an opinion.

4. Read the following quotation from paragraph two of the passage.

The teacher herself performs the exercise first, showing clearly how she places her feet, and the children imitate her without her even needing to speak.

This is an example of which of the following types of statements?

A) It is an opinion statement, because not everyone is a visual learner.
B) It is a factual statement, because it describes a step in the procedure for walking the line.
C) It is an opinion statement, because the author believes that the teacher should initiate walking the line, a belief that cannot be agreed upon unanimously.
D) It is a factual statement, because surveys to test this claim have been administered and analyzed.

Imagine living in the year 1800. The railroads then were very scarce. Gas lights were not yet invented, and electric lights were not even dreamed of. Even kerosene wasn't used at that point. This was the world into which Samuel Morse, the inventor of the telegraph, was born.

Samuel Morse was born in Charlestown, Massachusetts, shortly before the turn of the century, in 1791. When he was seven years old, he was sent to boarding school at Phillips Academy, Andover. While he was there, his father wrote him letters, giving him good advice. He told him about George Washington and about a British statesman named Lord Chesterfield, who was able to achieve many of his goals. Lord Chesterfield was asked once how he managed to find time for all of his pursuits, and he replied that he only ever did one thing at a time, and that he "never put off anything until tomorrow that could be done today."

Morse worked hard at school and began to think and act for himself at quite a young age. His biggest accomplishment was in painting, and he established himself as a successful painter after graduating from college at Yale. But he also had an interest in science and inventions. He was passionate about the idea of discovering a way for people to send messages to each other in short periods of time.

In the early 1800s, it took a long time to receive news of any sort, even important news. Whole countries had to wait weeks to hear word of the outcomes of faraway wars. The mail was carried by stagecoach. In emergency situations, such as when ships were lost at sea, there was no way to send requests for help. Electricity had been discovered, but little application had been made of it up until that point. This was about to change when Morse set his mind to his invention.

On October 1, 1832, Morse was sailing to America from a trip overseas on a ship called the *Sully*. He became preoccupied with the thought of inventing a machine that would later become the telegraph. Morse thought about the telegraph night and day. As he sat upon the deck of the ship after dinner one night, he took out a little notebook and began to create a plan.

If a message could be sent ten miles without dropping, he wrote, "I could make it go around the globe." He said this over and over again during the years after his trip.

One morning at the breakfast table, Morse showed his plan to some of the other *Sully* passengers. Five years later, when the model of the telegraph was built, it was exactly like the one shown that morning to the passengers on the *Sully*.

Once he arrived in America, Morse worked for twelve long years to get people to notice his invention. Though some supported the idea of the telegraph, many people scoffed at it. Morse persisted, and eventually a bill was passed by Congress in 1842. It authorized the funds needed to build the first trial telegraph line.

After two years, the telegraph line was complete. Morse and his colleagues tested it in May 1844. The device worked, and the telegraph became a huge success. Morse's persistence had finally paid off.

The next two questions are based on this passage.

5. Read the following quotation from the last paragraph of the passage.

The device worked, and the telegraph became a huge success.

This is an example of which of the following types of statements?

A) It is a factual statement, because the success of the telegraph can be documented with evidence.

B) It is a factual statement, because telegraphs are considered by most to be very useful.

C) It is an opinion statement, because some people do not think that the telegraph worked very well.

D) It is an opinion statement, because only the passage's author thinks that the telegraph was a success.

6. Which of the following quotations from the passage could be considered an opinion?

A) Though some supported the idea of the telegraph, many people scoffed at it.

B) "Never put off anything until tomorrow that could be done today."

C) On October 1, 1832, Morse was sailing to America from a trip overseas on a ship called the *Sully*.

D) Once he arrived in America, Morse worked for twelve long years to get people to notice his invention.

7. The Beatles influenced the genre of rock and roll just as Beethoven expanded the genre of the symphony. John Lennon, Paul McCartney, George Harrison, and Ringo Starr expanded the public's understanding of their musical genre and reclassified it as an anthem for rebellion. Their music transformed into the hippies' theme songs of the sixties. Beethoven similarly altered the public's understanding of the symphony. His addition of a chorus in the last movement of the Ninth Symphony attests to this feat.

Read the following quotation from the passage.

Beethoven similarly altered the public's understanding of the symphony.

Which of the following is true about the above quotation?

A) It is a factual statement, because everyone would agree that it is true.

B) It is a factual statement, because there is a verifiable example to back it up.

C) It is an opinion statement, because it reveals the author's bias towards Beethoven.

D) It is an opinion statement, because some people might not agree that Beethoven altered the public's understanding of the symphony.

8. Maslow's hierarchy postulates that human beings must have certain basic needs met before they can realize their potential by mastering more sophisticated and complex abilities. For example, people must be confident that they have reliable sources of food, clothing, and shelter before they can start to focus on needs such as being loved. This belief system serves as the foundation for early education programs like Head Start.

Read the following quotation from the passage.

For example, people must be confident that they have reliable sources of food, clothing, and shelter before they can start to focus on needs such as being loved.

Which of the following is true about the above quotation?

A) It is an opinion statement, because some people might believe that being loved should precede the obtainment of food, clothing, and shelter.

B) It is a factual statement, because it is common sense: people cannot live without food, clothing, and shelter, but they can live without being loved.

C) It is an opinion statement, because some people prefer food while others prefer love.

D) It is a factual statement, because a psychologist proposed it, and psychologists are authority figures in the area of human development.

9. Music can have a significant positive influence on individuals in many different circumstances. Persons who must spend time recuperating in the hospital are frequently soothed by the presence of soft music. Babies are trained to respond to auditory noises through the use of music. Persons going through emotional difficulties such as grief frequently listen to and create music as a means of dealing with the issues they are experiencing. Even people who simply need a short respite from the stresses of the day often use music as a calming and coping mechanism.

Read the following quotation from the passage.

Music can have a significant positive influence on individuals in many different circumstances.

Which of the following is true about the above quotation?

A) It is a factual statement, because it uses the qualifying phrase *can have*.

B) It is a factual statement, because no one would argue that music can have a negative influence.

C) It is an opinion statement, because some people might not be positively influenced by music.

D) It is an opinion statement, because only in some circumstances is music positive.

10. Athletes are extremely aware of how physical motion and its properties can affect the human body as well as the outcomes of competitions. Figure skating, for example, involves concentric motion for spins. Skaters learn how to use their arms to bring in their centers of gravity. In the same way that runners adopt a certain leg stance or swimmers use their arms to move quickly through the water, skaters also use their knowledge of physics to improve their skating.

Read the following quotation from the passage.

Athletes are extremely aware of how physical motion and its properties can affect the human body as well as the outcomes of competitions.

Which of the following revisions to the above statement would turn the statement into a fact?

A) Athletes are seldom aware of how physical motion and its properties can affect the human body as well as the outcomes of competitions.

B) All athletes are aware of how physical motion and its properties can affect the human body as well as the outcomes of competitions.

C) All athletes are extremely aware of how physical motion and its properties can affect the human body as well as the outcomes of competitions.

D) Some athletes are extremely aware of how physical motion and its properties can affect the human body as well as the outcomes of competitions.

11. Bees are a natural part of the pollination cycle of plants. Many plants require the assistance of bees in order to transfer their pollen so that flowers can be produced. Bees travel from flower to flower, and minuscule grains of pollen attach to the bees' legs. The pollen travels much more efficiently via bees than it might if it had to rely on the wind, for example. In this manner, bees assist in the natural pollination cycle through the action of gathering nectar from flowers. Bees are a critical component of this process; without them, plants would face much greater challenges in their reproduction.

Read the following quotation from the passage.

Bees are a critical component of this process; without them, plants would face much greater challenges in their reproduction.

Which of the following is true about the above quotation?

A) It is an opinion statement, because there is not enough evidence to support it.
B) It is an opinion statement, because only some people feel this way about bees.
C) It is a factual statement, because it can be verified empirically through scientific research.
D) It is a factual statement, because no one has found a way to prove or refute it.

12. As one of the most prolific female poets in nineteenth-century America, today Emily Dickinson is a household name. However, during her lifetime, she lived as a recluse and wrote most of her poetry from the solitude of her bedroom. She presents a unique perspective from this time period, when few women wrote about the themes she discusses. For this reason, critics are frequently interested in her perspective as a female author even beyond the contributions she made as an American nineteenth-century writer.

Read the following quotation from the passage.

She presents a unique perspective from this time period, when few women wrote about the themes she discusses.

Which of the following is true about the above quotation?

A) It is an opinion statement, because people have diverse feelings about Dickinson's work.
B) It is an opinion statement, because the author reveals a bias against female writers.
C) It is a factual statement, because people can read Emily Dickinson's poetry and decide for themselves.
D) It is a factual statement, because it can be backed up with verifiable evidence from the time period.

13. When artists achieve commercial successes, their emotional mindsets can be influenced by this experience. Claude Monet was one such example of this phenomenon. Monet's innovative style earned him considerable fame and public acclaim. In addition, he was extremely prolific as an artist because of his industrious work ethic. As a result, he was successful at his craft, and his paintings reflect a more contemplative and calm perspective than those of artists whose life experiences were fraught with poverty and struggle.

Read the following quotation from the passage.

When artists achieve commercial successes, their emotional mindsets can be influenced by this experience.

Which of the following most likely explains why the above quotation is a factual statement?

A) It is factual, because research has shown that celebrities tend to seek success.

B) It is factual, because it can be experienced with one of the senses, vision.

C) It is factual, because it can be proven by surveying a sample of celebrities.

D) It is factual, because it explains why celebrities prefer fame to struggle.

14. Arguably, the most well-known Siamese cat is the seal point. The dark brown ears, face, and tail are famous markers of this popular breed of cat. Many cats that appear in popular culture, including the mischievous Siamese cats in Disney animated films, are patterned after this type of Siamese. However, cat aficionados are well aware that other types of Siamese cats also exist. Two of these include the blue point and the snowshoe. Snowshoe Siamese are characterized by the white markings on their paws along with the dark "boots": these markings earn them their name and make the cats look as though they have been walking in the snow. Blue point Siamese cats do not have dark brown "points"; rather, their ears, paws, tails, and noses are characterized by bluish patches on their fur. Some Siamese cats are even hairless. They exhibit the darker pigment on their noses, tails, ears, and paws, similar to their fur-covered counterparts of the same breed. However, hairless Siamese cats exhibit these "points" on their skin instead of their fur. This type of Siamese is rather rare and not very well known. Despite the contrasts between the external appearances of these varying types of Siamese, all Siamese cats are known for being vocal, loyal, and rather mischievous.

Which of the following quotations from the above passage contains traces of the author's bias?

A) However, cat aficionados are well aware that other types of Siamese cats also exist.
B) Two of these include the blue point and the snowshoe.
C) Blue point Siamese cats do not have dark brown "points"; rather, their ears, paws, tails, and noses are characterized by bluish patches on their fur.
D) Some Siamese cats are even hairless.

15. The acoustics of various performance venues emerge as the result of careful planning and extensive decision making. Sound travels differently when it moves through air, and the objects it encounters in a particular environment strongly impact the way that listeners hear the sound. Venues that are designed primarily to house symphony orchestra performances require vastly different acoustic designs than do venues that cater to more intimate performances. Engineers must take into account a wide variety of variables during the design process, including vibration, sound, ultrasound, and infrasound.

A sound wave consists of a fundamental, followed by a series of sequential overtones. The way that listeners perceive these sound waves is impacted by the material used in the listening environment, the physical layout of the environment, the position of the stage relative to the audience's seating, and even the height of the ceiling. Many acoustic engineers also must take into consideration the manner in which transducers impact listening. Transducers include loudspeakers, microphones, and sonar projectors. The addition of these tools to an acoustic environment can strongly influence and transform how audience members in different locations in the room perceive any sound being transmitted.

Read the following quotation from the passage.

Venues that are designed primarily to house symphony orchestra performances require vastly different acoustic designs than do venues that cater to more intimate performances.

This statement is best characterized by which of the following?

A) It is a fact, because it can be supported by real-life examples drawn from the field of acoustic engineering.
B) It is an opinion, because the author states a preference for orchestra venues without supporting this position.
C) It is an opinion, because the statement cannot be supported with empirical data.
D) It is a fact, because the author has attended numerous performances and has noted the acoustic differences.

ANSWER KEY

1. B
2. A
3. One of the most important gymnastic exercises in the original Montessori school approach is that of the "line."
4. B
5. A
6. B
7. B
8. A
9. A
10. D
11. C
12. D
13. C
14. A
15. A

ANSWERS AND EXPLANATIONS

1. (B) The statement refers to the author's attitude—he or she finds this notion understandable. However, others might not agree with the author on this point, so choice A is incorrect. Choices C and D are incorrect because the statement is the author's viewpoint, not a fact.

2. (A) The author qualifies his or her statement by using the word *likely*, which indicates that there is a strong probability of low traffic on roads in sparsely populated areas. This probability can be documented with evidence, so it is a fact. Choice C is incorrect because scientific experimentation involves manipulating variables to test a particular outcome.

3. (One of the most important gymnastic exercises in the original Montessori school approach is that of the "line.") This sentence reflects a value judgment through its use of the word *important*, which can be refuted by anyone who believes that other exercises are more valuable than walking the line.

4. (B) The statement is a fact, which eliminates choices A and C. The statement describes a step in the exercise, so choice B is correct.

5. (A) In some cases, it is a matter of opinion whether something is or is not a *success*; however, in this sentence, the assertion is not based on a value judgment, but on an observable fact: the telegraph worked, which meant that Morse's intention was realized, and the widespread use of the telegraph can be documented with historical evidence. Thus, choices C and D are incorrect.

6. (B) Some people claim to work better under pressure and thrive on "putting things off" to the last minute; therefore, choice B is reflective of an opinion. Choices A, C, and D are facts that can be historically documented, so they are incorrect.

7. (B) While this statement looks like an opinion from the outset because people could technically argue against the validity of the statement, the statement is actually a fact. The music can be compared with other music from the time, and a conclusion can be drawn: the symphony was not like other symphonies of the time period, based on its inclusion of a chorus. This change altered the public's understanding of the symphony, so choice B is correct.

8. (A) The quotation is based on a postulation made by Maslow, not on experimental data, statistical research, or clearly observable information; therefore, it is an opinion. Choice B is incorrect because *common sense* is not a reliable enough factor on which to base truth. Choice C deals with preferences rather than viewpoints and is also incorrect.

9. (A) When statements include qualifiers such as *can have* or *may have,* they are not absolute; therefore, the author is not claiming that music will always have a positive influence, but that it *possibly* can. That statement can be verified and stands as a fact rather than an opinion.

10. (D) Referring to athletes as a group, without using a preceding qualifier such as *some* or *many,* suggests that *all* athletes are extremely aware of how physical motion can affect their bodies. This is not necessarily the case, however, so it would be impossible to prove. Choice D revises the sentence using the qualifying phrase *some athletes,* which turns the statement into a verifiable fact.

11. (C) This statement is a fact because it can be proven through scientific research; thus, choices A and B are incorrect. Choice D is incorrect because a fact is a statement that can be proven, not a statement that hasn't yet been proven or disproven.

12. (D) *Unique* means special or rare, which Dickinson's poetry was since there was so little poetry written by other women of the time period. The unique status of her poetry can be verified by evidence from the time period; therefore, the statement is a fact, eliminating choices A and B.

13. (C) A fact is a statement that can be proven using empirical evidence. This statement could be proven in several ways; conducting a survey of celebrities would be one of them.

14. (A) Not every reader is an expert and not every expert is necessarily "well aware" that there are different types of Siamese cats. Therefore, choice A reveals the author's bias. Choices B, C, and D are facts that can be readily observed.

15. (A) This quotation from the passage can be backed up by real-life examples from the field of acoustic engineering. The author provides some explanation of the different design variables that must be taken into account, and the differences could be further documented with case studies from actual venues, so choice A is correct.

CHAPTER 8

Point of View and Evaluating an Argument

POINT OF VIEW

Every author has a point of view. Previous chapters have discussed the various types of texts (narrative, informational, and persuasive) and the author's purpose for writing each of those types of texts. **Point of view** refers to how the author feels about the subject and the specific opinions the author holds about that subject. Sometimes the author's perspective on a subject will be obvious, but sometimes it may be quite subtle and you will need to think about it.

To determine point of view, look for and think about the following:

- The type of text: narrative, informational, or persuasive
- The author's purpose for writing the text (whether stated or unstated)
- The source of the text: In what type of source or context would this text appear?
- The author's identity: Who wrote the text?
- Facts versus opinions: Is this text based on verifiable facts or is it mostly just the author's opinions?

Here is an example of a question about point of view:

Before his famous voyage to the New World, it took some time for Christopher Columbus to convince Queen Isabella of Spain to support the journey. Eventually he did succeed, and she paid for the trip. Part of what led the queen to believe in Columbus was the way that he focused on his goal for such a long time with great intent. He spent the best years of his life working toward his dream, remaining persistent and determined. Legend has it that even during his first voyage, members of his crew became frightened and uncertain, wanting to return home, but Columbus pressed on. The eventual discovery of the Americas was the reward for his commitment.

Which of the following statements best describes the author's point of view about Columbus?

A) Columbus was not the first to sail around the world; he was only following in the footsteps of other ancient peoples.
B) Columbus was not widely respected by the geographers of his day.
C) Columbus was a master manipulator who could convince anyone of anything.
D) Columbus's skill at persuasion was largely due to his persistence.

The correct answer is **D**. The passage says that it took him a while to convince the queen to support him but that she agreed due to his persistence and drive.

TONE

A related term, **tone**, refers to the author's attitude toward the subject and the mood of the passage that is created by the author's choice of words in expressing his or her point of view. For example, look at the difference created by the choice of words in the following two sentences.

> *Jacques skipped merrily down the stairs.*
>
> *Jacques trudged reluctantly down the stairs.*

In both sentences, Jacques is going down some stairs, but the effect created by the choice of words is very different.

Here is a question about tone:

Michelangelo was arguably the most talented and prolific artist to emerge from the Italian Renaissance. Not only did he spend three years on his back lying on a scaffold to create the famous paintings adorning the Sistine Chapel, but he also created a sculpture of the Biblical hero David that has been emulated for centuries. Michelangelo himself reflected that he simply took a block of marble and removed all the pieces that did not belong to the David statue. Michelangelo is considered a consummate artist because he created works in so many different media, including painting and sculpture.

Which of the following most likely characterizes the author's attitude toward Michelangelo and his art?

A) Admiration
B) Disregard
C) Indifference
D) Tolerance

The correct answer is **A**. The passage describes Michelangelo's artistic contributions with a tone that communicates an admiration of the man and his work. Choice D is incorrect because the author's tone goes beyond mere tolerance.

EVALUATING AN ARGUMENT

The author's point of view, the tone of the passage, and the mode of writing are all important elements to understand when you evaluate a text. You may be asked about any of those elements, and each of them will help you to evaluate the author's argument. An "argument" in writing is not a fight between two people. The term **argument** refers to the point the author is trying to make. You can also think of it as the claim being made by the author. Claims must have evidence to back them up. When an author makes a claim, question it. What evidence does the author present to support the claim? How strong is that evidence and does it come from a credible source? You may be asked to identify the argument or to weaken or strengthen it.

Here is an example of an argument question:

The best method of treating individuals facing psychological difficulties is a blend of cognitive-behavioral therapy and medication. This approach not only serves to address the patient's potential chemical imbalances, but it also emancipates the patient by allowing him or her some autonomy in dealing with the issues associated with a possible malaise.

Cognitive-behavioral therapy requires the patient to examine his or her own behavior and to make moderations in a rational and well-thought-out manner. If a person's chemical makeup is preventing him or her from being able to carry out such a responsibility, then medication can help alleviate specific symptoms to allow the patient to deal with the underlying emotional and psychological issues in an effective manner. Nevertheless, psychologists have wide-ranging opinions on how to help these patients cope with challenges such as depression or anxiety.

Some trained professionals assert that medication alone can best serve psychological patients. Other psychologists believe that a utilization of Freud's psychoanalytic approach represents the best method for assisting persons with these emotional symptoms. Some counselors believe that each person's set of individual circumstances should be considered. Other counselors depend on the characteristics of behaviorism to modify the patients' behavior so that their behavioral patterns become more effective. Overall, however, many professionals agree that the combination of cognitive-behavioral therapy and medication will ultimately best serve the patient.

The author's argument regarding therapy and medication is most likely motivated by which of the following beliefs?

A) Those who suffer psychological issues are best treated in hospitals that can monitor their medication intake.
B) Patients with psychological issues often respond well to only one method of treatment: either therapy or medication.
C) Both therapy and medicine offer benefits, but using them in conjunction is most effective.
D) Medication-based treatment is the most effective option for all psychological patients.

The best answer is **C**. The author concedes the benefits of both therapy and medication and acknowledges their merits independently but states in the first sentence that "the best method of treating individuals . . . is a blend of cognitive-behavioral therapy and medication." The author later states that "many professionals agree" that using both methods is most effective.

REVIEW QUESTIONS

1. The way that scientists have envisioned the makeup of the universe has shifted and transformed as the centuries have passed. Prior to the work of Copernicus, people believed that the earth was at the center of the universe. The idea that the earth revolved around the sun was initially taken as heresy. The progression and gradual acceptance of these originally controversial ideas paved the way for the acceptance of later discoveries by Newton and Einstein. Their theories have revolutionized the ways in which science itself is conducted today.

What is the author's attitude toward scientific theory?

A) Skeptical regarding its potential pitfalls
B) Condescending about its inability to produce quick answers
C) Jovial about the possibilities that scientific theory presents
D) Earnestly appreciative of the work science has accomplished

2. Riggs's Toys has decided to open a second location in Kingwood. The store's first location near the town center achieved profitability in its first year, and profits have grown steadily in each subsequent year. A second location in the affluent suburb of Panther Creek should do equally well.

Which of the following, if true, would most strengthen the proposition to open a new location?

A) Kingwood is a suburb of Chicago.
B) The population of Kingwood has tripled over the past five years.
C) The average income of a family in Panther Creek is less than that of a family living near the town center.
D) Several new homes have been built in Panther Creek over the past year.

Questions 3–4 are based on the following conversation.

<u>Brie</u>: Compliance with the new homeowners' association regulations requiring the installation of sprinkler systems will cost the average homeowner $1,000 and increase property taxes as well! This new regulation will cause serious financial hardship to the average homeowner.

<u>Henri</u>: You have to look at the long-term goals of the plan. While there will be an initial investment in the systems, it will not constitute a serious financial hardship because the money spent on the sprinkler systems will be recovered through lower water bills. Less wasted water means less money spent.

3. Henri responds to Brie by

    A) Claiming that she does not understand the goals of the regulation
    B) Showing that she has based her conclusion on evidence that is not relevant
    C) Suggesting that she has overlooked a possible mitigating consequence
    D) Questioning her assessment of what constitutes serious financial hardship

4. Brie's argument would be most strengthened by which of the following statements, if true?

    A) Most homeowners in the neighborhood do not have the money needed for the initial investment in a sprinkler system.
    B) It would take approximately one year for the money it costs to install a sprinkler system to be recovered through lower water bills.
    C) The money it costs to install a sprinkler system is more than the average monthly water bill.
    D) The money saved by lower water bills with a sprinkler system more than makes up for the increase in property taxes.

Questions 5–7 are based on the following passage.

One of the most important gymnastic exercises in the original Montessori school approach is that of the "line." For this exercise, a line is drawn in chalk or paint on the floor. Instead of one line, there may also be two lines drawn. The children are taught to walk on these lines like tightrope walkers, placing their feet one in front of the other.

To keep their balance, the children must make efforts similar to those of real tightrope walkers, except that they have no danger of falling, since the lines are drawn only on the floor. The teacher herself performs the exercise first, showing clearly how she places her feet, and the children imitate her without her even needing to speak. At first it is only certain children who follow her, and when she has shown them how to walk the line, she leaves, letting the exercise develop on its own.

The children for the most part continue to walk, following with great care the movement they have seen, and making efforts to keep their balance so they don't fall. Gradually the other children come closer and watch and try the exercise. In a short time, the entire line is covered with children balancing themselves and continuing to walk around, watching their feet attentively.

Music may be used at this point. It should be a very simple march, without an obvious rhythm. It should simply accompany and support the efforts of the children. When children learn to master their balance in this way, Dr. Montessori believed, they can bring the act of walking to a remarkable standard of perfection.

5. What argument about how children learn is expressed by this passage?

    A) Children learn through individual instruction.
    B) Children learn through rhythmic exercises.
    C) Children learn through imitating others.
    D) Children learn through rote memorization.

6. Which of the following statements, if true, would most strengthen Dr. Montessori's argument about how children learn?

    A) In a recent survey, 83% of people surveyed reported that they learned to play basketball by watching other people play.
    B) Many children learn to cook by following written recipes.
    C) Most parents teach their child how to ride a bicycle by holding on to the back of the child's bicycle until the child has good balance and speed.
    D) In an experiment, a child was left alone with a new video game. After an hour of experimentation, the child had learned how to play the game.

7. Which of the following statements, if true, would most weaken Dr. Montessori's argument about how children learn?

    A) A girl watched how her father changed the tire on his car, and when she had a flat tire on her own car, she remembered how he had done it and changed her tire successfully.
    B) A boy read several books about ancient Egypt to study for his history test and received the highest score in the class.
    C) Dogs often go to the same spot at the same time to seek food.
    D) Babies with normal hearing will turn their heads toward the source of a sound.

8. The physician William Harvey was the first who discovered and demonstrated the true mechanism of the heart's action. No one before his time conceived that the movement of the blood was entirely due to the mechanical action of the heart as a pump. There were all sorts of speculations about the matter, but nobody had formed this conception. Harvey is as clear as possible about it. He says the movement of the blood is entirely due to the contractions of the walls of the heart—that it is the propelling apparatus—and all recent investigation tends to show that he was perfectly right.

Which of the following terms best describes the author's attitude toward William Harvey?

A) Scorn
B) Ridicule
C) Admiration
D) Envy

Questions 9–10 are based on the following passage:

Katherine Mansfield's short story "Prelude" was originally written in 1915 as "The Aloe" and was first published as "Prelude" by Virginia and Leonard Woolf's Hogarth Press in 1918. The impressionistic style of the story and the introspective natures of the characters shattered the traditional short story form. Mansfield foregrounds the family dynamic, deemphasizing the simple plot of a family moving to a new house. The characters of "Prelude" are not a stereotypical happy family with strong father, loving mother, and <u>sweet</u>, well-behaved children. Mansfield presents characters whose identities are impermanent and who have dual personas: the public selves they present to others and the private selves they <u>struggle</u> to hide. Every person in the household struggles to hold on to the threads of his or her individuality and experiences fear of losing that individuality to the family collective. Even the children desperately attempt to find something they can call their own and to be themselves. The element of strain that this produces drives each character nearly to the breaking point and creates <u>exquisite</u> moments of terror. Mansfield's narrative slides smoothly from conscious to unconscious to express this <u>tense</u> duality, and she frequently uses the images of glass and mirrors to symbolize the two worlds in which the characters exist.

9. Which of the words underlined in the passage does the author choose to illustrate that he or she enjoys the elements of fear in "Prelude"? Circle the correct word in the passage.

10. Which of the following best states the author's point of view on the story "Prelude"?

   A) "Prelude" proves that a female writer in the early twentieth century could be successful.
   B) "Prelude" undermines the traditional Victorian short story format with its emphasis on character rather than plot.
   C) "Prelude" presents a nuanced portrayal of family dynamic against which the individual ego struggles to assert itself.
   D) "Prelude" suggests the instability of the traditional family structure through its use of elements of fear.

ANSWER KEY

1. D	5. C	9. exquisite
2. B	6. A	10. C
3. D	7. B	
4. A	8. C	

ANSWERS AND EXPLANATIONS

1. (D) The question asks you to identify the author's attitude toward scientific theory. The author's choice of phrases such as *envisioned*, *paved the way*, and *revolutionized* indicates a sincere belief in and appreciation for the positive effects of scientific theory. Choice A is too negative and is not supported by any of the word choices the author makes. Choice B is also incorrect for a similar reason. Choice C contains a positive-tone word; however, the degree of positivity in *jovial* is too high. The author's word choices indicate an *appreciation* for scientific theory, not happiness about it.

2. (B) The argument's conclusion is that Riggs's Toys should open a new location in Kingwood. The evidence presented is a comparison with the business's success in a different location. The argument assumes that because the business is successful in one part of town, it will be successful in another part of town. Choices A and D are not relevant and choice C would weaken the proposal. Choice B shows that the population has grown, which makes it more likely that the company could support a second store.

3. (D) Henri responds to Brie by pointing out that she has not considered the positive effects a sprinkler system can provide. Choice D best expresses this.

4. (A) Choice A strengthens Brie's argument that the high initial cost would be a financial hardship. Choices B and C are not relevant and choice D would strengthen Henri's argument.

5. (C) The passage shows how the children initially imitate the teacher and then each other as they learn how to walk along the line. Although they may do this to music, the passage is clear in stating that the music does not have a distinct rhythm, which eliminates choice B.

6. (A) Choice A reinforces the idea that children learn by imitating what they see. The other choices weaken this idea.

7. (B) Choice B shows a situation in which children learn by reading and studying, not by imitating actions. Choice A strengthens the idea that children learn by imitating actions. Choices C and D are not relevant.

8. (C) The author writes about Harvey with admiration for his ability to discern the mechanisms of the heart before anyone else had and states that time has proven Harvey's theories correct.

9. (exquisite) The author describes the elements of fear as *exquisite moments of terror*. Exquisite means beautiful.

10. (C) The author shows in the passage how "Prelude" successfully portrays the complex family dynamic in which individuals struggle for identity. The best answer is C.

CHAPTER 9

Text Features and Sources

TEXT FEATURES

Text features are the elements that stand out in a text because the writer or designer of the text uses a tool or method to emphasize them. Text features are used for several purposes, such as to organize the text, to emphasize certain pieces of information, to provide tangential information, and to help the reader quickly locate vital information. Text features include the following:

> - Headings and subheadings
> - Formatting such as italicized text, bolded text, or underlined text
> - Footnotes
> - Sidebars
> - Graphic elements such as charts or graphs
> - Map features such as a key or legend
> - Index
> - Glossary
> - Table of contents

Text features are important elements of the text, so you should be aware of their use and ask yourself why they are being used. This knowledge can help you better understand the text. You may be asked for information that can only be found in a feature of the text such as a sidebar or graph. You may also be asked why certain features are used or should be used.

Look at this text and try the two practice questions that follow:

> **To Register for Camp**
>
> Parents must fill out the registration form prior to the first day of camp. Walk-in registrations will not be accepted. The chart below shows your options for registration.

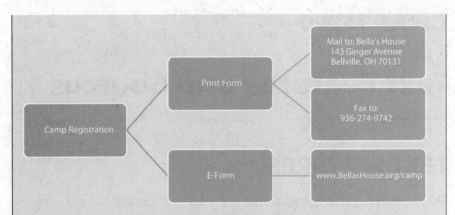

Make sure you fill out the activity selection form at the end of the registration document. Each afternoon there will be several activities available. Campers should choose only ONE activity per day. If you do not choose an activity, one will be assigned to you.

A deposit of $100 is due at time of registration, and the balance is due on the first day of camp. If you are registering online, payment may be made through the website with a credit card.

If you have any questions about the registration process, please call Sandy Elkins at 713-825-4692 or e-mail at SandyE@BellasHouse.org.

1. Which of the following techniques is used to stress important information in the text?

   A) Italicized text
   B) A numbered list
   C) All capital letters
   D) A sidebar

The correct answer is **C**. The text uses all capital letters to stress an important point: *Campers should choose only ONE activity per day.*

2. If a camper fills out a paper registration form, which of the following is an option for submitting the registration form?

   A) E-mail the form.
   B) Fax the form.
   C) Bring the form on the first day of camp.
   D) Only online registrations are accepted.

The correct answer is **B**. According to the chart, a paper form may be faxed or mailed.

You may be asked to identify a text feature that is not currently in the text but that could be added to the text to enhance it. Here is an example:

Making Slime

It is easy to make your own homemade slime from borax and white glue. You can make any color you like! First, get two bowls and two mixing spoons. In one bowl mix ½ cup (4 oz) glue and ½ cup (4 oz) water. If you want to make colored slime, add some food coloring to this mixture. You can even mix in glitter if you want! In the other bowl, mix 1 teaspoon borax with 1 cup water. Stir until the borax is dissolved. Add the glue mixture to the borax solution and stir slowly. The slime will begin to form very quickly. Stir the mixture until it becomes too thick, then just knead it with your hands until it gets less sticky. You may have some water that does not get absorbed into the slime—just pour it out.

Which of the following features could help organize the information in the text?

A) A numbered list of the steps
B) A picture of the finished product
C) Subheadings
D) Footnotes

The correct answer is **A**. Since this is a process, listing the steps in order by number would be useful. Any of the other listed features could be used in some way to enhance the text, but the question asks which feature could help *organize* the information.

SOURCES

You will be asked about one other important type of text feature: reference sources. There are many types of reference sources, as you probably know from writing research papers in your school courses. The TEAS is mostly concerned with your ability to categorize sources as primary, secondary, and tertiary and to be able to locate information within a primary source document. To simplify the concept, think of this example: The book *Moby Dick* is a primary source. A book about *Moby Dick* is a secondary source. A bibliography listing all the books and articles that have been written about *Moby Dick* is a tertiary source.

In general, a **primary source** is the original document or work created by the author. Examples of primary sources would include:

• Historical documents
• Literary texts
• Diaries or journals
• Letters or e-mails
• Autobiographies or memoirs
• Photographs
• Video or audio recordings
• Interviews or oral histories

- Speeches
- Original newspaper articles, advertisements, and so on
- Maps
- Artifacts
- Research data

A **secondary source** discusses or interprets information that was originally published elsewhere. Examples of secondary sources would include:

- Books, essays, and articles that interpret or review other works or data
- Biographies
- Reprints of artwork
- Literary criticism
- Book reviews
- Commentaries
- Encyclopedias
- Textbooks and reference books

A **tertiary source** is an index and/or textual consolidation of primary and secondary sources. A tertiary source provides an overview of a topic, a summary, or a guide to finding other sources. Examples of tertiary sources would include:

- Summaries
- Bibliographies
- Dictionaries
- Encyclopedias
- Textbooks
- Indexes
- Databases
- Travel guides and field guides
- Timelines
- Almanacs

It is sometimes difficult to identify whether a source is a primary, secondary, or tertiary source. As you can see above, encyclopedias and textbooks are listed under both secondary and tertiary sources because their categorization depends on their use. If an encyclopedia article is used as a source for an overview of a topic, it is a tertiary source. If it is used for a subjective analysis of a topic, then it would be a secondary source.

Here are two examples of questions about sources:

> Which of the following is a primary source?
>
> A) A book of photographs of Incan pottery
> B) An index of articles about Incan pottery
> C) A review of a museum exhibit of Incan pottery
> D) An Incan pottery shard on display in a museum

The correct answer is **D**. The pottery shard itself is the primary source, an original artifact.

Use the excerpt from the index below to answer the question.

A history student is writing a paper about Jefferson Davis's role as president of the Confederacy. If she wants to read about his inaugural address, on what page should she begin reading?

A) 961
B) 962
C) 963
D) 965

The correct answer is **D**. The index lists the inaugural address on page 965.

REVIEW QUESTIONS

The next two questions are based on the following graph.

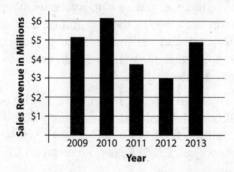

1. Based on the graph above, which of the following is true regarding sales revenue for the business shown?

A) The revenue of the business has been increasing.
B) The revenue of the business has been decreasing.
C) The business has seen fluctuating revenue between 2009 and 2013.
D) The business has brought in its best revenue in recent years.

2. Which of the following features of the graph could be omitted without significantly impacting viewers' understanding of the graph?

A) The dates shown (2009, 2010, and so on)
B) The vertical axis title
C) The wide black bars
D) The horizontal axis title

The RMS *Titanic* sank in the North Atlantic Ocean early on the morning of April 15, 1912.

3. Which of the following explains why the text above uses italicized print?

A) It is the title of a book.
B) It is the proper name of a ship.
C) It is a subheading.
D) It is a direct quotation.

The next three questions are based on these instructions.

Conference Registration Instructions

Time: Monday, 8:30 A.M. to 10:30 A.M.

Location: Wellings Ballroom

The Society for Associated Technologies is pleased to welcome our guests for the 2015 Annual Conference in San Jose, California. Upon checking in, please settle into your rooms and enjoy a complimentary Happy Hour on the hotel's East Deck. Cocktails and light appetizers will be served both Saturday and Sunday evenings from 5:00 to 7:00 P.M.

Conference registration begins promptly at 8:30 on Monday morning and will run until 10:30 A.M.

To register for the conference, please bring your membership ID card and payment confirmation with you to the registration area. Members with ID numbers 10000–20000 should register at Table 1; members with ID numbers 20001–30000 should register at Table 2; and members with ID numbers 30001–40000 should register at Table 3.

Members without a membership ID or payment confirmation should register in the Skylark Ballroom, located just down the corridor from the Wellings Ballroom, on the south side of the hotel. If you have questions regarding your registration, please call Liana Reyes, Registration Coordinator, at (669) 375-1700.

4. At which of the following tables should the member with ID number 39999 register?

A) Table 1
B) Table 2
C) Table 3
D) Table 4

5. At which of the following days and times should an attending conference member sign up for the conference?

A) Monday morning
B) Monday evening
C) Thursday morning
D) Saturday or Sunday evening

6. Which of the following features could help organize the information in this text?

A) An index of all the ID numbers
B) A chart showing the ID numbers and corresponding table assignments
C) A list of all the rooms in the building where the conference is held
D) A photo of Liana Reyes, the Registration Coordinator

7. Which of the following is a primary source document? Select all that apply.

A) A handwritten letter from Thomas Jefferson to James Madison
B) An excerpt from a journal entry made by Meriwether Lewis that is reprinted in a book
C) An autobiography of Virginia Woolf
D) An index of articles that have been written about quantum mechanics

Nutrition Facts

Serving size: 2/3 cup (55g)
Servings per container: about 8

Amount per serving	
Calories 230	Calories from fat 40

	% Daily Value*
Total Fat 8g	12%
Saturated Fat 1g	5%
Trans Fat 0g	
Cholesterol 0mg	0%
Sodium 160mg	7%
Total Carbohydrate 37g	12%
Dietary Fiber 4g	16%
Sugars 1g	
Protein 3g	
Vitamin A	10%
Vitamin C	8%
Calcium	20%
Iron	45%

*Percent Daily Values are based on a 2,000-calorie diet. Your daily value may be higher or lower depending on your caloric needs.

	Calories:	2,000	2,500
Total Fat	Less than	65g	80g
Sat Fat	Less than	20g	25g
Cholesterol	Less than	300mg	300mg
Sodium	Less than	2,400mg	2,400mg
Total Carbohydrate		300g	375g
Dietary Fiber		25g	30g

The next two questions are based on the following graphic.

8. A man who recently suffered from gallstones was instructed by his doctor to consume no more than one percent of his daily value of total fat in one meal. The man eats a 2,000-calorie diet each day. Is the above product a suitable choice for the man?

   A) No, because each serving of the product contains 12% of the daily fat value, which greatly exceeds the man's needs.
   B) Yes, because the product contains zero cholesterol, which is beneficial to a patient suffering from gallstones.
   C) Yes, because the food offers iron, which is considered an essential part of a balanced diet.
   D) No, because the product contains 230 calories, which is more than the man should consume in one meal.

9. "Dietary Fiber" is an example of which of the following text features?

   A) Title
   B) Footnote
   C) Italicized text
   D) Subheading

The next three questions are based on this price list.

COST OF COLOGNE

Company	City	Price per Case of 10	Shipping and Handling
Store 1	Albany, NY	$130.00	$15.00/case
Store 2	Washington, DC	$120.00	$20.00/case
Store 3	New York, NY	$150.00	Free shipping on all orders
Store 4	Hartford, CT	$135.00	$15.00/case (free in-state shipping)

10. A business owner from Connecticut is interested in purchasing 50 bottles of cologne to give as gifts to his employees this year. How much will he pay in total if he purchases the cologne from Store 4?

    A) $650.00
    B) $675.00
    C) $690.00
    D) $750.00

11. A woman from New York is interested in stocking her store with 90 bottles of cologne. Which store would save her the most money? Circle the number of the store in the chart above.

12. If a person living in Albany is purchasing a case of cologne from Store 1 and is considering picking up the case rather than having it shipped, which of the following would be the most accurate source to use to find the best route from the person's home to the store?

A) A world atlas
B) A phone call to the store to ask for directions
C) An Internet-based navigation application
D) The website for the Albany post office

ANSWER KEY

1. C	**5.** A	**9.** D
2. D	**6.** B	**10.** B
3. B	**7.** A and C	**11.** 2
4. C	**8.** A	**12.** C

ANSWERS AND EXPLANATIONS

1. (C) There is no general trend within the revenue data presented in the bar graph. Choice D is incorrect because the business saw declining revenue in 2011 and 2012.

2. (D) The horizontal axis title "Year" could be omitted because viewers would understand that 2009, 2010, and so on are the years being tracked.

3. (B) The text uses italicized print because *Titanic* is the proper name of a ship.

4. (C) The number 39999 falls between 30001 and 40000, so the member needs to register at Table 3; there is no Table 4 mentioned in the instructions.

5. (A) The instructions specifically mention 8:30 A.M.–10:30 A.M. on Monday morning as the designated conference sign-up period. While other times and days are also mentioned, they are not designated for conference sign-up.

6. (B) A chart showing the ID number ranges and table assignments would be helpful to registrants.

7. (A and C) A letter handwritten by Thomas Jefferson is a primary source, as is an autobiography of Virginia Woolf.

8. (A) The amount of total fat in this product is 12% of the suggested daily value, based on a 2,000-calorie diet. The man was instructed to eat less than one percent of his daily value of total fat in one meal, so this product is not suitable for him to consume.

9. (D) Dietary Fiber is shown as a subheading of the category Carbohydrates.

10. (B) Since the man is purchasing the cologne from the store in his home state, Connecticut, he does not have to pay any shipping charges. An order of five boxes of ten bottles of cologne each will be $135 times five, which comes to a total of $675, choice B.

11. (2) To obtain ninety bottles of cologne, the woman would have to order nine cases. Store 2 would provide the cases at the lowest total cost, which is $140 per case, including shipping. Store 1 would charge $145 per case, including shipping, while Store 3 and Store 4 would both charge $150 per case, including shipping.

12. (C) The best source to use to find the distance between two locations would be an Internet-based navigation system.

CHAPTER 10

Evaluating and Integrating Data

Data questions require you to identify information given in different types of resources. Some questions may also require you to identify the appropriate resources to consult in order to obtain specific types of information. Questions may test your ability to use a number of different skills, including following directions, recognizing steps in a sequence, reading labels and ingredient lists, analyzing outlines, identifying sources, and looking up information.

In **following directions questions**, a set of directions is given, and you are asked to identify the outcome that occurs when the directions are followed.

Here is an example of a following directions question:

Rachel walks out of the building shown on the map below at the corner of 4th and Maple. She takes a left on Maple Street, walks for two blocks, and then turns right. She walks one block. Circle the spot on the diagram that shows Rachel's current location.

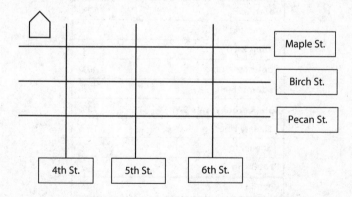

The correct answer is at the corner of Birch and 6th. From the corner of 4th and Maple, she walks down Maple for two blocks to the corner of Maple and 6th. She turns right onto 6th and goes one block to the corner of 6th and Birch.

Some questions may ask you to identify steps in a sequence. Here is an example:

Which of the following statements indicates the last step in a process?

A) Next take the wrench and loosen each bolt.
B) Take a left onto the highway after going three miles past the movie theater.
C) Finally, clean up your workstation, remembering to properly dispose of all waste.
D) The most important thing to remember is to wear goggles.

The correct answer is **C**. The word *finally* indicates that this is the last step.

In **reading labels and ingredient lists questions**, a nutritional label is provided or the ingredients of a recipe are listed. You might be asked to determine, for instance, whether this particular food or product would be suitable for an individual with certain dietary needs.

An example of a reading labels question is provided below:

Nutrition Facts

Serving size: 2/3 cup (55g)
Servings per container: about 8

Amount per serving	
Calories 230	Calories from fat 40

	% Daily Value*
Total Fat 8g	12%
Saturated Fat 1g	5%
Trans Fat 0g	
Cholesterol 0mg	0%
Sodium 160mg	7%
Total Carbohydrate 37g	12%
Dietary Fiber 4g	16%
Sugars 1g	
Protein 3g	
Vitamin A	10%
Vitamin C	8%
Calcium	20%
Iron	45%

*Percent Daily Values are based on a 2,000-calorie diet. Your daily value may be higher or lower depending on your caloric needs.

	Calories:	2,000	2,500
Total Fat	Less than	65g	80g
Sat Fat	Less than	20g	25g
Cholesterol	Less than	300mg	300mg
Sodium	Less than	2,400mg	2,400mg
Total Carbohydrate		300g	375g
Dietary Fiber		25g	30g

A hungry woman decides to eat four servings of the product. Her caloric needs are 2,000 calories per day. How many calories may she still eat for the rest of the day without exceeding her caloric needs?

A) 460 calories
B) 920 calories
C) 1,770 calories
D) 1,080 calories

The correct answer is **D**. Each serving of this product contains 230 calories. The number 230 multiplied by four servings is 920 calories already consumed. To find the amount of calories left to be eaten for the day, subtract 920 from 2,000 calories. The answer is 1,080.

In **analyzing outlines questions**, an outline is given, and you must identify patterns in the headings or subheadings of the outline. Here is an example:

Chapter 10 The Major Sports

1. Baseball

A) History
B) Rules
C) Notable Players

2. Basketball

A) History
B) Rules
C) Notable Players

3. Football

A) History
B) Rules
C) Notable Players

4. Hockey

A) History
B) Rules
C) Notable Players

5. Soccer

A) History
B) Rules
C) Notable Players

What is the organizational pattern reflected in the headings and subheadings?

A) The chapter discusses the history, rules, and notable players of five major sports.
B) The chapter discusses the history of five major sports played throughout the world.
C) The chapter discusses physical education activities and their rules.
D) The chapter discusses famous athletes' careers throughout history.

The correct answer is **A**. The chapter is arranged by major sport, and each sport covers the same three subtopics. No other choice offers this organizational option.

In **identifying sources questions**, a scenario is posed, and you must identify the correct information source to use to obtain the required information. Finally, in **looking up information questions**, an information source is provided, and you are asked to look up information and answer a question identifying that information. Information sources may be presented in text form or in graphic form. **Text information sources** include memos, advertisements, book indices, tables of contents, price lists, and yellow pages listings. **Graphic information sources** include graphs, charts, diagrams, and maps, among other possibilities.

Many data questions on the TEAS fall into the category of looking up information. To answer the question, you must look up the information requested and find the answer. Even though the sources provided may be vastly different—graphs and charts, for instance, versus yellow page ads—the skill used in answering these questions is the same.

The following three examples all test your skills at looking up information found in various sources:

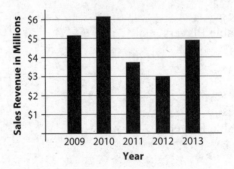

The bar graph above shows sales revenue for a business by the year. How much revenue did the business generate in 2013?

A) About $5.00
B) Almost $4,000
C) About $5,000
D) About $5,000,000

The correct answer is **D**. The bar graph compares the amount of revenue made by a business each year. The label on the left side of the graph indicates that the units are given in millions of dollars. The bar for 2013 extends to just below the 5 mark, which indicates almost five million dollars, or $5,000,000.

Consider this example:

Map of Lyndon B. Johnson State Park in Stonewall, Texas

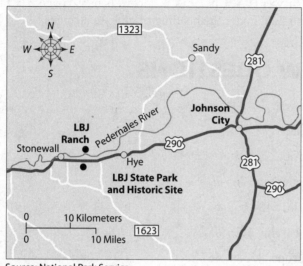

Source: National Park Service

Which of the following directions should someone who lives in the city of Sandy take in order to arrive at the LBJ State Park and Historic Site?

A)   Take HWY 281 N to 290 W.
B)   Take 1323 S to HWY 290 W.
C)   Take HWY 290 S to HWY 281 N.
D)   Take HWY 1323 W to 281 S.

The correct answer is **B**. The correct route to take is 1323 S to HWY 290 W. The other routes offer incorrect ordinal directions.

Let's look at one more example related to looking up information.

Climate

Africa, 722–4

Antarctica, 765–7

Asia, 543–7

Australia, 669–70

Europe, 453–5, 467

North America, 363, 379–81

South America, 497–9

Climate changes, 203–23

A student would like to compare climate changes in the sixteenth and twenty-first centuries. On which of the following pages might she find this information?

A) Page 221
B) Page 232
C) Page 453
D) Page 723

The correct answer is **A**. Choice A is correct because page 221 falls between pages 203 and 223, under the heading of climate changes.

REVIEW QUESTIONS

1.

Climate

    Africa, 722–4

    Antarctica, 765–7

    Asia, 543–7

    Australia, 669–70

    Europe, 453–5, 467

    North America, 363, 379–81

    South America, 497–9

Climate changes, 203–23

In which of the following resources would the above index most likely be found?

A) Biology textbook
B) History textbook
C) Ecology textbook
D) Chemistry textbook

2.

Chapter 10: The Major Sports

1. Baseball

    A) History
    B) Rules
    C) Notable Players

2. Basketball

    A) History
    B) Rules
    C) Notable Players

3. Football

    A) History
    B) Rules
    C) Notable Players

4. Hockey

    A) History
    B) Rules
    C) Notable Players

5. Soccer

    A) History
    B) Rules
    C) Notable Players

If the title of the above outline were changed to read "Chapter 10: Ball Sports," which of the following sections would not belong in the chapter?

A) Hockey
B) Football
C) Tennis
D) Soccer

Apple Pie

3 cups all-purpose flour

1¼ cup sugar

1 cup butter

4-5 Granny Smith apples

3 egg yolks

1 lemon

¼ cup cold water

3 Tbsp heavy cream

1 Tbsp cinnamon

The next two questions are based on this ingredients list.

3. Are the ingredients in the recipe above suitable for an individual with diabetes?

   A) Yes, because egg yolks are a staple of any diabetic diet.
   B) Yes, because diabetes is a disorder for which the body requires extra sugar ingestion.
   C) No, because diabetics are allergic to products containing fruit.
   D) No, because the ingredients include sugar, which is not appropriate for people with diabetes.

4. In which of the following cookbooks are you most likely to find a recipe using the ingredients list above?

   A) *Halloween Candies and Confections*
   B) *Egg-Based Entrees for Entertaining*
   C) *Healthy Living for Longevity*
   D) *Delicious Desserts to Die For*

Map of Lyndon B. Johnson State Park in Stonewall, Texas

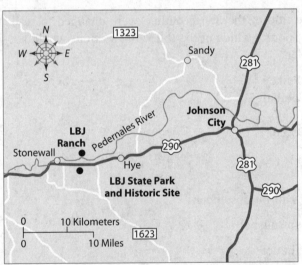

Source: National Park Service

The next two questions are based on this map.

5. In which of the following guides would you most likely find the map above?

   A) *World Atlas*
   B) *Johnson City Street Guide*
   C) *Map of California*
   D) *Texas Roads and Recreation Atlas*

6. Which of the following could be the second step in a list of directions for traveling from Sandy to Johnson City?

    A) Turn left from LBJ Ranch onto the highway access road.
    B) Follow Highway 290 for 22 miles.
    C) Take Highway 1323 southeast for 12 miles.
    D) Go south on Highway 281.

7. A woman is concerned that her dog's leg might be broken. Which resource should the woman consult?

    A) A website about pet care
    B) A zoology textbook
    C) An anatomy textbook
    D) *The Yellow Pages,* under V for veterinarian

Units Produced by Teams A–E

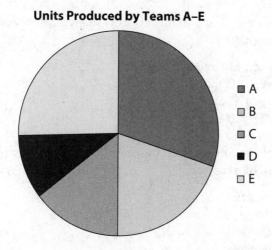

The next two questions are based on this pie chart.

8. In the key above, circle the letter of the team that produced the most units.

9. About how many units were produced without Team E?

    A) Four-fifths of the units
    B) Half of the units
    C) Three-fourths of the units
    D) One-fourth of the units

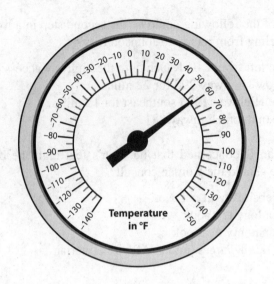

10. A temperature of approximately how many degrees is represented on the thermometer?

A) Between 110 and 110 degrees
B) Between 60 and 65 degrees
C) Between 55 and 60 degrees
D) Between 50 and 55 degrees

11. Which of the following resources would be most helpful for finding the length of a car?

A) A protractor
B) A ruler
C) A yardstick
D) A calculator

Marcia decided to run a trail 3.5 miles every other day and to run a different path 3.9 miles on her off days. The chart below demonstrates the number of miles she ran over two weeks' time.

Sunday	Monday	Tuesday	Wednesday	Thursday	Friday	Saturday
3.5	3.9	3.5	3.9	3.9	3.5	3.9
3.5	3.9	3.5	3.9	3.9	3.5	3.9

The next three questions are based on this passage and chart.

12. How many times did Marcia run a trail, and how many times did she run a path?

A) Marcia ran a trail five times and a path nine times.
B) Marcia ran a trail six times and a path eight times.
C) Marcia ran a trail eight times and a path six times.
D) Marcia ran a trail seven times and a path seven times.

13. Which of the following is a true statement, based on the chart?

    A) Marcia ran the trail two more times than she ran the path.
    B) Marcia ran the path and the trail an equal number of times.
    C) Marcia ran the path two more times than she ran the trail.
    D) Marcia ran the path three more times than she ran the trail.

14. How many times did Marcia deviate from her typical routine?

    A) One
    B) Two
    C) Three
    D) Four

ANSWER KEY

1. C	**6.** D	**11.** C
2. A	**7.** D	**12.** B
3. D	**8.** A	**13.** C
4. D	**9.** C	**14.** B
5. D	**10.** C	

ANSWERS AND EXPLANATIONS

1. (C) Climate is a subtopic of the ecology discipline. Biology textbooks are concerned with life processes, while history textbooks are concerned with social and political events of the past, and chemistry textbooks are concerned with chemical processes, so choices A, B, and D are incorrect.

2. (A) Hockey does not belong in the chapter because the chapter is about ball sports; a puck is used in hockey. Balls are used in all of the other sports listed.

3. (D) Diabetics produce insufficient insulin to break down sugar, so their sugar intake should be limited; this apple pie recipe calls for 1¼ cups of sugar, which is not suitable for a diabetic.

4. (D) Apple pie is a dessert and would likely be included in a cookbook about desserts. Choice A is incorrect because apple pie is not a candy, and it is not traditionally served on Halloween. Choice B is incorrect because, while the recipe calls for eggs, apple pie is not considered an *egg-based* dish—such as quiche—and it is not an *entrée*, or main dish. Choice C is incorrect, because while apples are healthy, an apple pie made with sugar would not be considered to be a particularly healthy dish.

5. (D) This map is too specific to be found in a world atlas, and it is too large-scale to be found in a city guidebook. Choice C is incorrect because this map excerpt shows points of interest in Texas, not California.

6. (D) To get from Sandy to Johnson City, you would first take Highway 1323 southeast and then go south on Highway 281.

7. (D) An animal's broken bone requires a veterinarian for treatment; all of the other options given are too broad and would be inappropriate for a dog owner to consult for help in treating such a major injury.

8. (A) Team A shows the largest shaded area on the pie chart.

9. (C) The shaded area for Team E on the pie chart represents approximately 25%, or one-fourth, of the pie graph. Without this one-fourth, the rest of the teams' production makes up 75%, or three-fourths, of the total number of units produced.

10. (C) The gauge of the thermometer is just under the 60 degree mark, which falls between 55 and 60 degrees.

11. (C) A car would be best measured with a yardstick, which is 3 feet, or 36 inches long; a ruler would be too small, at 12 inches. A calculator is used to calculate, while a protractor is used to measure angles.

12. (B) The chart demonstrates that Marcia ran 3.5 miles six times. The trail is 3.5 miles long, so she ran a trail six times. She ran 3.9 miles eight times, so she ran the path eight times.

13. (C) The chart demonstrates that Marcia ran the path eight times and the trail six times. Therefore, she ran the path two more times than she ran the trail.

14. (B) The chart demonstrates that Marcia deviated from her usual running schedule twice, on both Thursdays. The other days, she adhered to her usual schedule.

CHAPTER 11

Comparing and Contrasting Themes

The **themes** of a passage are broad ideas or concepts that weave throughout the passage and frequently recur. A passage regarding key battles of the Civil War might contain themes of heroism, bravery, or strategic prowess, for instance. Theme and main idea are related, but think of the theme as a lesson or universal truth rather than a specific point the author is trying to make. For example, the main idea of a passage may be that Columbus had to ask may people for funding before Queen Isabella agreed, but the theme is that perseverance pays off. Theme is also related to topic. For example, the topic of a passage may be a company policy about unisex bathrooms, while the theme is gender equality in the workplace.

Themes are present in all types of media, not just literature. Photographers, painters, sculptors, and filmmakers all have themes for their work. Even nonfiction works have themes. Once you are adept at finding the theme of a work, pay attention to how different works treat the same theme. Even the same author may treat a theme differently in two separate works. For example, Shakespeare explores the theme of love very differently in *Othello* versus in *As You Like It*.

Look at this text and try the practice question that follows:

Saltwater fish and freshwater fish are related, but their natural environments prove rather distinctive. In terms of being kept as pets, freshwater fish require less maintenance. They live in water that can be adapted from tap water, and they can be kept in many different types of containers in addition to aquariums. Saltwater fish, on the other hand, require a specific type of salt-infused water. The water's pH balance must also be carefully monitored and maintained.

Is the phrase *maintenance requirements* a topic, main idea, supporting detail, or theme of the above passage?

A) Main idea
B) Topic
C) Supporting detail
D) Theme

The correct answer is **D**. *Maintenance requirements* is a theme of this passage. The passage compares and contrasts saltwater and freshwater fish (the topic), with a focus on their respective maintenance requirements. The main idea is that saltwater and freshwater fish have different maintenance requirements.

Try another example:

Published in 1719, nearly a century before Britain passed the Abolition of the Slave Trade Act in 1807, *Robinson Crusoe* is an overtly racist novel that seems to celebrate slavery and imperialism. Despite that, there are hints of a change in the prevailing Western attitude toward nonwhite people. While never questioning his superiority to Friday, Crusoe does acknowledge his honorable characteristics: he is loyal, he is brave, he is useful, and he helps cheerfully. Sure, Friday was a cannibal, but it was culturally acceptable among his people and he did not know any better. As soon as the Western, Christian Crusoe teaches him how wrong it is, he immediately swears it off. Defoe doesn't exactly lay the groundwork for nonwhite characters who are equal to their white counterparts, but he does plant a tiny seed of possibility.

Which of the following is a theme introduced in the passage above?

A) Western superiority
B) Loyalty
C) Cannibalism
D) The value of literature

The correct answer is **A**. The passage explores the idea that racist Western attitudes may be starting to change slightly. Loyalty and cannibalism are mentioned, but are not repeated or expanded upon in the way a theme should be. The value of literature is not mentioned.

The TEAS will also ask you to compare and contrast themes across different texts. To do this, you will need to be able to find what two texts have in common and how they differ in presenting the same theme. Here is an example:

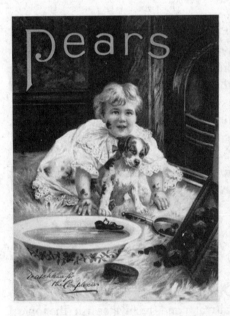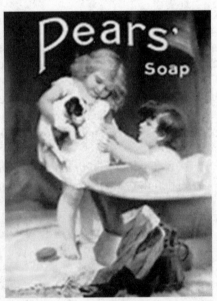

Source: for ad on left: https://commons.wikimedia.org/wiki/File:Pears_Soap_1900.jpg; for ad on right: https://commons.wikimedia.org/wiki/File:Frederick_Morgan02.jpg

What theme is common to both these soap ads?

A) Motherhood
B) Youth
C) Beauty
D) Honesty

The correct answer is **B**. Both ads feature both children and puppies. The implied message is that the soap preserves youth.

Try another question:

Which of the following is a way in which both photographers and film-makers might express a theme?

A) By repeating the same word multiple times
B) By showing their work at the same gallery
C) By using a certain camera angle
D) By using imagery to describe a landscape

The correct answer is **C**. Using a certain camera angle is something both filmmakers and photographers can do to influence how a subject is viewed and thus can express theme. Choices A and D both refer to written works and choice B is unclear as to how this could express a theme.

REVIEW QUESTIONS

1. The way that scientists have envisioned the makeup of the universe has shifted and transformed as the centuries have passed. Prior to the work of Copernicus, people believed that the earth was at the center of the universe. The idea that the earth revolved around the sun was initially taken as heresy. The progression and gradual acceptance of these originally controversial ideas paved the way for the acceptance of later discoveries by Newton and Einstein. Their theories have revolutionized the ways in which science itself is conducted today.

   Is *changing mindsets* a topic, main idea, supporting detail, or theme of the above passage? Write your answer in the blank: _____

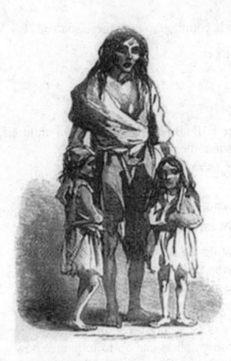

Source: Illustrated London News, December 22, 1849 (public domain)

2. What theme is expressed in the political cartoon above?

A) The Irish potato famine
B) Poverty
C) The rich should help the poor
D) Adoption

Questions 3–4 are based on the passage and photo below.

Now they were to witness one of the most impressive ceremonies of the United States Navy.

Division after division of the crew was formed in line and marched aft, in rhythmic tread, to the stern deck, on which stood Captain Dunham and a group of his officers in full uniform, the last rays of the sun glinting on their gold braid.

The men stood facing the flag and grouped on each side of the deck. Their hands raised uniformly in salute to the flag as at the last notes of the bugle it slowly descended the staff.

As it reached the deck, the band, stationed with their shining instruments on the starboard side of the ship, burst forth into the "Star-Spangled Banner."

The eyes of every man on that deck shone as the emblem for which they were pledged to fight fluttered down and the band blared forth the inspiring strains of the national anthem. Their officers stood in a little group, bare-headed, the chaplain conspicuous among them in his plain braided garb.

"First division, right about face!"

The sharp command of the ensign in charge of that division broke the impressive silence.

"March!"

Division after division, the men melted away from the after deck and left the little group of officers standing chatting alone. In all their after years in the navy, the two Dreadnought Boys never forgot that ceremony. Its recollection remained with them long after the annoying incidents and trials of their first year of service had faded.

(from *The Dreadnought Boys on Battle Practice* by John Henry Goldfrap)
Source: Project Gutenberg http://www.gutenberg.org/files/
47776/47776-h/47776-h.htm

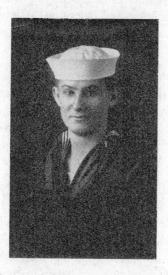

Source: James Voelkle, *photo of Otto Meinhart*, U.S. Navy

3. Which of the following themes does the phrase *their hands raised uniformly in salute to the flag* represent?

   A) Patriotism
   B) Rebellion
   C) Bravery
   D) Sacrifice

4. What theme do the passage and photo have in common?

   A) Men's fashion
   B) Loyalty
   C) Navy pride
   D) War

Questions 5–6 are based on the passage below.

Imagine living in the year 1800. The railroads then were very scarce. Gas lights were not yet invented, and electric lights were not even dreamed of. Even kerosene wasn't used at that point. This was the world into which Samuel Morse, the inventor of the telegraph, was born.

Samuel Morse was born in Charlestown, Massachusetts, shortly before the turn of the century, in 1791. When he was seven years old, he was sent to boarding school at Phillips Academy, Andover. While he was there, his father wrote him letters, giving him good advice. He told him about George Washington and about a British statesman named Lord Chesterfield, who was able to achieve many of his goals. Lord Chesterfield was asked once how he managed to find time for all of his pursuits, and he replied that he only ever did one thing at a time, and that he "never put off anything until tomorrow that could be done today."

Morse worked hard at school and began to think and act for himself at quite a young age. His biggest accomplishment was in painting, and he established himself as a successful painter after graduating from college at Yale. But he also had an interest in science and inventions. He was passionate about the idea of discovering a way for people to send messages to each other in short periods of time.

In the early 1800s, it took a long time to receive news of any sort, even important news. Whole countries had to wait weeks to hear word of the outcomes of faraway wars. The mail was carried by stagecoach. In emergency situations, such as when ships were lost at sea, there was no way to send requests for help. Electricity had been discovered, but little application had been made of it up until that point. This was about to change when Morse set his mind to his invention.

On October 1, 1832, Morse was sailing to America from a trip overseas on a ship called the *Sully*. He became preoccupied with the thought of inventing a machine that would later become the telegraph. Morse thought about the telegraph night and day. As he sat upon the deck of the ship after dinner one night, he took out a little notebook and began to create a plan.

If a message could be sent ten miles without dropping, he wrote, "I could make it go around the globe." He said this over and over again during the years after his trip.

One morning at the breakfast table, Morse showed his plan to some of the other *Sully* passengers. Five years later, when the model of the telegraph was built, it was exactly like the one shown that morning to the passengers on the *Sully*.

Once he arrived in America, Morse worked for twelve long years to get people to notice his invention. Though some supported the idea of the telegraph, many people scoffed at it. Morse persisted, and eventually a bill was passed by Congress in 1842. It authorized the funds needed to build the first trial telegraph line.

After two years, the telegraph line was complete. Morse and his colleagues tested it in May of 1844. The device worked, and the telegraph became a huge success. Morse's persistence had finally paid off.

5. Which of the following describes the word *perseverance* as it relates to the passage?

   A) Main idea
   B) Topic
   C) Supporting detail
   D) Theme

6. Which of the following lines from the passage is an example of Morse's perseverance?

   A) Morse worked for twelve long years to get people to notice his invention.
   B) Morse was sailing to America from a trip overseas on a ship called the *Sully*.
   C) One morning at the breakfast table, Morse showed his plan to some of the other *Sully* passengers.
   D) He took out a little notebook and began to create a plan.

7. Shelley's poem "Mont Blanc" focuses on the Romantic notion of the sublime. The Romantic poets believed that when people interacted with nature, it sometimes caused them to be in a state of wonder—or it caused them to be awestruck. For example, when a person gazed at a mountain, the huge size of the mountain could cause the person to become speechless with wonder. This was the effect that the sublime quality of nature could have on a viewer.

In "Mont Blanc," Shelley describes the mountain in a way that attempts to explain its effects on the viewer's mind. According to Shelley, the mountain itself causes the viewer's thoughts to enter a kind of strange trance, and to be affected in a way that resembles how a poet or an artist feels whenever he or she is caught in the midst of a creative inspiration. In the poem, Shelley draws a comparison between the effect of the mountain on the viewer and the power that the imagination has over the artist's mind.

What theme is expressed in the passage above?

   A) Shelley's poem "Mont Blanc"
   B) Effects of the sublime
   C) Romantic poetry
   D) Nature can inspire imagination.

Questions 8–10 are based on the two paragraphs below.

A: The part that the wild life of America played in the settlement and development of this continent was so far-reaching in extent, and so enormous in potential value, that it fairly staggers the imagination. From the landing of the Pilgrims down to the present hour the wild game has been the mainstay and the resource against starvation of the pathfinder, the settler, the prospector, and at times even the railroad-builder. In view of what the bison millions did for the Dakotas, Montana, Wyoming, Kansas and Texas, it is only right and square that those states should now do something for the perpetual preservation of the bison species and all other big game that needs help. (excerpt from *Our Vanishing Wild Life*, by William T. Hornaday)

Source: Project Gutenberg http://www.gutenberg.org/files/13249/13249-h/13249-h.htm

B: Till quite recently Nature had her own sanctuaries, where man either did not go at all or only as a tool-using animal in comparatively small numbers. But now, in this machinery age, there is no place left where man cannot go with overwhelming forces at his command. He can strangle to death all the nobler wild life in the world today. Tomorrow he certainly will have done so, unless he exercises due foresight and self-control in the mean time. There is not the slightest doubt that birds and mammals are now being killed off much faster than they can breed. And it is always the largest and noblest forms of life that suffer most. (excerpt from *Animal Sanctuaries in Labrador*, by William Wood)

Source: Project Gutenberg http://www.gutenberg.org/files/14866/14866-h/14866-h.htm

8. What theme is evoked in Passage A by the phrase *it is only right and square*?

    A) Using corrals to protect bison
    B) Ownership of land
    C) Reciprocity
    D) Revenge

9. What is the common theme expressed by both passages?

    A) The American West
    B) Conservation of wildlife
    C) Nature preserves
    D) Bison

10. If Passage B was being written for an ecotourism advertisement, which of the following sentences would be most appropriate to add to the end of the passage?

    A) The best way to protect these animals is to leave them in peace.
    B) You can do your part to protect them by donating to animal protection agencies.
    C) Humans will continue to destroy their habitats until these beautiful creatures no longer inhabit the earth.
    D) Learn what you can do to protect these animals while seeing them in their natural habitats.

ANSWER KEY

1. theme	**5.** D	**9.** B
2. B	**6.** A	**10.** D
3. A	**7.** B	
4. C	**8.** C	

ANSWERS AND EXPLANATIONS

1. (theme) *Changing mindsets* is a theme of this passage. Be careful not to confuse the theme with the topic. The topic is not focused on changing mindsets but, more specifically, on scientific views of the universe.

2. (B) The theme of the cartoon is poverty. The main idea might be the rich should help the poor. The topic could possibly be the Irish potato famine.

3. (A) The phrase is about saluting the flag, so patriotism is the theme.

4. (C) The photo is of a man in a navy uniform, and the passage is about a navy flag ceremony and the pride the men felt about it and how they never forgot it. Both evoke the theme of navy pride.

5. (D) *Perseverance* is a theme of this passage. The passage discusses Morse's perseverance throughout, while the topic of the passage is the telegraph.

6. (A) Working for twelve years certainly shows perseverance.

7. (B) The theme expressed in the passage is the effects of the sublime. The topic is Shelley's poem "Mont Blanc" and the main idea is that nature can inspire imagination.

8. (C) Passage A, in saying *it is only right and square*, uses the reasoning of reciprocity. The author says that since wildlife has done so much for the people in the western states, the people in those states should repay the debt by helping the endangered animals there.

9. (B) Both passages stress the importance of conserving natural resources, specifically wildlife. Only the first passage mentions the American West and bison. Only passage B discusses nature preserves.

10. (D) Only choice D involves the idea of travel, so it would be the most appropriate for a tourism advertisement.

CHAPTER 12

Vocabulary

Vocabulary questions on the TEAS ask you to define the meaning of a vocabulary word based on the context of the passage. The chosen vocabulary word is often one that might have an unusual meaning or might be interpreted as having several meanings. The correct meaning must be clarified based on your understanding of the surrounding text.

The context surrounding the vocabulary word is particularly important because words may have different denotative and connotative meanings.

Denotation refers to the literal definition of a word that you would find in a dictionary. Since many words also have more than one literal definition, be sure you know which one is being used in the text.

Connotation refers to what the word suggests or implies. Connotation is often a function of the culture in which the word is used and may be a symbolic meaning rather than a literal one. For example, the word *snake* has a literal denotative meaning, the reptile, but it also has a connotative meaning of deception or trickery.

You also should be familiar with **figurative language**, in which the meaning is imparted through creative figurative devices such as similes, metaphors, personification, hyperbole, and so on. If your brother cheats at cards and you say "You are such a snake!" then you are using figurative language (a metaphor) to signify the connotative meaning that your brother is a cheater. Be familiar with these figurative devices:

- Simile: a comparison using *like* or *as*
  She runs like the wind.
- Metaphor: a comparison without *like* or *as*
  My brother is such a snake.
- Hyperbole: exaggeration
  He jumped as high as the sky.
- Personification: giving inanimate objects human characteristics
  The moon smiled down on us.
- Imagery: using descriptive language that appeals to the senses
  The pizza crust was thin as a cracker, buttery, and fragrant with garlic and rosemary.

Here is an example:

Shelley was born in England in 1792, as a member of the <u>aristocracy</u>. He was educated at two prestigious English schools, Eton College and Oxford University.

Based on context, which of the following is the definition of the underlined word in the sentences above?

A) A worker's union
B) A Republican consortium
C) The upper class
D) A lower socioeconomic class

The correct answer is **C**. The word *aristocracy* means the wealthy or the upper class of a society. The context clue about Shelley's education at *prestigious* schools indicates that his family was wealthy enough to afford such select schools, so choice C is correct.

The sentences are about education and not employment or labor, so we can rule out choice A. Choice B can also be eliminated because, like with choice A, there is no discussion of politics or political groups in the sentences surrounding the word. Finally, choice D is the opposite of the correct answer. The context clues lead the reader to believe that Shelley was wealthy. The phrase *lower socioeconomic class* would indicate someone who was poor and thus unable to afford expensive schooling.

The following example includes a selection from the same passage on Shelley:

Shelley's ideas were heavily influenced by the politics of his time. He grew up at a time when governments were under <u>transformation</u>. In fact, he came of age in the shadow of the French Revolution. This war was very violent, and since France was so close to England, Shelley was acutely aware of the violence that was occurring there.

Based on context, which of the following is the definition of the underlined word in the passage above?

A) Change
B) Suspicion
C) Surveillance
D) Regrowth

The correct answer is **A**. *Change*, which can be synonymous with *transformation*, is the best fit with the context of this passage. *Transformation* is followed in the next sentence by the mention of a revolution, which would indicate a shift or change in governments. Therefore, the context clues given indicate that the author was describing the transforming or changing political landscape of the time.

Choice B can be eliminated because *suspicion* indicates doubt or skepticism. The paragraph does not discuss doubt or skepticism either on the part of the government or on Shelley's part. Choice C, *surveillance*, indicates that the governments were being watched closely by an entity or person. While this may have been true historically, there are no surrounding context clues in the passage to support this interpretation. Finally, choice D is incorrect because *regrowth* would mean that the governments were destroyed or eliminated and would need to be built again. There is nothing in the passage to suggest that this was the case.

Let's look at another example.

As one of the most prolific female poets in nineteenth-century America, today Emily Dickinson is a household name. However, during her lifetime, she lived as a recluse and wrote most of her poetry from the <u>solitude</u> of her bedroom. She presents a unique perspective from this time period, when few women wrote about the themes she discusses. For this reason, critics are frequently interested in her perspective as a female author even beyond the contributions she made as an American nineteenth-century writer.

> Based on the context of the passage above, which of the following is the definition of the underlined word?
>
> A) Happiness
> B) Misery
> C) Crowdedness
> D) Privacy

The correct answer is **D**. In this question, the author uses the word *solitude* to describe the atmosphere of Dickinson's writing space, her bedroom. Since the passage previously describes Dickinson as a *recluse*—a person who prefers to be alone—it is logical to conclude that Dickinson would prefer a space of *privacy* that would allow her to be alone.

Choice A is incorrect because *happiness* is irrelevant to the topic. The passage does not comment on Dickinson's moods but rather on how she lived her life. Regarding choice B, the passage specifically states that Dickinson preferred to be alone: she was a recluse. This preference does not indicate *misery*. Choice C is also incorrect because *crowdedness* is the opposite of reclusiveness, which the passage has already established that Dickinson preferred.

The next two passages contain additional examples of vocabulary words similar to those that might be tested.

Gardner has postulated an alternative theory concerning the existence of multiple intelligences. He <u>posits</u> that individuals can possess intelligence in particular areas, including linguistic intelligence, spiritual intelligence, spatial intelligence, intrapersonal intelligence, interpersonal intelligence, musical intelligence, mathematical intelligence, and kinesthetic intelligence, among others. Gardner asserts that individuals can be extremely intelligent and exhibit talent in one area, while failing to demonstrate the same level of prowess in another area.

> Based on the context of the passage above, which of the following is the definition of the underlined word?
>
> A) Claims
> B) Questions
> C) Evades
> D) Disagrees

The correct answer is **A**. The word *posits* indicates that someone, in this case Howard Gardner, has made a *claim* or argument about a particular topic.

The preceding and following sentences contain similar words, such as *postulated* and *asserts,* which also indicate a claim or argument.

Choice B is incorrect because if the word *posits* were replaced by the word *questioned,* the new sentence would indicate that Gardner was unsure of the statement that followed. However, the statement was his idea, so choice B does not make sense in this context. Choice C is incorrect because the purpose of the paragraph is to identify what Gardner thinks about IQ measurement; a person who has an opinion or argument on the subject would not logically be portrayed as *evading* the topic. Similar to choice B, choice D can be eliminated because if it were used to replace the word *posits,* the sentence would have the opposite of its intended meaning. Gardner does believe that people have multiple intelligences, so saying that he *disagrees* with the information in the statement would not make sense here.

Now consider this final passage:

The best method of treating individuals facing psychological difficulties is a blend of cognitive-behavioral therapy and medication. This approach not only serves to address the patient's potential chemical imbalances, but it also emancipates the patient by allowing him or her some autonomy in dealing with the issues associated with a possible malaise.

Based on the context of the passage above, which of the following is the definition of the underlined word?

A) Traps
B) Inspires
C) Frees
D) Confuses

The correct answer is **C**. Discussion of the patient's *emancipation* is immediately followed by mention of the patient's *autonomy* or independence. A person who is independent is *free*, so choice C is correct. Choice A is incorrect because it is the opposite of the meaning indicated. A patient cannot be *autonomous* if he or she is *trapped*. Choice B is incorrect because the passage does not describe the *inspiration* that therapy and medicine can produce. The focus is instead on the well-being of the patient and his or her ability to take ownership in dealing with psychological issues. Choice D is incorrect because if you plug *confuses* into the sentence to replace *emancipates*, the sentence no longer makes sense.

REVIEW QUESTIONS

1. Shelley's ideas were heavily influenced by the politics of his time. He grew up at a time when governments were under transformation. In fact, he came of age <u>in the shadow of</u> the French Revolution.

   Which figurative device is used in the underlined part of the sentence above?

   A) Hyperbole
   B) Simile
   C) Personification
   D) Metaphor

2. Shelley's poem "Mont Blanc" focuses on the Romantic notion of the <u>sublime</u>. The Romantic poets believed that when people interacted with nature, it sometimes caused them to be in a state of wonder—or it caused them to be awestruck.

   Based on the context, which of the following is the definition of the underlined word in the sentences above?

   A) Below par
   B) Truly inspirational
   C) Submerged
   D) Quietly introspective

3. Almost all approaches to CPR suggest that a person begin resuscitation efforts with chest <u>compressions</u>. To perform a chest compression, the individual places both hands flat on the patient's chest and then begins pushing down carefully but firmly, most likely at equal intervals.

   Based on the context, which of the following is the definition of the underlined word in the sentences above?

   A) Actions that remove items
   B) Actions that decrease density
   C) Actions that condense files
   D) Actions that press together

4. The lifesaver should start first by checking the patient's airway. He or she might also <u>administer</u> mouth-to-mouth rescue breathing.

   Which of the following is a synonym for <u>administer</u> in the sentences above?

   A) Supervise
   B) Apply
   C) Preach
   D) Teach

5. In planning improvements of highway systems, several different types of traffic may be encountered. These range from business traffic to agricultural shipping to residential transportation. Improvement activities must meet the requirements of all <u>classes</u> of traffic, with the most important provided for first.

   Based on the context of the passage above, which of the following is the definition of the underlined word?

   A) Groups of students taught by a professor
   B) Rankings in society based on economics
   C) Groups of items with similar qualities
   D) Individuals who maintain an elegant appearance

6. To keep their balance, the children must make efforts similar to those of real tightrope walkers, except that they have no danger of falling, since the lines are drawn only on the floor. The teacher herself performs the <u>exercise</u> first, showing clearly how she places her feet, and the children imitate her without her even needing to speak.

   Based on the context, which of the following is the correct definition of the word <u>exercise</u> in the sentences above?

   A) Freedom
   B) Process
   C) Removal
   D) Physical fitness

7. Personality is the combination of traits that make up an individual's sense of self. Traits can range from descriptors of behavior, such as "calm" or "emotional," to <u>modes</u> of experiencing the world, such as "thinking" or "sensing."

   Based on the context, which of the following is the definition of the underlined word in the sentences above?

   A) Ways
   B) Fashions
   C) Numbers
   D) Cuisines

8. Freud believed that as a child, an individual's actions are driven by hidden impulses—and that repression or denial of those impulses by parents or society can lead to fixations or personality disorders. Alternatively, if the child's impulses are accepted as normative to his or her development, then a functional adult behavioral pattern should <u>take root</u>.

Based on the context, which of the following is the definition of the underlined phrase in the sentences above?

A) Grow in the ground
B) Steal
C) Disappear
D) Develop

9. Freud often worked with highly distressed female clients, repressed in their natural modes of expression; this is how he developed many of his theories, which some people believe are not very scientific. By today's standards, they are not, but Freud's idea that unconscious urges drive our behavior was <u>revolutionary</u> for his time.

Based on the context of the sentences above, which of the following is the definition of the underlined word?

A) Referring to a political advocate
B) Referring to an early war in American history
C) Referring to an innovative idea
D) Referring to overthrowing a government

10. Close to the Guildhall is the <u>site</u> of a house known as New Place, which was bought by Shakespeare himself. Here Shakespeare lived during the later part of his life, until his death in 1616.

Based on the context, which of the following is the definition of the underlined word in the sentences above?

A) A position or location
B) The sense of looking
C) To officially summon
D) To refer to as an example

11. Although Shakespeare spent most of his career in London, with trips back to Stratford, he moved permanently to his home at New Place in the last years of his life and is believed to have written some of his later works there. Only the <u>foundations</u> of the New Place house now remain.

Based on the context, which of the following is the definition of the underlined word in the sentences above?

A) States of being established
B) The physical bases that buildings are built upon
C) Institutions engaged in philanthropy
D) The conceptual underpinnings of an idea

12. Christopher Columbus was particularly influenced by the maps of the ancient geographer Ptolemy. Ptolemy argued that the world was round, which went against the belief of the day that the world was flat. Columbus sided with Ptolemy on this question and <u>set out</u> to prove that it was so.

Based on the context of the passage above, which of the following is the definition of the underlined phrase?

A) To reflect upon an upcoming event
B) To act against one's own beliefs
C) To begin sailing on a voyage abroad
D) To begin working toward a plan

13. To make the journey westward, Columbus would require the help of a generous financial backer, so he went to seek the aid of the king of Portugal. Columbus asked the king for ships and sailors to make the journey.

Based on the context, which of the following is the definition of the underlined phrase in the sentences above?

A) A person who hoards resources in secret
B) A wealthy and resourceful travel partner
C) A person who provides money for a cause
D) An athlete who donates his income to charity

14. Once he arrived in America, Morse worked for twelve long years to get people to notice his invention. Though some supported the idea of the telegraph, many people scoffed at it. Morse persisted, and eventually a bill was passed by Congress in 1842.

Which of the following words are synonyms for the underlined word in the sentences above? Select all that apply.

A) Derided
B) Mocked
C) Condoned
D) Ridiculed

15. Persons going through emotional difficulties such as grief frequently listen to and create music as a means of dealing with the issues they are experiencing. Even people who simply need a short respite from the stresses of the day often use music as a calming and coping mechanism.

Based on the context of the passage above, which of the following is the definition of the underlined word?

A) A sudden awakening
B) A change in perspective
C) A way to get even
D) A pause for relief

ANSWER KEY

1. C	**6.** B	**11.** B
2. B	**7.** A	**12.** D
3. D	**8.** D	**13.** C
4. B	**9.** C	**14.** A, B, and D
5. C	**10.** A	**15.** D

ANSWERS AND EXPLANATIONS

1. (C) *In the shadow of* the French Revolution is an example of personification. The French Revolution is not a person and thus cannot cast an actual shadow.

2. (B) While *sub* is often used as a prefix meaning "under" or "below" in such words as *subpar* or *submarine*, this is not the way the prefix is being used in this excerpt, as indicated by the second sentence, which speaks of *awe* and *wonder*. Since *sublime* is equated with causing *awe* and *wonder*, its definition in this context most nearly means *truly inspirational*.

3. (D) The common definition of *compression* is an increase (not a decrease) in density, which eliminates choice B. The word *compression* in this context means to press down on the chest to enable circulation, so choice D is the only option that makes sense here. Choice C refers to the context of the computer field and is incorrect.

4. (B) The word *administer* typically means either "to manage" or "to apply." In this case, a person may administer, or *apply*, mouth-to-mouth breathing, deeming choice B correct and choice A incorrect. Choice C offers the word *preach*, the activity of *ministers*, which does not fit the context here.

5. (C) *Classes of traffic* refers to categories of traffic with similar qualities, such as cars or big trucking rigs, deeming choice C correct. While all of the other answer choices are definitions of *classes* in other contexts, they are incorrect in this sentence.

6. (B) For this sentence, choice B is the correct answer in that "performing an exercise" refers to the process of the teacher placing her feet on the line. Choice D is one definition of *exercise,* but it does not fit in this sentence. Choice A's definition, *freedom,* does not make sense in this context and is, therefore, incorrect. Choice C is related to the word *excise,* not *exercise.*

7. (A) The phrase *"modes* of experiencing the world" can be replaced with *"ways* of experiencing the world," so choice A fits the context here. While *modes* can also refer to *fashions* or *numbers,* choices B and C are not the correct definitions in this context.

8. (D) Choice A is incorrect, since it is a literal definition of *take root* instead of an idiom, which is figurative. Choices B and C do not fit the context and are therefore incorrect, while choice D, in the context of this passage, makes sense: a functional adult behavioral pattern should *develop.*

9. (C) While each of the answer choices refers to a definition of *revolutionary,* only choice C makes sense in the context of this sentence; Freud's ideas about the unconscious were *innovative* during the time he was living.

10. (A) The word *site* is used as a noun in this sentence, since it is preceded by the word *the,* deeming the verb definitions in choices C and D incorrect. Choices C and D are definitions of a homophone for *site,* spelled *cite.* Choice B is also the definition of a homophone for *site* that is spelled *sight.* Hence, the correct answer is choice A.

11. (B) Each of these choices offers a possible definition of the word *foundations,* but only choice B makes sense, as the last sentence of the selection refers to a *house,* which is a *building.*

12. (D) Columbus *set out to,* or *began working toward,* proving Ptolemy correct, choice D. Choices A and B are not definitions of *set out,* and neither of them makes sense in the context of this sentence. Choice C, *to begin sailing on a voyage,* is one possible definition for *set out,* but it does not make sense in this sentence.

13. (C) *A person who provides money for a cause,* choice C, is a *generous financial backer;* Columbus hoped that the king of Portugal would be that person, but he was not. Choices A, B, and D do not fit the context and are therefore incorrect.

14. (A, B, and D) This sentence contrasts the words *supported* and *scoffed,* revealing that some people supported Morse's idea, but others did not. Scoff means to show contempt, so *derided, mocked,* and *ridiculed* are all synonyms.

15. (D) A synonym for the word *respite* in this sentence would be the word *break. Break* can be substituted for *respite* in the sentence without a change in meaning. The word *break* means *a pause for relief,* so choice D is the correct answer.

PART II

MATHEMATICS

Math questions on the TEAS are designed to test your skills in four different areas: numbers and operations, data interpretation, measurement, and algebraic applications. In this section, we'll review some math fundamentals as well as more advanced skills you'll need to correctly answer questions involving word problems and algebra.

CHAPTER 13

Basic Operations

Basic operations questions on the TEAS involve addition, subtraction, multiplication, and division with whole numbers. You cannot use a calculator on the test, so you must know how to perform these operations by hand.

MULTIPLICATION TABLES

The operations of multiplication and division on the TEAS generally require that you know the multiplication tables of numbers from 1 through 12 by heart. To answer the test questions in the time allotted, you'll need to be able to draw these numbers quickly from memory. Here is a multiplication table of the numbers through 12 × 12:

1	2	3	4	5	6	7	8	9	10	11	12
2	4	6	8	10	12	14	16	18	20	22	24
3	6	9	12	15	18	21	24	27	30	33	36
4	8	12	16	20	24	28	32	36	40	44	48
5	10	15	20	25	30	35	40	45	50	55	60
6	12	18	24	30	36	42	48	54	60	66	72
7	14	21	28	35	42	49	56	63	70	77	84
8	16	24	32	40	48	56	64	72	80	88	96
9	18	27	36	45	54	63	72	81	90	99	108
10	20	30	40	50	60	70	80	90	100	110	120
11	22	33	44	55	66	77	88	99	110	121	132
12	24	36	48	60	72	84	96	108	120	132	144

ESTIMATING AND ROUNDING

Estimating is an important skill since an estimated answer to a real-world problem can tell you whether your detailed, calculated answer is likely correct. When doing calculations, people sometimes make mistakes such as

167

putting the decimal point in the wrong place. An estimation done by rounding to whole numbers would quickly show you whether your calculation was wrong.

On the TEAS, you cannot use a calculator, so rounding and estimation are valuable skills that can help you find the correct answer quickly and more easily.

First you must understand place value. If you are going to round a number to the nearest hundred, you will need to be able to find the number in the hundreds place.

Look at this number: 123,456

In expanded form, the number is $100,000 + 20,000 + 3,000 + 400 + 50 + 6$.

6 = ones' or units' place
5 = tens' place
4 = hundreds' place
3 = thousands' place
2 = ten thousands' place
1 = hundred thousands' place

If the number to the right of the one you are rounding is a 0, 1, 2, 3, or 4, then leave the number you are rounding alone and make all digits to its right zeros. For example, to round 234 to the nearest hundred, find the digit in the hundreds' place: 2. Since the digit to the right is a 3, leave the 2 alone and make the digits to its right zeros: 200.

If the number you are rounding is a 5, 6, 7, 8, or 9, then round up. For example, to round 567 to the nearest hundred, find the digit in the hundreds' place: 5. Since the digit to the right is a 6, round the 5 up to a 6 and make the digits to its right zeros: 600.

Most of the calculations you will do on the TEAS and in healthcare professions will be in the metric system, so be sure you are familiar with metric units. For estimation purposes, it may be helpful to have a real-world reference for common metric amounts.

Metric Unit	Real-World Example
milliliter	A dropperful of liquid
liter	Half of a two-liter bottle of soda
gram	The mass of a paper clip
kilogram	The mass of half of a 2-liter bottle of soda
millimeter	The thickness of a credit card
centimeter	The width of a pencil
meter	The height of a doorknob from the floor
kilometer	2.5 times around an indoor running track or 11 football field lengths

Try an example question:

Which of the following estimates the answer to 52.83 + 12.98?

A) 60
B) 66
C) 65.81
D) 70

The best answer is **B**. Rounding the numbers to the closest whole number gives you 53 + 13 = 66. Choice C is the actual answer, not an estimation.

ORDER OF OPERATIONS

Performing basic operations requires using the correct order of operations. In math, the **order of operations** is the set of rules that govern the sequence in which operations are performed.

The order of operations can be remembered using the phrase PEMDAS. **PEMDAS** stands for Parentheses, Exponents, Multiplication, Division, Addition, and Subtraction. Here's an example:

Simplify the expression: $4 \times (2 + 3)$.

To simplify this question, we would first perform the operation in parentheses:

$$2 + 3 = 5$$

Next, we would perform multiplication:

$$4 \times 5 = 20$$

The correct answer is **20**. When performing a series of operations, the order of operations is crucial to the accuracy of your result. If you don't follow the sequence exactly, your answer will be incorrect. In the example above, if we had multiplied 4×2 first, the answer would have been 6 + 3, or 9, which is incorrect.

The chart below summarizes the PEMDAS rules:

	Step	Explanation
1.	Parentheses	Perform all operations in parentheses first.
2.	Exponents	Next, perform all operations involving exponents.
3.	Multiplication & Division	Perform all multiplication and division in order from left to right.
4.	Addition & Subtraction	Perform all addition and subtraction in order from left to right.

Note that there are six letters in the word PEMDAS and six operations to be performed, but there are only four steps in the process. This is because multiplication and division are performed together in the same step, and addition and subtraction are performed together in the step after that. Here's an example:

Simplify the expression: $5 + 7 \times 2 - 12 \div 3$.

To solve this problem, follow the rules of PEMDAS. There are no parentheses or exponents in this expression, so we'll go straight to step 3, multiplication and division. All multiplication and division must be performed first, in order from left to right, before any addition or subtraction. So we first multiply 7×2 and divide $12 \div 3$:

$$5 + 7 \times 2 - 12 \div 3 = 5 + 14 - 4$$

Next, we perform addition and subtraction in order from left to right:

$$5 + 14 - 4 = 19 - 4$$
$$= 15$$

The correct answer is **15**. If we had multiplied 7×2 and then subtracted 12 right away, without dividing by 3 first, this would have given an incorrect answer, as shown in the example below:

Simplify the expression: $5 + 7 \times 2 - 12 \div 3$.

$$5 + 7 \times 2 - 12 \div 3 = 5 + 14 - 12 \div 3$$
$$= 19 - 12 \div 3$$
$$= 7 \div 3 \qquad \text{✗ INCORRECT}$$
$$= \frac{7}{3}$$

By performing the order of operations incorrectly, we reached the incorrect answer of $\frac{7}{3}$.

The correct approach is to perform all multiplication and division first, in order from left to right. Only then should you proceed to addition and subtraction, again in order from left to right:

Simplify the expression: $5 + 7 \times 2 - 12 \div 3$.

$$5 + 7 \times 2 - 12 \div 3 = 5 + 14 - 4$$
$$= 19 - 4 \qquad \text{✓ CORRECT}$$
$$= 15$$

REVIEW QUESTIONS

1. Which of the following is the most appropriate unit of measure to use for the mass of a baseball?

   A) Grams
   B) Kilograms
   C) Centimeters
   D) Liters

2. $10,741 \div 23$

   Simplify the expression above. Which of the following is correct?

   A) 365
   B) 397
   C) 467
   D) 489

3. $8 \times (4 + 3)$

   Simplify the expression above. Write your answer in the blank:

   _____

4. $5,614 + 373$

   Simplify the expression above. Which of the following is correct?

   A) 5,987
   B) 5,997
   C) 6,017
   D) 6,097

5. $17 + 6^2 - (4 + 2)$

   Simplify the expression above. Which of the following is correct?

   A) 23
   B) 36
   C) 47
   D) 51

6. 324×37

   Simplify the expression above. Which of the following is correct?

   A) 3,240
   B) 4,768
   C) 11,968
   D) 11,988

7. $473 - 67$

Simplify the expression above. Which of the following is correct?

A) 404
B) 406
C) 416
D) 429

8. $13,325 \div 25$

Simplify the expression above. Which of the following is correct?

A) 400
B) 425
C) 533
D) 535

9. $3 \times 5^2 \div (9 - 4)$

Simplify the expression above. Which of the following is correct?

A) -25
B) 3
C) 15
D) 27

10. 267×49

Round each number to the nearest ten, and then multiply.

A) 8,000
B) 13,083
C) 13,500
D) 15,000

11. $2 + (4 - 5) \times (12 \div 3)$

Simplify the expression above. Which of the following is correct?

A) -2
B) 1
C) 3
D) 4

12. $3^2 \times 2 + 6 \times 4^2$

Simplify the expression above. Which of the following is correct?

A) 96
B) 114
C) 268
D) 384

13. A nail salon owner is building a shelf to hold a single row of nail polish bottles. If the shelf is 1.5 meters long and the nail polish bottles are 4.8 centimeters wide, which of the following shows the best approximation of how many bottles of nail polish will fit on the shelf?

A) 0.31 because $1.5 \div 4.8 = 0.3125$.

B) 30 because a meter is 100 centimeters, so the shelf is 150 centimeters. Round the width of each bottle to 5 centimeters, and $150 \div 5 = 30$.

C) 31.25 because a meter is 100 centimeters, so the shelf is 150 centimeters. $150 \div 4.8 = 31.25$.

D) 40 because a meter is 100 centimeters, so the shelf is 150 centimeters. Round that to 200 centimeters. The width of each bottle is 5 centimeters, and $200 \div 5 = 40$.

14. $5 \times (4 + 2) \div 10 + 9$

Simplify the expression above. Write your answer in the blank:

_____

15. $2^3 \times 3 \div 24 + (1 - 4)$

Simplify the expression above. Which of the following is correct?

A) −3
B) −2
C) 1
D) 14

ANSWER KEY

1. A	**6.** D	**11.** A
2. C	**7.** B	**12.** B
3. 56	**8.** C	**13.** B
4. A	**9.** C	**14.** 12
5. C	**10.** C	**15.** B

ANSWERS AND EXPLANATIONS

1. (A) The most appropriate unit of measure for a baseball would be in grams. Kilograms could be used, but since a baseball has a mass significantly less than one kilogram, using grams would be better.

2. (C) Perform the indicated long division, as follows:

$$
\begin{array}{r}
467 \\
23\overline{)10{,}741} \\
-92 \\
\hline
154 \\
-138 \\
\hline
161 \\
-161 \\
\hline
0
\end{array}
$$

To check your work, multiply 23×467. The result is the original number, 10,741. The correct answer is 467.

3. (56) To simplify the expression $8 \times (4 + 3)$, use the order of operations. Following PEMDAS, first perform operations in parentheses: $4 + 3 = 7$. Next, multiply 8×7. The correct answer is 56.

4. (A) Perform the indicated addition, as follows:

$$
\begin{array}{r}
5{,}\ 6\ \ 1\ \ 4 \\
+\ \ \ 3\ \ 7\ \ 3 \\
\hline
5{,}\ 9\ \ 8\ \ 7
\end{array}
$$

The correct answer is 5,987.

5. (C) To simplify the expression $17 + 6^2 - (4 + 2)$, use the correct order of operations. Following PEMDAS, first perform all operations in parentheses:

$$17 + 6^2 - (4 + 2) = 17 + 6^2 - (6)$$

Next, simplify all exponents:

$$
\begin{aligned}
17 + 6^2 - (6) &= 17 + (6 \times 6) - (6) \\
&= 17 + (36) - (6)
\end{aligned}
$$

There is no multiplication or division to perform, so we move to the final step. Perform all addition and subtraction in order from left to right:

$$
\begin{aligned}
17 + (36) - (6) &= 17 + 36 - 6 \\
&= 53 - 6 \\
&= 47
\end{aligned}
$$

The correct answer is 47.

6. (D) Perform the indicated multiplication, as follows:

$$
\begin{array}{r}
3\ \ 2\ \ 4 \\
\times\ \ 3\ \ 7 \\
\hline
2{,}\ 2\ \ 6\ \ 8 \\
9{,}\ 7\ \ 2\ \ 0 \\
\hline
1\ 1{,}\ 9\ \ 8\ \ 8
\end{array}
$$

The correct answer is 11,988.

7. (B) Perform the indicated subtraction, as follows:

$$
\begin{array}{r}
{\scriptstyle 6\ \ \ 13} \\
4\ \ \not{7}\ \ \not{3} \\
-\ 6\ \ \ 7 \\
\hline
4\ \ 0\ \ 6
\end{array}
$$

To check your work, add $406 + 67$. The result is the original number, 473. The correct answer is 406.

8. (C) Perform the indicated long division, as follows:

$$
\begin{array}{r}
533 \\
25\overline{)13{,}325} \\
-125 \\
\hline
82 \\
-75 \\
\hline
75 \\
-75 \\
\hline
0
\end{array}
$$

To check your work, multiply 25×533. The result is the original number, 13,325. The correct answer is 533.

9. (C) To simplify the expression $3 \times 5^2 \div (9 - 4)$, use the order of operations. Following PEMDAS, first perform all operations in parentheses:

$$3 \times 5^2 \div (9 - 4) = 3 \times 5^2 \div (5)$$

Next, perform all operations involving exponents:

$$3 \times 5^2 + (5) = 3 \times 25 \div 5$$

Next, perform all multiplication and division in order from left to right:

$$
\begin{aligned}
3 \times 25 \div 5 &= 75 \div 5 \\
&= 15
\end{aligned}
$$

The correct answer is 15.

10. (C) Round the numbers as instructed. 267 rounded to the nearest 10 is 270. 49 rounded to the nearest 10 is 50. $270 \times 50 = 13{,}500$. Choice B is incorrect because the numbers were not rounded before they were multiplied. Choice D has the first term rounded to the hundreds' place. The correct answer is 13,500.

11. (A) To simplify the expression $2 + (4 - 5) \times (12 \div 3)$, use the order of operations. Following PEMDAS, we first perform all operations in parentheses:

$$2 + (4 - 5) \times (12 \div 3) = 2 + (-1) \times (4)$$

There are no exponents in this expression, so we move to the next step. Perform all multiplication and division in order from left to right:

$$2 + (-1) \times (4) = 2 + (-4)$$

Finally, perform all addition and subtraction in order from left to right:

$$2 + (-4) = -2$$

The correct answer is −2.

12. (B) To simplify the expression $3^2 \times 2 + 6 \times 4^2$, use the order of operations. There are no parentheses in this expression, so we skip to the next step—simplify all exponents:

$$3^2 \times 2 + 6 \times 4^2 = 9 \times 2 + 6 \times 16$$

Next, perform all multiplication and division in order from left to right:

$$9 \times 2 + 6 \times 16 = 18 + 96$$

Finally, perform all addition and subtraction in order from left to right:

$$18 + 96 = 114$$

The correct answer is 114.

13. (B) The best answer is B because the width of the bottles has been rounded and the question asks for an approximation. Choice C does not estimate. Choice A does not convert meters to centimeters. Choice D unnecessarily rounds the length of the board.

14. (12) To simplify the expression $5 \times (4 + 2) \div 10 + 9$, use the order of operations. Following PEMDAS, we first perform all operations in parentheses:

$$5 \times (4 + 2) \div 10 + 9 = 5 \times (6) \div 10 + 9$$

There are no exponents in this expression, so we move to the next step. Perform all multiplication and division in order from left to right:

$$5 \times 6 \div 10 + 9 = 30 \div 10 + 9$$
$$= 3 + 9$$

Finally, perform all addition and subtraction in order from left to right. The correct answer is $3 + 9$, or 12.

15. (B) To simplify the expression $2^3 \times 3 \div 24 + (1 - 4)$, use the order of operations. Following PEMDAS, we first perform all operations in parentheses:

$$2^3 \times 3 \div 24 + (1 - 4) = 2^3 \times 3 \div 24 + (-3)$$

Next, simplify all exponents:

$$2^3 \times 3 \div 24 + (-3) = 8 \times 3 \div 24 + (-3)$$

Next, perform all multiplication and division in order from left to right:

$$8 \times 3 \div 24 + (-3) = 24 \div 24 + (-3)$$
$$= 1 + (-3)$$

Finally, perform all addition and subtraction in order from left to right. The correct answer is $1 - 3$, or -2.

CHAPTER 14

Fractions

Fractions questions on the TEAS test your ability to add, subtract, multiply, and divide fractions. To perform these operations, you must understand how to convert fractions to different forms.

WORKING WITH FRACTIONS

Working with fractions requires knowledge of certain vocabulary. A fraction represents a part of a whole. **Proper fractions** consist of two numbers:

Proper Fraction

$$\frac{1}{2} \begin{array}{l} \longleftarrow \text{Numerator} \\ \longleftarrow \text{Denominator} \end{array}$$

The top number of the fraction is the **numerator**, and the bottom number is the **denominator**. In a proper fraction, the numerator is smaller than the denominator.

A fraction can also contain a numerator that is larger than the denominator. These fractions are called **improper fractions**.

Improper Fraction

$$\frac{4}{3} \begin{array}{l} \longleftarrow \text{Numerator} \\ \longleftarrow \text{Denominator} \end{array}$$

Improper fractions can be converted to a whole number plus a proper fraction. These combinations are called **mixed numbers**. The fraction above, for example, can be converted into 1 plus $\frac{1}{3}$. To write $\frac{4}{3}$ as a mixed number, we would write $1\frac{1}{3}$.

Proper Fraction	Improper Fraction	Mixed Number
$\frac{1}{2}$	$\frac{4}{3}$	$1\frac{1}{3}$

To perform math with fractions, we must first convert mixed numbers to improper fractions.

COMPARING FRACTIONS

When comparing fractions with the same denominator, we look at the numerator to determine which fraction is larger:

Which fraction is larger, $\frac{1}{3}$ or $\frac{2}{3}$?

In the example above, the fractions both have the same denominator, 3. When we compare the numerators, we see that $\frac{2}{3}$ is larger than $\frac{1}{3}$.

Comparing numerators works well if the fractions have the same denominator. If the fractions have different denominators, however, the comparison requires another step:

Which fraction is larger, $\frac{2}{3}$ or $\frac{5}{6}$?

In the example above, the fractions $\frac{2}{3}$ and $\frac{5}{6}$ have different denominators. To compare them, we must first change them both to fractions with the same denominator. For this, we look for the least common denominator of the two fractions.

The **least common denominator** of two fractions is the smallest number that can be divided equally by the denominators of both fractions. In this case, the number 6 is the least common denominator of the two fractions. We know this because 6 can be divided by 3 exactly 2 times, and 6 can be divided by 6 exactly 1 time. Convert both fractions to fractions over 6:

$$\frac{2}{3} = \frac{?}{6}$$

$$\frac{2}{3} \times \frac{2}{2} = \frac{4}{6}$$

Since we must multiply the denominator by 2 to produce 6, we also multiply the numerator by 2 to produce 4. The fraction $\frac{2}{3}$ is then converted to the fraction $\frac{4}{6}$. Now we can compare numerators and see that $\frac{5}{6}$ has the greatest value.

ADDITION

When adding fractions with the same denominator, simply add the numerators:

Simplify the expression: $\frac{1}{4} + \frac{2}{4}$.

The correct answer to this problem is $\frac{3}{4}$. We simply added the numerators, $1 + 2$, to produce 3.

When adding fractions with different denominators, first convert the fractions to fractions with the same denominator:

Simplify the expression: $\frac{3}{4} + \frac{5}{6}$.

In this case, we can't simply add the numerators because the denominators are different. To convert the fractions, we must find the least common denominator. The least common denominator is the smallest number that can be divided evenly by both 4 and 6. The number 6 won't work because 6 cannot be divided evenly by 4. The number 12 will work, however, because it can be divided evenly by both 6 and 4.

Convert both fractions to fractions with 12 as the denominator:

$$\frac{3}{4} = \frac{?}{12}$$

$$\frac{3}{4} \times \frac{3}{3} = \frac{9}{12}$$

The fraction $\frac{3}{4}$ converts to $\frac{9}{12}$. Next, convert the fraction $\frac{5}{6}$:

$$\frac{5}{6} = \frac{?}{12}$$

$$\frac{5}{6} \times \frac{2}{2} = \frac{10}{12}$$

The fraction $\frac{5}{6}$ converts to $\frac{10}{12}$. Now we can add the numerators:

$$\frac{9}{12} + \frac{10}{12} = \frac{19}{12}$$

The sum is an improper fraction, $\frac{19}{12}$. We can also convert this to a mixed number, $1\frac{7}{12}$.

SUBTRACTION

Subtraction of fractions works the same way as addition. When subtracting fractions with the same denominator, simply subtract the numerators:

Simplify the expression: $\dfrac{6}{8} - \dfrac{3}{8}$.

Here, the denominators are the same, so we subtract 6 − 3 to produce 3. The correct answer is $\dfrac{3}{8}$.

If the fractions have different denominators, we must convert the fractions to fractions over the same denominator:

Simplify the expression: $\dfrac{8}{12} - \dfrac{5}{8}$.

To convert the fractions, first find the least common denominator of $\dfrac{8}{12}$ and $\dfrac{5}{8}$. The least common denominator is 24. The number 24 is the smallest number that can be divided evenly by both 12 and 8. Convert both fractions to fractions over 24:

$$\frac{8}{12} = \frac{?}{24}$$

$$\frac{8}{12} \times \frac{2}{2} = \frac{16}{24}$$

The fraction $\dfrac{8}{12}$ converts to $\dfrac{16}{24}$. Next, convert the fraction $\dfrac{5}{8}$:

$$\frac{5}{8} = \frac{?}{24}$$

$$\frac{5}{8} \times \frac{3}{3} = \frac{15}{24}$$

The fraction $\dfrac{5}{8}$ converts to $\dfrac{15}{24}$. Now we can perform subtraction with the numerators:

$$\frac{16}{24} - \frac{15}{24} = \frac{1}{24}$$

The correct answer is $\dfrac{1}{24}$.

MULTIPLICATION

Multiplying fractions is relatively simple compared to adding and subtracting. This is because we don't have to convert the fractions, even if they have different denominators. To multiply fractions, multiply the numerator by the numerator and the denominator by the denominator, as follows:

Simplify the expression: $\frac{1}{6} \times \frac{3}{5}$.

These fractions have different denominators, but we can simply multiply them to get the result:

$$\frac{1}{6} \times \frac{3}{5} = \frac{1 \times 3}{6 \times 5}$$

$$= \frac{3}{30}$$

The fraction $\frac{3}{30}$ can be further reduced to the fraction $\frac{1}{10}$. This is the correct answer in its simplest form.

DIVISION

Dividing fractions is slightly more complicated than multiplying. To divide fractions, you turn first turn the division into multiplication, and then multiply as shown above. Here's an example:

Simplify the expression: $\frac{2}{8} \div \frac{3}{4}$.

When dividing fractions, you turn the divisor upside down and multiply it by the first fraction. The **divisor** is the fraction that the first fraction is being divided by:

$$\frac{2}{8} \div \boxed{\frac{3}{4}} \longleftarrow \text{Divisor}$$

In the following example, the divisor is $\frac{3}{4}$. Flip the divisor over and multiply the fractions:

$$\frac{2}{8} \div \frac{3}{4} = \frac{2}{8} \times \frac{4}{3}$$

$$= \frac{2 \times 4}{8 \times 3}$$

$$= \frac{8}{24}$$

The correct answer is $\dfrac{8}{24}$. This can be further reduced to $\dfrac{1}{3}$. The fraction $\dfrac{1}{3}$ is the correct answer in its simplest form.

FRACTION SUMMARY

Here's a summary of the most important steps you need to know:

Addition   Convert to fractions with the same denominator.

Add the numerators.

$$\frac{3}{4} + \frac{5}{6} = \frac{9}{12} + \frac{10}{12}$$

$$= \frac{19}{12} \text{ or } 1\frac{7}{12}$$

Subtraction   Convert to fractions with the same denominator.

Subtract the numerators.

$$\frac{8}{12} - \frac{5}{8} = \frac{16}{24} - \frac{15}{24}$$

$$= \frac{1}{24}$$

Multiplication   Multiply the numerators and denominators.

$$\frac{1}{6} \times \frac{3}{5} = \frac{1 \times 3}{6 \times 5}$$

$$= \frac{3}{30} \text{ or } \frac{1}{10}$$

Division   Flip the divisor over.

Perform multiplication.

$$\frac{2}{8} \div \frac{3}{4} = \frac{2}{8} \times \frac{4}{3}$$

$$= \frac{2 \times 4}{8 \times 3}$$

$$= \frac{8}{24} \text{ or } \frac{1}{3}$$

REVIEW QUESTIONS

1. $3\frac{1}{4} \times 2\frac{2}{3}$

Simplify the expression above. Which of the following is correct?

A) $8\frac{2}{3}$

B) $6\frac{1}{4}$

C) $6\frac{1}{6}$

D) $5\frac{2}{7}$

2. $\frac{2}{3} \div \frac{5}{9}$

Simplify the expression above. Which of the following is correct?

A) $\frac{10}{27}$

B) $\frac{7}{12}$

C) $1\frac{1}{5}$

D) $1\frac{2}{3}$

3. Put the following fractions in correct order, from least to greatest value.

$\frac{2}{3}, \frac{3}{4}, \frac{7}{12}, \frac{1}{6}$

4. $6\dfrac{1}{2} \times 3\dfrac{3}{8}$

Simplify the expression above. Which of the following is correct?

A) $18\dfrac{3}{16}$

B) $18\dfrac{3}{10}$

C) $20\dfrac{2}{5}$

D) $21\dfrac{15}{16}$

5. $\dfrac{6}{10} - \dfrac{1}{3}$

Simplify the expression above. Which of the following is correct?

A) $\dfrac{7}{30}$

B) $\dfrac{4}{15}$

C) $\dfrac{3}{10}$

D) $\dfrac{11}{12}$

6. $5\dfrac{1}{6} + 4\dfrac{7}{8}$

Simplify the expression above. Which of the following is correct?

A) $10\dfrac{1}{24}$

B) $10\dfrac{1}{48}$

C) $9\dfrac{1}{2}$

D) $9\dfrac{4}{7}$

7. $\dfrac{3}{8} - \dfrac{1}{4}$

Simplify the expression above. Which of the following is correct?

A) $\dfrac{3}{32}$

B) $\dfrac{1}{16}$

C) $\dfrac{1}{8}$

D) $\dfrac{1}{2}$

8. $\dfrac{6}{8} \div \dfrac{4}{10}$

Simplify the expression above. Which of the following is correct?

A) $1\dfrac{7}{8}$

B) $1\dfrac{15}{16}$

C) $2\dfrac{1}{4}$

D) $2\dfrac{3}{4}$

9. $5\dfrac{5}{6} \times 4\dfrac{2}{5}$

Simplify the expression above. Which of the following is correct?

A) $20\dfrac{1}{3}$

B) $20\dfrac{3}{10}$

C) $25\dfrac{1}{5}$

D) $25\dfrac{2}{3}$

10. $2\dfrac{1}{4} + 6\dfrac{5}{12}$

Simplify the expression above. Which of the following is correct?

A) $8\dfrac{3}{8}$

B) $8\dfrac{2}{3}$

C) $8\dfrac{11}{12}$

D) $8\dfrac{15}{16}$

11. Put the following fractions in correct order, from least to greatest value.

$6\dfrac{1}{6}, \ 4\dfrac{2}{3}, \ 2\dfrac{1}{3}, \ 4\dfrac{5}{6}$

12. $5\dfrac{1}{3} - 4\dfrac{1}{6}$

Simplify the expression above. Which of the following is correct?

A) $\dfrac{7}{12}$

B) $1\dfrac{1}{6}$

C) $1\dfrac{1}{3}$

D) $1\dfrac{2}{3}$

13. $\dfrac{4}{9} + \dfrac{7}{10}$

Simplify the expression above. Which of the following is correct?

A) $1\dfrac{13}{90}$

B) $1\dfrac{4}{9}$

C) $1\dfrac{7}{10}$

D) $1\dfrac{13}{16}$

14. $\dfrac{6}{8} \div \dfrac{3}{12}$

Simplify the expression above. Which of the following is correct?

A) $\dfrac{7}{24}$

B) 2

C) 3

D) $3\dfrac{1}{2}$

15. $\dfrac{7}{15} - \dfrac{1}{5}$

Simplify the expression above. Which of the following is correct?

A) $\dfrac{1}{15}$

B) $\dfrac{1}{5}$

C) $\dfrac{4}{15}$

D) $\dfrac{6}{15}$

ANSWER KEY

1. A	7. C	13. A
2. C	8. A	14. C
3. $\frac{1}{6}, \frac{7}{12}, \frac{2}{3}, \frac{3}{4}$	9. D	15. C
	10. B	
4. D		
5. B	11. $2\frac{1}{3}, 4\frac{2}{3}, 4\frac{5}{6}, 6\frac{1}{6}$	
6. A	12. B	

ANSWERS AND EXPLANATIONS

1. (A) Convert the mixed numbers to improper fractions, and then multiply:

$$3\frac{1}{4} \times 2\frac{2}{3} = \frac{13}{4} \times \frac{8}{3}$$

$$= \frac{104}{12}$$

$$= 8\frac{8}{12}$$

$$= 8\frac{2}{3}$$

2. (C) Flip the divisor over, and then multiply:

$$\frac{2}{3} \div \frac{5}{9} = \frac{2}{3} \times \frac{9}{5}$$

$$= \frac{18}{15}$$

$$= 1\frac{3}{15}$$

$$= 1\frac{1}{5}$$

3. When the fractions are all converted to fractions over 12, they can be written as follows: $\frac{8}{12}, \frac{9}{12}, \frac{7}{12}, \frac{2}{12}$. The correct order from smallest to largest is therefore $\frac{1}{6}, \frac{7}{12}, \frac{2}{3}, \frac{3}{4}$.

4. (D) Convert the mixed numbers to improper fractions, and then multiply:

$$6\frac{1}{2} \times 3\frac{3}{8} = \frac{13}{2} \times \frac{27}{8}$$

$$= \frac{351}{16}$$

$$= 21\frac{15}{16}$$

5. (B) Find the least common denominator of the two fractions. In this case, the least common denominator is 30. Convert both fractions so that they have the same denominator, and then perform subtraction on the numerators:

$$\frac{6}{10} - \frac{1}{3} = \frac{18}{30} - \frac{10}{30}$$

$$= \frac{8}{30}$$

$$= \frac{4}{15}$$

6. (A) Convert the mixed numbers to improper fractions. Convert both fractions so that they have the same denominator, and then add the numerators:

$$5\frac{1}{6} + 4\frac{7}{8} = \frac{31}{6} + \frac{39}{8}$$

$$= \frac{124}{24} + \frac{117}{24}$$

$$= \frac{241}{24}$$

$$= 10\frac{1}{24}$$

7. (C) Find the least common denominator of the two fractions. In this case, the least common denominator is 8. Convert both fractions so that they have the same denominator, and then perform subtraction on the numerators:

$$\frac{3}{8} - \frac{1}{4} = \frac{3}{8} - \frac{2}{8}$$

$$= \frac{1}{8}$$

8. (A) Flip the divisor over, and then multiply:

$$\frac{6}{8} \div \frac{4}{10} = \frac{6}{8} \times \frac{10}{4}$$

$$= \frac{60}{32}$$

$$= \frac{15}{8}$$

$$= 1\frac{7}{8}$$

9. (D) Convert the mixed numbers to improper fractions, and then multiply:

$$5\frac{5}{6} \times 4\frac{2}{5} = \frac{35}{6} \times \frac{22}{5}$$

$$= \frac{770}{30}$$

$$= 25\frac{20}{30}$$

$$= 25\frac{2}{3}$$

10. (B) Convert the mixed numbers to improper fractions. Convert both fractions so that they have the same denominator, and then add the numerators:

$$2\frac{1}{4} + 6\frac{5}{12} = \frac{9}{4} + \frac{77}{12}$$

$$= \frac{27}{12} + \frac{77}{12}$$

$$= \frac{104}{12}$$

$$= 8\frac{8}{12}$$

$$= 8\frac{2}{3}$$

11. These mixed numbers begin with the whole numbers 2, 4, and 6. The fraction $\frac{2}{3}$ can be converted to $\frac{4}{6}$. The fraction $\frac{4}{6}$ is smaller than the fraction $\frac{5}{6}$, so the correct order of the fractions is $2\frac{1}{3}, 4\frac{2}{3}, 4\frac{5}{6}, 6\frac{1}{6}$.

12. (B) Convert the mixed numbers to improper fractions. Convert both fractions so that they have the same denominator, and then perform subtraction on the numerators:

$$5\frac{1}{3} - 4\frac{1}{6} = \frac{16}{3} - \frac{25}{6}$$

$$= \frac{32}{6} - \frac{25}{6}$$

$$= \frac{7}{6}$$

$$= 1\frac{1}{6}$$

13. (A) Find the least common denominator of the fractions. In this case, the least common denominator is 90. Convert both fractions so that they have the same denominator, and then add the numerators:

$$\frac{4}{9} + \frac{7}{10} = \frac{40}{90} + \frac{63}{90}$$

$$= \frac{103}{90}$$

$$= 1\frac{13}{90}$$

14. (C) Flip the divisor over, and then multiply:

$$\frac{6}{8} \div \frac{3}{12} = \frac{6}{8} \times \frac{12}{3}$$

$$= \frac{72}{24}$$

$$= \frac{24}{8}$$

$$= 3$$

15. (C) Find the least common denominator of the two fractions. In this case, the least common denominator is 15. Convert both fractions so that they have the same denominator, and then perform subtraction on the numerators:

$$\frac{7}{15} - \frac{1}{5} = \frac{7}{15} - \frac{3}{15}$$

$$= \frac{4}{15}$$

CHAPTER 15

Decimals

Decimals questions on the TEAS test your ability to add, subtract, multiply, and divide decimals. You may also be asked to compare the values of decimal numbers.

WORKING WITH DECIMALS

A **decimal** is a number that expresses part of a whole. Decimals are similar to fractions, but instead of showing a numerator over a denominator, decimals show portions of a number using a decimal point.

Each number to the right or left of a decimal point has a certain place value. In the figure below, the numbers to the left of the decimal point are 3, 1, and 4. The number 3 is in the hundreds place, the number 1 is in the tens place, and the number 4 is in the ones place, as shown:

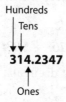

The numbers to the right of the decimal have specific place values as well. In the figure shown, the numbers to the right of the decimal are 2, 3, 4, and 7:

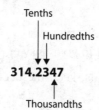

The number 2 is in the tenths place, the number 3 is in the hundredths place, the number 4 is in the thousandths place, and so on.

COMPARING DECIMALS

To compare decimals, look at the numbers in the same place value.

> Which of the following decimals is larger: 0.2 or 0.3?

In the example above, both of the decimals have numbers only in the tenths place. Since 3 is larger than 2, the decimal 0.3 is larger.

If decimal numbers contain more than one place value, look at the numbers in each place value to compare them. In the following example, both numbers have the number 2 in the tenths place:

Which of the following decimals is larger: 0.22 or 0.27?

When we look at the hundredths place, however, the numbers are different. In this case, 7 is larger than 2, so 0.27 is larger.

Here is one more example with longer decimals:

Which of the following decimals is larger: 0.22463 or 0.22419?

In this example, both of the numbers have 2 in the tenths place. Both also have 2 in the hundredths place and 4 in the thousandths place. In the ten thousandths place, however, the numbers are different. The first number has a 6 in the ten thousandths place, and the second number has a 1 in the ten thousandths place. The number 6 is greater than 1, so 0.22463 is larger.

ADDITION AND SUBTRACTION

To add and subtract decimals, perform addition and subtraction as you would with whole numbers. You must keep the decimal points of the two numbers lined up as you add.

Simplify the expression: 1.763 + 2.93.

Line the two numbers up by their decimals:

```
    1
    1 .7 6 3
  + 2 .9 3
  ─────────
    4 .6 9 3
```

Be sure to include the decimal in your answer. The correct answer is **4.693**.

When subtracting two decimals, keep the decimal points lined up as well. Here is an example:

Simplify the expression: 36.15 − 3.323.

To solve this problem, line up the decimal points as shown:

```
      5  11   4  10
  3  6̶  .1̶  5̶  0̶
  −    3  .3   2   3
  ──────────────────
  3  2  .8   2   7
```

In this case, we added a 0 to the right of the 5, so that we could subtract the 3 on the far right. Always be sure to add the decimal to your result. The correct answer is **32.827**.

MULTIPLICATION

To multiply decimals, perform multiplication as you would for whole numbers. Then count up the number of decimal places in the numbers being multiplied, and insert the decimal point correctly in your result.

Simplify the expression: 0.02×0.4.

In this case, multiply 2 times 4, which produces 8. Then count the number of decimal places in the numbers being multiplied. The decimal 0.02 has two decimal places to the right of the decimal, 0 and 2. The number 0.4 has one decimal place to the right of the decimal, 4. Added together, there are 3 decimal places in these two numbers. So the final answer must also have 3 decimal places. Starting with the number 8, count to the left 3 decimal places. Add zeros as you go:

0.008

This result has 3 decimal places. The correct answer is **0.008**.

DIVISION

To divide with decimals, perform division as you normally would, paying attention to the placement of decimals. The procedure is slightly different depending on whether you are dividing by a whole number or a decimal number.

If you are dividing by a whole number, be sure to put the decimal point directly above the number being divided. Consider this example:

Simplify the expression: $16.236 \div 18$.

Set up the long division problem and divide by 18:

$$
\begin{array}{r}
.902 \\
18{\overline{\smash{\big)}\,16.236}} \\
\underline{-162} \\
3 \\
\underline{-0} \\
36 \\
\underline{-36} \\
0
\end{array}
$$

The correct answer is **0.902**.

If you are dividing by a decimal number, change the divisor to a whole number first by moving the decimal to the right. Also be sure to move the decimal the same number of places on the number being divided as well:

Simplify the expression: $270.48 \div 9.2$.

To solve this problem, we must divide by a decimal number. Set up the long division problem:

$$9.2\overline{)\ 270.48}$$

Before going further, move the decimal points to the right one place. Do this for both numbers:

$$92\overline{)\ 2{,}704.8}$$

Now divide as normal. Keep the decimal point in your answer directly above the decimal point in the number 2,704.8:

$$
\begin{array}{r}
29.4 \\
92\overline{)\ 2{,}704.8} \\
-184 \\
\hline
864 \\
-828 \\
\hline
368 \\
-368 \\
\hline
0 \\
\end{array}
$$

The correct answer is **29.4**.

REVIEW QUESTIONS

1. 0.11×0.07

Simplify the expression above. Which of the following is correct?

A) 0.00077
B) 0.0077
C) 0.077
D) 0.77

2. $227.65 + 320.4$

Simplify the expression above. Which of the following is correct?

A) 230.85
B) 259.69
C) 547.69
D) 548.05

3. Which of the following lists the decimal numbers in correct order, from smallest to largest?

   A) 0.0007, 0.007, 0.07, 0.7
   B) 0.007, 0.7, 0.07, 0.0007
   C) 0.7, 0.07, 0.007, 0.0007
   D) 0.07, 0.0007, 0.007, 0.7

4. $3.20 \div 0.40$

Simplify the expression above. Which of the following is correct?

   A) 0.08
   B) 0.8
   C) 8
   D) 80

5. $12.92 - 7.6$

Simplify the expression above. Write your answer in the blank:

_____

6. 41.1×0.06

Simplify the expression above. Which of the following is correct?

   A) 0.2466
   B) 2.466
   C) 24.66
   D) 246.6

7. Put the following decimal numbers in correct order, from largest to smallest.

7.04, 6.97, 7.24, 7.54

8. $0.00393 + 0.0241$

Simplify the expression above. Which of the following is correct?

   A) 0.00634
   B) 0.02803
   C) 0.0634
   D) 0.2803

9. $72 \div 0.12$

Simplify the expression above. Which of the following is correct?

   A) 0.06
   B) 6
   C) 600
   D) 6,000

10. Which of the following lists the decimal numbers in correct order, from smallest to largest?

A) 0.0413, 0.0513, 0.0613, 0.0713
B) 0.0713, 0.0613, 0.0513, 0.0413
C) 0.0613, 0.0413, 0.0713, 0.0513
D) 0.0513, 0.0413, 0.0713, 0.0613

11. $0.045 - 0.0037$

Simplify the expression above. Which of the following is correct?

A) 0.0008
B) 0.0413
C) 0.0467
D) 0.054

12. $5.327 + 0.0229$

Simplify the expression above. Which of the following is correct?

A) 5.3499
B) 5.556
C) 5.762
D) 5.9476

13. $0.015 \div 0.3$

Simplify the expression above. Which of the following is correct?

A) 0.00005
B) 0.0005
C) 0.005
D) 0.05

14. $0.0602 - 0.001$

Simplify the expression above. Which of the following is correct?

A) 0.0502
B) 0.0592
C) 0.0601
D) 0.602

15. 0.25×0.075

Simplify the expression above. Which of the following is correct?

A) 0.001875
B) 0.01875
C) 0.1875
D) 1.875

ANSWER KEY

1. B	**6.** B	**11.** B
2. D	**7.** 7.54, 7.24, 7.04, 6.97	**12.** A
3. A	**8.** B	**13.** D
4. C	**9.** C	**14.** B
5. 5.32	**10.** A	**15.** B

ANSWERS AND EXPLANATIONS

1. (B) First, multiply 11 times 7 without the decimals:

$$11 \times 7 = 77$$

Now count the number of decimal places in the two numbers being multiplied. There are two decimal places in each number, for a total of four decimal places. The correct answer must also have four decimal places. Count back four decimal places from the right of 77, adding zeros if necessary, and insert a decimal. The correct answer is 0.0077.

2. (D) Add up the numbers, being sure to keep the decimal points aligned:

$$
\begin{array}{r}
1 \\
2\ 2\ 7\ .6\ 5 \\
+\ 3\ 2\ 0\ .4\ 0 \\
\hline
5\ 4\ 8\ .0\ 5 \\
\end{array}
$$

The correct answer is 548.05.

3. (A) In this set of numbers, the largest number is 0.7. It has a 7 in the tenths place, while the other numbers have zeros in the tenths place. The number 0.07 is the next largest number. It has a 7 in the hundredths place, while 0.007 and 0.0007 have zeros in the hundredths place.

The number 0.007 is larger than 0.0007, so choice A is correct.

4. (C) Set up the long division problem:

$$0.40\overline{)\ 3.20}$$

Move the decimal points two places to the right in both numbers:

$$40\overline{)\ 320}$$

Perform long division:

$$
\begin{array}{r}
8 \\
40\overline{)\ 320} \\
-320 \\
\hline
0 \\
\end{array}
$$

The correct answer is 8.

5. (5.32) Perform subtraction as you normally would, lining up the decimal points in the two numbers:

$$
\begin{array}{r}
\overset{12}{} \\
\not{1}\ \not{2}\ .9\ 2 \\
-\quad 7\ .6\ 0 \\
\hline
5\ .3\ 2
\end{array}
$$

The correct answer is 5.32.

6. (B) First, multiply 411 times 6 without the decimals:

$$411 \times 6 = 2{,}466$$

Now count the number of decimal places in the two numbers being multiplied. There is one decimal place in 41.1, and there are two decimal places in 0.06, which gives a total of three decimal places. The correct answer must also have three decimal places. Count back three decimal places from the right of 2,466, and insert a decimal. The correct answer is 2.466.

7. (7.54, 7.24, 7.04, 6.97) In this set of numbers, the largest number is 7.54. It has a 7 in the tens place and a 5 in the tenths place. The other numbers with 7 in the tens place have smaller numbers in the tenths place. The number 7.24 is the next largest number. It has a 2 in the tenths place, while 7.04 has a 0 in the tenths place. The number 6.97 is the smallest of the four numbers.

8. (B) Add up the numbers 0.00393 and 0.0241, being sure to keep the decimal points aligned:

$$
\begin{array}{r}
1 \\
0\ .0\ 0\ 3\ 9\ 3 \\
+\ 0\ .0\ 2\ 4\ 1\ 0 \\
\hline
0\ .0\ 2\ 8\ 0\ 3
\end{array}
$$

The correct answer is 0.02803.

9. (C) First, set up the problem:

$$0.12\overline{)\ 72}$$

Next, for both numbers, move the decimal points to the right two places. Add two zeros to the right of 72, to create 7,200:

$$12\overline{)\ 7{,}200}$$

Now divide as normal:

$$
\begin{array}{r}
600 \\
12\overline{)\ 7{,}200} \\
-7{,}200 \\
\hline
0
\end{array}
$$

The correct answer is 600.

10. (A) In this set of numbers, the only difference between the numbers is the number in the hundredths place. The numbers in the hundredths place are 4, 5, 6, and 7. So the decimals should be placed in that order: 0.0413, 0.0513, 0.0613, and 0.0713. Choice A is correct.

11. (B) Set up the subtraction problem, lining up the two numbers based on their decimal points as shown:

```
            4  10
   0 .0  4  5̶  0̶
 − 0 .0  0  3  7
   0 .0  4  1  3
```

The correct answer is 0.0413.

12. (A) Add up the numbers 5.327 and 0.0229. Be sure to line up the decimal points:

```
   5 .3  2  7  0
 + 0 .0  2  2  9
   5 .3  4  9  9
```

The correct answer is 5.3499.

13. (D) Set up the long division problem:

$$0.3\overline{)\,0.015}$$

Next, move the decimal points for both numbers one place to the right:

$$0.3\overline{)\,0.015}$$

Now divide as normal. Keep the decimal point in your answer directly above the decimal point in the number being divided:

```
       .05
  3) 00.15
     − 15
        0
```

The correct answer is 0.05.

14. (B) Align the two numbers based on their decimal points and subtract:

```
            5  10
   0 .0  6̶  0̶  2
 − 0 .0  0  1  0
   0 .0  5  9  2
```

The correct answer is 0.0592.

15. (B) Multiply 25 times 75 without the decimals:

$$25 \times 75 = 1,875$$

Next, count the number of decimal places in the two numbers being multiplied. There are two decimal places in 0.25 and three decimal places in 0.075, for a total of five decimal places. The correct answer must therefore also have five decimal places. Count back five decimal places from the right of 1,875, adding zeros if necessary, and insert a decimal. The correct answer is 0.01875.

CHAPTER 16

Percentages

Percentage questions on the TEAS test your ability to calculate percentages based on information given. You will also be asked to determine the percentage increase or decrease that is represented by a change in certain numbers. In addition, you may be asked to calculate original or final numbers when provided with information regarding a specific percentage change.

CALCULATING PERCENTAGES

A **percentage** is a portion of an amount. Any percentage can be expressed as a fraction over 100. Another way to write 20%, for instance, is $\frac{20}{100}$.

To take the percentage of a number, multiply that number by the percentage given. Let's look at an example:

What is 30% of 250?

To solve this problem, we must multiply 250 by 30%. To do this, first convert the percentage to a decimal number. Start with the percentage given, and move the decimal point to the left two places:

30% = 0.30

Now that we've converted the percentage to a decimal, we can multiply 250 by 0.30:

$250 \times 0.30 = 75.00$

The correct answer is **75**.

Percentages can be numbers less than 1, and they can also be numbers greater than 100. The process for solving problems with these percentages is the same. Here's an example involving a percentage less than 1:

What is 0.10% of 170?

Notice the question did not ask for 10% of 170; instead, it asked for 0.10%. It is important to be clear about this, because the decimal point will make a big difference in your answer.

Solve this problem the same way as shown in the first example in this section. First, convert the percentage to a decimal number. Start with the percentage given, and move the decimal point two places to the left:

.10% = 0.0010

In this case, we added two zeros to the left of the 1 in order to move the decimal point two places to the left.

Next, multiply 170 by 0.0010:

$$170 \times 0.0010 = 0.1700$$

The correct answer is **0.17**.

In the following example, we'll see a problem involving a percentage that is greater than 100:

What is 400% of 12?

Although this time the percentage is a large one, we still solve the problem as we did in the first two examples in this section. First, convert the percentage to a decimal number. Start with the percentage given (400%), and move the decimal point two places to the left:

$$400\% = 4.00$$

Now multiply 12 by 4:

$$12 \times 4 = 48$$

The correct answer is **48**.

PERCENTAGE INCREASE OR DECREASE

Another type of problem that is likely to appear on the TEAS involves the percent increase or decrease of a given quantity. Consider this example:

A sweater went on sale for 20% off its original price. The original price of the sweater was $40. What is the sale price?

To answer this question, first determine the amount of the discount. Then subtract the discount from the original price of the sweater.

The sweater originally cost $40 and went on sale for 20% off. Thus, the discount represents 20% of the original price. To calculate 20% of $40, we first convert 20% to a decimal number:

$$20\% = 0.20$$

Now we can multiply $40 by 0.20 to determine the amount of the discount:

$$\$40 \times 0.20 = \$8.00$$

The amount of the discount is $8.00. Next, subtract $8.00 from the original price:

$$\$40.00 - \$8.00 = \$32.00$$

The sale price of the sweater is **$32.00**.

In the example above, you were given the percent decrease and asked to find the amount of the decrease. Sometimes, you may be asked to do the opposite. You may be given the amount of the decrease (or increase) and asked to find the percentage it represents:

A store increases its sales from $5,000 to $6,000 in one month. What is the percent increase in sales?

To find the percent increase, first find the amount of the increase in sales. Subtract the original sales ($5,000) from the final amount ($6,000):

$6,000 − $5,000 = $1,000

The amount of the increase in sales is $1,000. Next, to find the percent increase, divide the amount of the increase by the original amount:

$$\text{percent increase} = \frac{\text{amount of increase}}{\text{original amount}}$$

In this case, the amount of increase is $1,000, and the original amount is $5,000. Plug these values into the formula:

$$\text{percent increase} = \frac{\text{amount of increase}}{\text{original amount}}$$
$$= \frac{\$1,000}{\$5,000}$$
$$= 0.20 \text{ or } 20\%$$

The percent increase turns out to be 0.20, which can be converted to 20%. To convert a decimal to a percentage, we move the decimal point to the right two places:

0.20 = 20%

The percent increase is **20%**.

REVIEW QUESTIONS

1. 304.9% of 23 = _____

Which of the following completes the equation above?

A) 70.127
B) 701.27
C) 7,012.7
D) 70,127

2. A car went on sale for 80% of its original price. If the sales price of the car was $20,000, which of the following was the car's original price?

A) $16,000
B) $25,000
C) $27,000
D) $32,000

3. A bookstore inventory increases from 120,000 to 170,000 books over one year. Which of the following is the percent increase of the books? (Round the solution to the nearest tenth of a percent.)

A) 29.4%
B) 33.2%
C) 41.4%
D) 41.7%

4. The number of patients seen at a medical clinic decreased from 460 to 375 in the month of January. Which of the following is the percent decrease to the nearest tenth of a percent?

A) 18.5%
B) 22.7%
C) 35.9%
D) 81.5%

5. 23.5% of 906 = _____

Which of the following completes the equation above?

A) 2.1291
B) 21.291
C) 212.91
D) 2,129.1

6. A plumber increased his hourly rate by 10%, which added a total of $8.00 to his rate. What was the plumber's original rate? Write your answer in the blank (you do not need to include the dollar sign):

_____

7. 33.2% of 17.4 = _____

Which of the following completes the equation above?

A) 0.0057768
B) 0.057768
C) 0.57768
D) 5.7768

8. Which of the following represents 32% of 1,700?

   A) 5.44
   B) 54.4
   C) 544
   D) 5,440

9. The temperature in a greenhouse increases from 77 degrees to 85 degrees overnight. Which of the following is the percent increase of the temperature? (Round the solution to the nearest tenth of a percent.)
   A) 8.1%
   B) 10.4%
   C) 16.3%
   D) 21.2%

10. The number of residents at an animal shelter went down from 179 to 127 over a six-month period. Which of the following is the percent decrease to the nearest tenth of a percent?

    A) 5.2%
    B) 13.6%
    C) 17.9%
    D) 29.1%

11. A school increased its student enrollment by 32% over a two-year period. At the beginning of the period, a total of 7,000 students were enrolled. How many students were enrolled at the school at the end of the two-year period?

    A) 9,240
    B) 10,060
    C) 10,350
    D) 11,480

12. 417.6% of 275 = _____

    Round to the nearest tenth and write your answer in the blank.

13. A flock of birds increases in size from 60 birds to 200. Which of the following is the percent increase of the birds? (Round the solution to the nearest tenth of a percent.)

    A) 367.7%
    B) 233.3%
    C) 140%
    D) 70%

14. Which of the following represents 0.5% of 32?

   A) 160
   B) 16
   C) 1.6
   D) 0.16

15. A television show's audience decreased by 26% in one week. The original size of the audience was 12.5 million viewers. What was the number of viewers after one week? (Round the solution to the nearest tenth of a percent.)

   A) 3.3 million
   B) 7.6 million
   C) 9.3 million
   D) 10.4 million

ANSWER KEY

1. A	**6.** 80.00	**11.** A
2. B	**7.** D	**12.** 1,148.4
3. D	**8.** C	**13.** B
4. A	**9.** B	**14.** D
5. C	**10.** D	**15.** C

ANSWERS AND EXPLANATIONS

1. (A) Change the percentage to a decimal number by moving the decimal to the left two places: 304.9% = 3.049. Then multiply 23 × 3.049. The correct answer is 70.127.

2. (B) This question asks you to find the original price of the car. We know that 80% of this price is $20,000. We can use this information to find the original price. First, change the percentage to a decimal number by moving the decimal to the left two places: 80% = 0.80. Next, use the formula for calculating percentage: original price × 0.80 = $20,000. Divide $20,000 by 0.80 to find the original price. The correct answer is $25,000.

3. (D) To find the percent increase, first find the amount of the increase in books. Subtract the original number of books from the final amount: 170,000 − 120,000 = 50,000. The amount of the increase in books is 50,000. Next, to find the percent increase, divide the amount of the increase by the original number of books: 50,000 ÷ 120,000 = 0.4167. The percent increase is 0.4167, which can be converted to 41.67% and rounded up to 41.7%.

4. (A) First, find the amount of the decrease in patients seen. Subtract the final number of patients from the original number: 460 − 375 = 85. The number of patients seen decreased by 85. Now divide the amount of the decrease by the original number of patients: 85 ÷ 460 is approximately 0.1848.

The percent decrease is about 0.1848, which can be converted to 18.48% and rounded up to 18.5%.

5. (C) Change the percentage to a decimal number by moving the decimal to the left two places: 23.5% = 0.235. Then multiply 906 × 0.235. The correct answer is 212.91.

6. (80.00) First, change the percentage to a decimal number by moving the decimal to the left two places: 10% = 0.10. Next, use the formula for calculating percentages: original rate × 0.10 = $8.00. Divide $8 by 0.10 to find the original rate. The correct answer is $80.00.

7. (D) Change the percentage to a decimal number by moving the decimal to the left two places: 33.2% = 0.332. Then multiply 17.4 × 0.332. The correct answer is 5.7768.

8. (C) Change the percentage to a decimal number by moving the decimal to the left two places: 32% = 0.32. Then multiply 1,700 × 0.32. The result is 544.

9. (B) To find the percent increase in temperature, first find the amount of the increase. Subtract the original temperature from the final temperature: 85 − 77 = 8. The temperature in the greenhouse increased by 8 degrees. Next, to find the percent increase, divide the amount of the increase by the original temperature: 8 ÷ 77 equals approximately 0.1039. The percent increase is about 0.1039, which can be converted to 10.39% and rounded up to 10.4%.

10. (D) First, find the amount of the decrease in residents at the shelter. Subtract the final number of animals from the original number: 179 − 127 = 52. The number of animals decreased by 52. Now divide the amount of the decrease by the original number of animals: 52 ÷ 179 is approximately 0.2905. The percent decrease is about 0.2905, which can be converted to 29.05% and rounded up to 29.1%.

11. (A) First, determine the amount of the increase. Then add the increased amount to the original number of enrolled students. At the beginning of the period, a total of 7,000 students were enrolled. In two years, the enrollment increased by 32%. To calculate 32% of 7,000, first convert 32% to a decimal number: 32% = 0.32. Then multiply 7,000 by 0.32 to determine the amount of the increase: 7,000 × 0.32 = 2,240. The enrollment increased by 2,240 students. Next, add 2,240 to the original number of enrolled students: 7,000 + 2,240 = 9,240. At the end of the two-year period, the number of enrolled students was 9,240.

12. (1,148.4) Change the percentage to a decimal number by moving the decimal to the left two places: 417.6% = 4.176. Then multiply 275 × 4.176. The correct answer is 1,148.4.

13. (B) First, find the amount of the increase. Subtract the original number of birds from the final number: 200 − 60 = 140. The flock increased by 140 birds. Now divide the amount of the increase by the original number of birds: 140 ÷ 60 equals approximately 2.3334. The percent increase is about 2.3334, which can be converted to 233.34% and rounded down to 233.3%.

14. (D) The question is asking for 0.5% of 32, not 5%. Starting with the percentage of 0.5, move the decimal to the left two places: 0.5% = 0.005. In this case, you must add two zeros before the 5 to move the decimal point two places to the left. Now multiply 32 × 0.005. The result is 0.16.

15. (C) First, determine the amount of the decrease. Then subtract the decreased amount from the original number of viewers. The original size of the audience was 12.5 million viewers. In one week, the audience decreased by 26%. To calculate 26% of 12.5 million, first convert 26% to a decimal number: 26% = 0.26. Then multiply 12.5 million by 0.26 to determine the amount of the decrease: 12.5 million × 0.26 = 3.25 million. The audience decreased by 3.25 million viewers. Next, subtract 3.25 million from the original size of the audience: 12.5 million − 3.25 million = 9.25 million. After one week, the number of viewers was about 9.3 million.

CHAPTER 17

Converting Fractions, Decimals, and Percentages

Conversion questions on the TEAS ask you to recognize equivalent values in different forms. You may be asked to convert between decimals and percentages, fractions and decimals, fractions and percentages, and vice versa.

DECIMALS AND PERCENTAGES

In the preceding chapter, we have seen how to convert between decimals and percentages and vice versa. To convert a percentage to a decimal, move the decimal point to the left two places.

$$41.7\% = 0.417$$

To convert a decimal to a percentage, move the decimal point to the right two places.

$$0.0635 = 6.35\%$$

FRACTIONS AND DECIMALS

To convert a fraction to a decimal, divide the numerator of the fraction by the denominator:

$$\frac{5}{20} = 0.25$$

To convert a decimal to a fraction, remove the decimal point and use the remaining number as the numerator of the fraction. Here is an example:

What fraction is equivalent to 0.36?

Start by removing the decimal point and placing the number 36 in the numerator of the fraction:

$$0.36 = \frac{36}{\text{denominator}}$$

Use the following method to determine the denominator. Start with the number 1 and add a zero for every decimal place in the original number. In this case, 0.36 has two decimal places, so we start with 1 and add two zeros:

$$0.36 = \frac{36}{100}$$

Next, simplify the fraction. The fraction $\frac{36}{100}$ reduces to $\frac{9}{25}$.

FRACTIONS AND PERCENTAGES

To convert a fraction to a percentage, first convert the fraction to a decimal number. Then move the decimal to the left two places:

What percentage is equivalent to $\frac{2}{5}$?

Divide the numerator of the fraction by the denominator:

$$\frac{2}{5} = 0.40$$

Then move the decimal two places to the right:

$$0.40 = 40\%$$

The correct answer is **40%**.

To convert a percentage to a fraction, first convert the percentage to a decimal number. Then convert the decimal number to a fraction:

What fraction is equivalent to 80%?

Move the decimal to the left two places:

$$80\% = 0.80$$

Then follow the steps to convert a decimal to a fraction. Place the number in the numerator of the fraction, without the decimal:

$$0.80 = \frac{80}{\text{denominator}}$$

For the denominator, start with the number 1. Then add a zero for every decimal place in the original number. The decimal 0.80 has two decimal places, so we add two zeros:

$$0.80 = \frac{80}{100}$$

This fraction simplifies to $\frac{8}{10}$, which further reduces to $\frac{4}{5}$. The correct answer is $\frac{4}{5}$.

CONVERSION CHART

Some conversions are so common that it would be worth your time to memorize them. If you can convert easily among 20%, 0.2, and $\frac{1}{5}$, for example, it will save you valuable time on the actual exam. Here is a chart with the most common conversions, some of which you probably already know:

Fraction	Decimal	Percent
1/2	0.5	50%
1/3	0.333…	33.333…%
2/3	0.666…	66.666…%
1/4	0.25	25%
3/4	0.75	75%
1/5	0.2	20%
1/6	0.1666…	16.666…%
1/8	0.125	12.5%
3/8	0.375	37.5%
5/8	0.625	62.5%
1/10	0.1	10%
1/12	0.08333…	8.333…%
1/16	0.0625	6.25%
1/32	0.03125	3.125%

Knowing these conversions can also help you quickly figure out others. For example, if you know $\frac{1}{5} = 20\%$, then you can easily figure out that $\frac{2}{5}$ will be double that, or 40%. You can also increase that to $\frac{3}{5} = 60\%$, and $\frac{4}{5} = 80\%$.

WORD PROBLEMS

You may also encounter word problems that require you to convert among fractions, decimals, and percentages. The hardest part about these is figuring out which calculations to do, so read the questions slowly and carefully.

Dr. Li wants to reduce a patient's medication by 30%. The current dose is 25 mg. What will the new dose be?

First, let's make sure we understand what the question is asking. We need to find 30% of 25 mg and then subtract that amount from 25 mg to find the new dose.

Calculate the reduction. Find 30% of 25. We can do that either by converting the percent to a fraction or to a decimal.

$$\frac{30}{100} \times \frac{25}{1} = \frac{3}{10} \times \frac{25}{1} = \frac{75}{10} = 7.5$$

or $0.3 \times 25 = 7.5$

The reduction is 7.5 mg. Now subtract the amount of the reduction from the original 25 mg amount.

$$25 - 7.5 = 17.5$$

The new dose is 17.5 mg.

There is another way to do this type of question that is a bit faster. Remember that percents are out of 100. A reduction of 30% is 100% − 30%, which is 70%. A reduction of 30% from the original 100% means we are using 70% of the original amount. To find the reduced amount, we could just find 70% of 25 mg and not have to subtract anything.

$$0.7 \times 25 = 17.5$$

REVIEW QUESTIONS

1. $-7, -\dfrac{17}{3}, -7.2, -\dfrac{43}{6}$

   Arrange the numbers above from least to greatest. Which of the following is correct?

   A) $-7, -\dfrac{43}{6}, -7.2, -\dfrac{17}{3}$

   B) $-7.2, -7, -\dfrac{43}{6}, -\dfrac{17}{3}$

   C) $-7.2, -\dfrac{43}{6}, -7, -\dfrac{17}{3}$

   D) $-\dfrac{43}{6}, -7, -\dfrac{17}{3}, -7.2$

2. Which of the following is equivalent to 60%?

A) $\dfrac{3}{5}$

B) $\dfrac{2}{3}$

C) $\dfrac{5}{6}$

D) $\dfrac{7}{8}$

3. Which of the following percentages is equivalent to 0.017?

A) 0.17%
B) 1.7%
C) 17%
D) 170%

4. Which of the following is the decimal equivalent of $\dfrac{3}{8}$?

A) 0.375
B) 2.667
C) 5
D) 11

5. Sarah correctly answered 83 out of 90 questions on a test. What percent of the questions did she answer correctly?

A) 83%
B) 90%
C) 92%
D) 93%

6. Order the following list of numbers from least to greatest.

$5, \dfrac{9}{2}, -1, 4.1$

7. Rashid tossed a coin 12 times, and 9 times the result was heads. Which of the following is the decimal equivalent of the fraction of tosses that were heads?

A) 0.60
B) 0.75
C) 1.333
D) 3

8. Which of the following is the decimal equivalent of 834%?

A) 0.0834
B) 0.834
C) 8.34
D) 83.4

9. Which of the following percentages is equivalent to 7.237?

   A) 0.07237%
   B) 0.7237%
   C) 72.37%
   D) 723.7%

10. A cleaning solution is 30% bleach. How many ounces of bleach will need to be used to fill a 48-oz bottle of cleaning solution?

   A) 14.4 oz
   B) 19.2 oz
   C) 20 oz
   D) 33.6 oz

ANSWER KEY

1. C
2. A
3. B
4. A

5. C
6. $-1, 4.1, \frac{9}{2}, 5$
7. B

8. C
9. D
10. A

ANSWERS AND EXPLANATIONS

1. (C) Convert the fractions to decimals. The fraction $-\frac{17}{3}$ is equivalent to $-17 \div 3$, or approximately -5.667. The fraction $-\frac{43}{6}$ is equivalent to $-43 \div 6$, or approximately -7.167. The correct answer is $-7.2, -\frac{43}{6}, -7, -\frac{17}{3}$.

2. (A) To convert a percentage to a fraction, first convert the percentage to a decimal number. Move the decimal to the left two places: $60\% = 0.60$. Next, convert the decimal number to a fraction. Place the number in the numerator of the fraction, without the decimal:

$$0.60 = \frac{60}{\text{denominator}}$$

For the denominator, start with the number 1 and add a zero for every decimal place in the original number:

$$0.60 = \frac{60}{100}$$

The fraction $\frac{60}{100}$ reduces to $\frac{3}{5}$.

3. (B) To convert a decimal to a percentage, move the decimal point to the right two places: $0.017 = 1.7\%$.

4. (A) To convert a fraction to a decimal number, divide the numerator of the fraction by the denominator: $\dfrac{3}{8} = 0.375$.

5. (C) First, write Sarah's score as a fraction: 83 points out of 90 can be written as $\dfrac{83}{90}$. Now divide the numerator of the fraction by the denominator: $83 \div 90$ equals approximately 0.922. Convert that to a percentage by moving the decimal two places to the right to get 92%.

6. Convert the fraction to a decimal number. The fraction $\dfrac{9}{2}$ is equivalent to 4.5. The numbers, in order from least to greatest, are -1, 4.1, $\dfrac{9}{2}$, and 5.

7. (B) Write the number of heads as a fraction of all the coin tosses: 9 heads out of 12 throws can be written as $\dfrac{9}{12}$. This fraction reduces to $\dfrac{3}{4}$. Now divide the numerator of the reduced fraction by the denominator: $3 \div 4 = 0.75$.

8. (C) To convert a percentage to a decimal, move the decimal point to the left two places: $834\% = 8.34$.

9. (D) To convert a decimal to a percentage, move the decimal point to the right two places: $7.237 = 723.7\%$.

10. (A) As a fraction: $\dfrac{30}{100} \times 48 = \dfrac{3}{10} \times 48 = \dfrac{144}{10} = 14.4$. As a decimal: $0.3 \times 48 = 14.4$.

CHAPTER 18

Ratios and Proportions

Ratios and proportions questions test your ability to identify ratios and to use proportions to solve problems regarding ratios.

Ratios are a means of comparing numbers. They express the relationship of one number to another. Let's look at an example:

Adrian received 4 toys and 6 pieces of clothing for his birthday. What is the ratio of toys to pieces of clothing that Adrian received?

The ratio of toys to clothing can be expressed as 4 to 6. It can also be written as 4:6, using a colon, or as $\frac{4}{6}$ in fractional form.

To solve problems regarding ratios, we use proportions. **Proportions** are equations in which two ratios are set equal to each other.

Brianna buys 4 pizzas for a total cost of $25.00. How much does it cost her to buy 6 more pizzas if she buys them at the same price per pizza?

To solve this problem, we set up a proportion. Create two ratios and set them equal to each other:

$$\frac{4 \text{ pizzas}}{\$25} = \frac{6 \text{ pizzas}}{c}$$

We are looking for the cost, c, of the 6 pizzas. Cross multiply $4 \times c$ and $\$25 \times 6$. Set the values equal to one another:

$$\frac{4 \text{ pizzas}}{\$25} = \frac{6 \text{ pizzas}}{c}$$
$$4 \times c = \$25 \times 6$$
$$4c = \$25 \times 6$$

Now solve for c:

$$4c = \$25 \times 6$$
$$4c = \$150$$
$$c = \frac{\$150}{4}$$
$$c = \$37.50$$

It will cost $37.50 to buy 6 pizzas at the same rate. We will discuss more about solving equations in the Algebra chapter.

RATE OF CHANGE

Rate of change describes how one quantity changes in relation to another. Think of it like finding the slope of a line between two points.

$$\text{slope} = \frac{y_2 - y_1}{x_2 - x_1}$$

For example, let's find the rate of change in bank deposits over a six-month period. The starting balance is $500 and the ending balance is $1,700. Those will be your y-coordinates. The x-coordinates are the months 0 to 6. Your equation will be

$$\text{Rate of change} = \frac{1,700 - 500}{6 - 0} = \frac{1,200}{6} = 200$$

This tells you that the average deposit each month was $200.

REVIEW QUESTIONS

1. A sleepaway camp had 120 campers last year divided evenly into 8 squads. This year, the number of campers will rise to 165. If each squad has the same number of students as last year, how many squads will the camp have this year?

   A) 8
   B) 10
   C) 11
   D) 15

2. Jenna reads 360 pages in 180 minutes. How many pages can she read in 30 minutes if she reads at the same rate of speed? Write your answer in the blank: _____

3. A model of a skyscraper is built according to a 1:2,000 scale. If the model skyscraper measures 30 centimeters in height, which of the following is the actual height of the skyscraper?

   A) 6,000 centimeters
   B) 15,000 centimeters
   C) 60,000 centimeters
   D) 66,667 centimeters

4. The Doll Collector's Store has an inventory of 420 dolls. A total of 70 dolls are made of porcelain, and the remainder are made of plastic. Which of the following is the ratio of the plastic dolls to the total number of dolls in the store's inventory?

A) $\dfrac{1}{6}$

B) $\dfrac{3}{8}$

C) $\dfrac{5}{6}$

D) $\dfrac{7}{8}$

5. The scale on a trail map indicates that 1 centimeter on the map represents 10 miles. Lilah walks a distance of 12 miles on the trail. Which of the following represents the measure of that distance on the map?

A) 0.6 centimeters
B) 1.2 centimeters
C) 6.4 centimeters
D) 12 centimeters

6. Geraldo has 180 marbles. Of these, 120 are solid colors, and the rest are multicolored. Which of the following is the ratio of the multicolored marbles to the total number of marbles in Geraldo's collection?

A) $\dfrac{1}{3}$

B) $\dfrac{1}{2}$

C) $\dfrac{2}{3}$

D) $\dfrac{4}{5}$

7. The families on a neighborhood block have 14 dogs and 20 cats altogether. What is the ratio of dogs to cats on the block?

A) $\dfrac{7}{17}$

B) $\dfrac{10}{17}$

C) $\dfrac{7}{10}$

D) $\dfrac{10}{7}$

8. A replica of a radio tower is built based on a 1:300 scale. If the replica measures 9 inches in diameter across its base, which of the following is the diameter of the base of the radio tower?

A) 1,200 inches
B) 1,500 inches
C) 1,800 inches
D) 2,700 inches

9. An interior designer brings 16 textured fabric samples and 18 smooth fabric samples to a job site. What is the ratio of textured to smooth fabric samples that she brings?

A) $\dfrac{8}{9}$

B) $\dfrac{15}{16}$

C) $\dfrac{17}{18}$

D) $\dfrac{5}{4}$

10. A map contains a scale showing that every 1 inch on the map represents 12 kilometers. A cyclist wishes to travel a distance measuring 4 inches on the map. Which of the following represents the distance the cyclist will travel in kilometers?

A) 3.0
B) 4.8
C) 30
D) 48

11. Two hours into his hike, Isaac was at an altitude of 300 feet. Six hours into the hike, he was at an altitude of 900 feet. What is the average rate of change?

A) 900
B) 600
C) 300
D) 150

12. Find the rate of change in miles between Tuesday and Thursday using the chart below.

Day	Miles Walked
Monday	2.3
Tuesday	2.8
Wednesday	1.9
Thursday	4.6
Friday	3.1

A) −0.2
B) 1.8
C) 0.9
D) 0.6

ANSWER KEY

1. C   **5.** B   **9.** A
2. 60   **6.** A   **10.** D
3. C   **7.** C   **11.** D
4. C   **8.** D   **12.** C

ANSWERS AND EXPLANATIONS

1. (C) Create a proportion using two ratios. The first ratio is the number of campers to squads last year: $\dfrac{120 \text{ campers}}{8 \text{ squads}}$. The second ratio is the number of campers to squads this year: $\dfrac{165 \text{ campers}}{? \text{ squads}}$. Set the ratios equal to each other:

$$\frac{120 \text{ campers}}{8 \text{ squads}} = \frac{165 \text{ campers}}{? \text{ squads}}$$

Use the letter s to represent the missing number of squads:

$$\frac{120 \text{ campers}}{8 \text{ squads}} = \frac{165 \text{ campers}}{s}$$

Cross multiply to solve for s, the missing number of squads:

$$\frac{120}{8} = \frac{165}{s}$$

$$120s = 165 \times 8$$

$$120s = 1{,}320$$

$$s = \frac{1{,}320}{120}$$

$$s = 11$$

This year, the camp will have 11 squads.

2. (60) Create a proportion using two ratios. The first ratio is the number of pages read in 180 minutes: $\dfrac{360 \text{ pages}}{180 \text{ minutes}}$. The second ratio is the number of pages read in 30 minutes: $\dfrac{? \text{ pages}}{30 \text{ minutes}}$. Set the ratios equal to each other:

$$\frac{360 \text{ pages}}{180 \text{ minutes}} = \frac{? \text{ pages}}{30 \text{ minutes}}$$

Use the letter p to represent the missing number of pages:

$$\frac{360 \text{ pages}}{180 \text{ minutes}} = \frac{p}{30 \text{ minutes}}$$

Cross multiply to solve for p:

$$\frac{360}{180} = \frac{p}{30}$$

$$180p = 360 \times 30$$

$$180p = 10{,}800$$

$$p = \frac{10{,}800}{180}$$

$$p = 60$$

Jenna can read 60 pages in 30 minutes.

3. (C) Create a proportion, setting the two ratios equal to each other:

$$\frac{1}{2{,}000} = \frac{30 \text{ centimeters}}{\text{actual height}}$$

Cross multiply to solve for *h,* the actual height:

$$\frac{1}{2,000} = \frac{30 \text{ centimeters}}{h}$$

$$1h = 2,000 \times 30$$

$$h = 60,000$$

The actual height of the skyscraper is 60,000 centimeters.

4. (C) The store has 420 dolls total. The number of porcelain dolls is 70. Subtract 70 from the total to find the number of plastic dolls: $420 - 70 = 350$. The ratio of plastic dolls to the total dolls is $\frac{350}{420}$, which reduces to $\frac{5}{6}$.

5. (B) Create a proportion, setting the two ratios equal to each other:

$$\frac{1 \text{ centimeter}}{10 \text{ miles}} = \frac{? \text{ centimeters}}{12 \text{ miles}}$$

Cross multiply to solve for *c,* the missing number of centimeters:

$$\frac{1}{10} = \frac{c}{12}$$

$$10c = 1 \times 12$$

$$10c = 12$$

$$c = \frac{12}{10}$$

$$c = 1.2$$

The measure of the distance on the map is 1.2 centimeters.

6. (A) Geraldo has 180 marbles total. The number of solid colored marbles is 120. Subtract 120 from the total to find the number of multicolored marbles: $180 - 120 = 60$. The ratio of multicolored marbles to the total number of marbles is $\frac{60}{180}$, which reduces to $\frac{1}{3}$.

7. (C) The ratio of dogs to cats on the block is $\frac{14}{20}$, which reduces to $\frac{7}{10}$.

8. (D) Create a proportion, setting the two ratios equal to each other:

$$\frac{1}{300} = \frac{9}{\text{diameter}}$$

Cross multiply to solve for d, the missing length of the diameter:

$$\frac{1}{300} = \frac{9}{d}$$
$$1d = 9 \times 300$$
$$d = 2,700$$

The measure of the diameter of the base is 2,700 inches.

9. (A) The ratio of textured fabrics to smooth fabrics is $\frac{16}{18}$, which reduces to $\frac{8}{9}$.

10. (D) Create a proportion, setting the two ratios equal to each other:

$$\frac{1 \text{ inch}}{12 \text{ kilometers}} = \frac{4 \text{ inches}}{? \text{ kilometers}}$$

Cross multiply to solve for k, the missing number of kilometers:

$$\frac{1}{12} = \frac{4}{k}$$
$$1k = 12 \times 4$$
$$k = 48$$

The cyclist will travel 48 kilometers.

11. (D) Set up the slope formula. The y-values are the altitudes, and the x-values are the hours.

$$\frac{900 - 300}{6 - 2} = \frac{600}{4} = 150$$

12. (C) Set up the slope formula. The y-values are the miles walked on Tuesday and Thursday, and the x-values are the days (let Tuesday = day 0 and Thursday = day 2).

$$\frac{4.6 - 2.8}{2 - 0} = \frac{1.8}{2} = 0.9$$

CHAPTER 19

Algebra

Algebra questions on the TEAS test your ability to simplify expressions and to solve equations containing unknown quantities. You may also be asked to solve inequalities and absolute value equations or inequalities.

SIMPLIFYING EXPRESSIONS

To simplify algebraic expressions, we must combine like terms. **Like terms** in algebra are terms that contain the same variables raised to the same power (or no variables at all):

Simplify the expression: $(x^2 + 2x + 1) + (2x^2 + x + 4)$.

To simplify this expression, combine like terms. In this expression, x^2 and $2x^2$ are like terms. They both contain the variable x raised to the second power (x^2). The terms $2x$ and x are also like terms. They both contain the variable x, with no exponent.

Finally, the terms 1 and 4 are like terms. They contain no variables at all. Combine the three sets of like terms. It may be helpful to put the like terms next to each other in the equation:

$$(x^2 + 2x + 1) + (2x^2 + x + 4) = x^2 + 2x^2 + 2x + x + 1 + 4$$

$$= (x^2 + 2x^2) + (2x + x) + (1 + 4)$$

$$= 3x^2 + 3x + 5$$

The simplified expression is $\mathbf{3x^2 + 3x + 5}$.

FOIL

Some expressions require you to multiply two binomials. **Binomials** contain exactly two terms, such as $x + 3$ or $2x + 5$:

Simplify the expression: $(x + 3)(2x + 5)$.

Here you are being asked to multiply the binomial $x + 3$ by the binomial $2x + 5$. To perform this multiplication, we use a process known as FOIL. The letters in **FOIL** stand for First, Outer, Inner, and Last. This tells you the order of terms to multiply in the two binomials.

First, multiply the first two terms of each binomial:

First: $x \times 2x = 2x^2$

Then multiply the outer two terms:

Outer: $x \times 5 = 5x$

Then multiply the inner two terms:

Inner: $3 \times 2x = 6x$

Then multiply the last two terms:

Last: $3 \times 5 = 15$

Now add the results together:

$2x^2 + 5x + 6x + 15$

This expression can be further simplified to $\mathbf{2x^2 + 11x + 15}$.

SOLVING EQUATIONS

Algebra equations contain at least one unknown variable. This unknown variable is represented by a letter, such as x or y. The purpose of solving the equation is to find the value of the unknown variable.

To solve equations, we must isolate the variable on one side of the equation. Let's consider an example:

Solve the equation: $2x + 4 = 8$.

To solve this equation, we must isolate the variable x on one side of the equation. First, subtract the number 4 from both sides:

$$2x + 4 = 8$$
$$2x + 4 - 4 = 8 - 4$$
$$2x + 0 = 4$$
$$2x = 4$$

Subtracting 4 from both sides leaves only the term $2x$ on the left side of the equation. Now divide both sides by 2 to isolate the variable x:

$$2x = 4$$
$$\frac{2x}{2} = \frac{4}{2}$$
$$x = 2$$

The value of x is **2**.

SOLVING INEQUALITIES

In algebra, **inequalities** express relationships between quantities where one quantity is greater than or less than another. The symbols > and < are used to express "greater than" and "less than." A quantity may also be greater than or equal to another quantity. The symbol ≥ is used to represent "greater than or equal to," and the symbol ≤ represents "less than or equal to."

Inequality Symbols

>   greater than

<   less than

≥   greater than or equal to

≤   less than or equal to

Inequalities are solved in the same way as equations, with one exception. When multiplying or dividing both sides of an inequality by a negative number, you must reverse the direction of the inequality sign.

Solve the inequality: $-3x > 6$.

To solve this inequality, we must isolate x on one side of the equation. This means we must divide both sides of the inequality by -3. Therefore, we must reverse the direction of the inequality sign:

$$-3x > 6$$

$$\frac{-3x}{-3} < \frac{6}{-3}$$

$$x < -2$$

Notice that when we divide by -3, we change the direction of the inequality sign from greater than (>) to less than (<). The correct answer is **$x < -2$**.

ABSOLUTE VALUE EQUATIONS

Absolute value equations may also appear on TEAS Math. The **absolute value** of a number is the distance that number lies from zero on a number line. Absolute value is indicated by two vertical bars, as shown:

$$\left| x \right| = 5$$

If the absolute value of x equals 5, then x must lie exactly 5 units away from zero on the number line. The value of x could be positive (5) or it could be negative (-5). Both 5 and -5 lie exactly 5 units away from zero on the number line. So the value of x is 5 or -5. Here is another example:

Solve the equation: $\left| x - 1 \right| = 6$.

In this equation, the absolute value of $x - 1$ is 6. This tells us that the quantity $x - 1$ lies exactly 6 units away from zero on the number line. So $x - 1$ could equal 6 or -6. Set up two equations and solve for both possibilities:

$$x - 1 = 6 \qquad\qquad x - 1 = -6$$
$$x - 1 + 1 = 6 + 1 \qquad x - 1 + 1 = -6 + 1$$
$$x = 7 \qquad\qquad\qquad x = -5$$

The value of x is 7 or -5. In set notation, this would be written as $\{7, -5\}$.

REVIEW QUESTIONS

1. $12 - \dfrac{x}{4} = 8$

Solve the equation above. Which of the following is correct?

A) $x = 6$
B) $x = 8$
C) $x = 12$
D) $x = 16$

2. $(3x + 2)(x + 1)$

Simplify the expression above. Which of the following is correct?

A) $4x + 2$
B) $3x^2 + 2$
C) $3x^2 + 5x + 2$
D) $3x^2 + 6x + 1$

3. $\left| x + 2 \right| > 4$

Solve the inequality above. Which of the following is correct?

A) $x > 2$ or $x < -6$
B) $x > 4$ or $x > -6$
C) $x > 6$
D) $x < 8$

4. Cassandra's height, x, is 3 inches greater than twice her brother's height, y.

Which of the following algebraic equations best represents the statement above?

A) $x = 3x + y$
B) $x = 2y + 3$
C) $y = 2x + 3$
D) $x = 3y + 2$

5. $4(x + 7) = 2(x + 15)$

Solve the equation above. What is the value of x? Write your answer in the blank: _____

6. $(2x^2 + 4x - 7) - (2x^2 + 3x - 4)$

Simplify the expression above. Which of the following is correct?

A) $2x + 8$
B) $x - 3$
C) $7x - 3$
D) $4x^2 + 1$

7. The value of x is 5 less than $\dfrac{3}{4}$ the value of y.

Which of the following algebraic expressions correctly represents the sentence above?

A) $x - 5 = \dfrac{3}{4}y$

B) $y = \dfrac{3}{4}x + 5$

C) $x = 5 - \dfrac{3}{4}y$

D) $x = \dfrac{3}{4}y - 5$

8. $-4x - 9 > 3$

Solve the inequality above. Which of the following is correct?

A) $x < -3$
B) $x > 2$
C) $x < 3$
D) $x > 4$

9. $(2x^2 - 3x + 7) + (3x^2 + 2x + 6)$

Simplify the expression above. Which of the following is correct?

A) $5x^2 - x + 13$
B) $5x^2 + 5x - 1$
C) $6x^2 + x + 13$
D) $6x^2 + 5x - 1$

10. $|9 - x| = 4$

Which of the following is the solution set for the equation above?

A) $\{5, -13\}$
B) $\{5, 13\}$
C) $\{-5, 13\}$
D) $\{-5, -13\}$

ANSWER KEY

1. D   **5.** 1   **9.** A
2. C   **6.** B   **10.** B
3. A   **7.** D
4. B   **8.** A

ANSWERS AND EXPLANATIONS

1. (D) Isolate the variable x on one side of the equation. First, subtract the number 12 from both sides:

$$12 - \frac{x}{4} = 8$$

$$-\frac{x}{4} = 8 - 12$$

$$-\frac{x}{4} = -4$$

Then, multiply both sides by -4 to isolate the variable x:

$$-\frac{x}{4} = -4$$

$$-4 \times \left(-\frac{x}{4}\right) = -4 \times -4$$

$$x = 16$$

The value of x is 16.

2. (C) Use the process of FOIL to multiply the binomials $(3x + 2)(x + 1)$. First, multiply the first two terms of each binomial:

First: $3x \times x = 3x^2$

Then multiply the outer two terms:

Outer: $3x \times 1 = 3x$

Then multiply the inner two terms:

Inner: $2 \times x = 2x$

Then multiply the last two terms:

Last: $2 \times 1 = 2$

Now add the results together:

$3x^2 + 3x + 2x + 2$

This expression can be further simplified to $3x^2 + 5x + 2$.

3. (A) In this inequality, the absolute value of $x + 2$ is greater than 4. This tells us that the quantity $x + 2$ lies more than 4 units away from zero on the number line. So the value of $x + 2$ could be greater than 4, or it could be less than −4. Set up two inequalities and solve for both possibilities:

$$x + 2 > 4 \qquad\qquad x + 2 < -4$$
$$x + 2 - 2 > 4 - 2 \qquad x + 2 - 2 < -4 - 2$$
$$x > 2 \qquad\qquad\qquad x < -6$$

The solution is $x > 2$ or $x < -6$.

4. (B) Start with Cassandra's height, x. Then set up an equation:

$$x = ?$$

Cassandra's brother's height is denoted by y. Cassandra's height is equal to 3 more than twice y, which can be written as $2y + 3$. Add this expression to the equation:

$$x = 2y + 3$$

5. (1) Isolate the variable x on one side of the equation. First, perform the multiplication on both sides of the equation:

$$4(x + 7) = 2(x + 15)$$
$$4x + 28 = 2x + 30$$

Then subtract 28 from both sides:

$$4x + 28 = 2x + 30$$
$$4x + 28 - 28 = 2x + 30 - 28$$
$$4x = 2x + 2$$

Next, subtract $2x$ from both sides:

$$4x = 2x + 2$$
$$4x - 2x = 2$$
$$2x = 2$$

Now divide both sides by 2 to isolate the variable x:

$$2x = 2$$

$$\frac{2x}{2} = \frac{2}{2}$$

$$x = 1$$

The value of x is 1.

6. (B) To simplify this expression, combine like terms:

$$
\begin{aligned}
(2x^2 + 4x - 7) - (2x^2 + 3x - 4) &= 2x^2 - 2x^2 + 4x - 3x - 7 - (-4) \\
&= (2x^2 - 2x^2) + (4x - 3x) - (7 + 4) \\
&= 0 + x - 3 \\
&= x - 3
\end{aligned}
$$

The simplified expression is $x - 3$.

7. (D) Start with the value of x, and set up an equation:

$$x = ?$$

The question tells us that x is 5 less than $\frac{3}{4}$ the value of y, which can be written as $\frac{3}{4}y - 5$. Add this expression into the equation:

$$x = \frac{3}{4}y - 5$$

8. (A) To solve this inequality, we must isolate x on one side of the equation. To do this, first add 9 to both sides of the equation:

$$-4x - 9 > 3$$

$$-4x - 9 + 9 > 3 + 9$$

$$-4x > 12$$

Next, divide both sides of the equation by -4:

$$-4x > 12$$

$$\frac{-4x}{-4} < \frac{12}{-4}$$

$$x < -3$$

Because we are dividing by a negative number, we must change the direction of the inequality sign. The correct answer is therefore $x < -3$.

9. (A) To simplify this expression, combine like terms: $(2x^2 - 3x + 7) + (3x^2 + 2x + 6)$

$$(2x^2 - 3x + 7) + (3x^2 + 2x + 6) = 2x^2 + 3x^2 - 3x + 2x + 7 + 6$$
$$= (2x^2 + 3x^2) - (3x + 2x) + (7 + 6)$$
$$= 5x^2 - x + 13$$

The simplified expression is $5x^2 - x + 13$.

10. (B) In this equation, the absolute value of $9 - x$ is 4. This tells us that the quantity $9 - x$ lies exactly 4 units away from zero on the number line. So $9 - x$ could equal 4 or −4. Set up two equations and solve for both possibilities:

$$9 - x = 4 \qquad\qquad 9 - x = -4$$
$$9 - 9 - x = 4 - 9 \qquad\qquad 9 - 9 - x = -4 - 9$$
$$-x = -5 \qquad\qquad -x = -13$$
$$x = 5 \qquad\qquad x = 13$$

The value of x is 5 or 13. In set notation, this is written as {5, 13}.

CHAPTER 20

Word Problems

WRITING EXPRESSIONS

An expression is simply a mathematical symbol or group of symbols that represent a value. These might be variables, operations, or numbers. Each of the following is an expression:

x
$3y$
$4x + 2$

You will need to be able to translate word problems into expressions to write equations that you can solve. Use variables to represent unknown quantities. For example, the phrases in the left column below can be written as the algebraic expressions on the right.

Twice a number	$2x$
Half of the boys	$\frac{1}{2}b$
Two less than the total	$t - 2$

WRITING EQUATIONS

An equation is multiple expressions combined with an equals sign. Each of the following is an equation:

$x = 234$
$x + 2y = 30$
$4x^2(3-y) = 49$

You will need to be able to translate word problems into equations to solve them. Use variables to represent unknown quantities. For example, the sentences in the left column below can be written as the algebraic equations on the right.

There are four times as many boys as girls.	$b = 4g$
She paid $143 for three shirts and two pairs of pants.	$3s + 2p = 143$
The square of a number is also twice the number.	$x^2 = 2x$

239

WRITING INEQUALITIES

An inequality is multiple expressions combined with an inequality symbol ($<$, $>$, $\leq$, or $\geq$). Each of the following is an inequality:

$x \geq 234$
$x + 2y < 30$
$4x^2(3-y) > 49$

You will need to be able to translate word problems into equations to solve them. Use variables to represent unknown quantities. For example, the sentences in the left column below can be written as the algebraic equations on the right.

There are more than four times as many boys as girls.	$b > 4g$
She paid less than $143 for three shirts and two pairs of pants.	$3s + 2p < 143$
The total must be no more than half of your allowance.	$t \leq \dfrac{1}{2}a$

SOLVING ALGEBRA WORD PROBLEMS

To solve algebra word problems, you must put all these skills together. Take your time and make sure you have written your equations or inequalities correctly. Be sure that you have used all the relevant information and identified any extraneous information that you do not need. Once you have solved your equation, reread the question to be sure you are answering the right question. For example, if you solved for x, don't get tricked by a question that asks for $2x$.

Try an example:

The square of a number increased by 3 is greater than 7. Which of the following could be the number?

A) -3
B) -2
C) 0
D) 2

The correct answer is **A**. Write the expressions to build the inequality: $x^2 + 3 > 7$. Now solve for x. Subtract 3 from both sides to get $x^2 > 4$. Take the square root of both sides to get $x > 2$ or $x < -2$ since x could be negative as well. The only answer choice that fits this is A. Be sure to check your work: $(-3)^2 + 3 > 7$ gives $9 + 3 > 7$ gives $12 > 7$.

REVIEW QUESTIONS

1. A hammer costs x dollars and a box of nails costs y dollars. Before tax, which of the following represents the cost to purchase the hammer and two boxes of nails?

A) xy
B) $x + y$
C) $xy + 2$
D) $x + 2y$

2. If $5q + r = 27$ and $r = 2$, then what is the value of q?

A) -5
B) 2
C) 5
D) 25

3. Gabe and Kevin both collect model train cars. Together they have a total of 46 cars. If Gabe has 12 more cars than Kevin, how many cars does Gabe have in his collection? Write your answer in the blank:

_____

4. At a dental office, hygienists earn $14 per hour and lab technicians earn $12 per hour. If there are x hygienists and y lab technicians, which of the following represents their total hourly pay, in dollars?

A) $14x + 12y$
B) $14y + 12x$
C) $x + y$
D) $26xy$

5. Alexia has a total of 58 science textbooks. She has only biology and chemistry books, and she has 14 more chemistry books than biology books. How many biology books does Alexia have?

A) 44
B) 40
C) 36
D) 22

6. Kendra is saving up to buy a snowboard. She has $90 so far. If she saves $30 per week, which of the following shows how many more weeks until she has at least $300?

A) $30x + 90 > 300$
B) $30x + 90 = 300$
C) $30x = 210$
D) $90 + 30x < 300$

7. In a toy box, there are x dolls, y trucks, and z blocks. Which of the following expressions shows the percentage of blocks on the shelf?

A) $\dfrac{z}{100(x + y + z)}\%$

B) $\dfrac{100z}{x + y}\%$

C) $\dfrac{100z}{x + y + z}\%$

D) $\dfrac{z}{100}\%$

8. A bakery pays a delivery driver a flat fee of x dollars, plus y dollars per hour to deliver baked goods. If the delivery driver takes z hours to make a delivery, which of the following shows how much the bakery pays the driver?

A) $x + y + z$
B) $x + yz$
C) $z(x + y)$
D) $x + y$

9. The student-to-teacher ratio at a private school is 12:1. If there are 364 students enrolled for the next semester, which of the following shows how to find the number of teachers that will be needed to maintain the ratio?

A) $\dfrac{364}{12} \leq \dfrac{t}{1}$

B) $\dfrac{364}{t} = \dfrac{12}{1}$

C) $\dfrac{364}{t} \leq \dfrac{12}{1}$

D) $364t = 12$

10. Which of the following shows that twelve less than a certain number is greater than ten more than another number?

A) $x - 12 < y + 10$
B) $y - 12 > x + 10$
C) $x - 10 > y + 12$
D) $x - 12 > y + 10$

ANSWER KEY

1. D	**5.** D	**9.** C
2. C	**6.** A	**10.** D
3. 29	**7.** C	
4. A	**8.** B	

ANSWERS AND EXPLANATIONS

1. (D) The cost of a hammer is x. The cost of two boxes of nails would be $2y$. The total cost would be $x + 2y$.

2. (C) Plug in 2 for r to get $5q + 2 = 27$. Now subtract 2 from both sides to get $5q = 25$. Divide both sides by 5 to get $q = 5$.

3. (29) Let k = the number of cars Kevin has and g = the number of cars Gabe has. Now you can write the equations $g + k = 46$ and $g = k + 12$. You can substitute the second equation into the first to get $k + 12 + k = 46$. Simplify that to $2k + 12 = 46$. Subtract 12 from both sides to get $2k = 34$. Divide both sides by 2 to get $k = 17$. Since the question asks for the number of train cars Gabe has, you need to solve for g. $g = k + 12$, so $g = 17 + 12 = 29$.

4. (A) The salary of the hygienists would be $14x$. The salary of the lab technicians would be $12y$. The total salary would be $14x + 12y$.

5. (D) Let b = the number of biology books and c = the number of chemistry books. The total then is $b + c = 58$. You also know that Alexia has 14 more chemistry books than biology books, so $c = 14 + b$. Substitute the second equation into the first to get $b + 14 + b = 58$. Simplify that to $14 + 2b = 58$. Subtract 14 from both sides to get $2b = 44$. Divide both sides by 2 to get $b = 22$.

6. (A) Let x = the number of weeks. Kendra saves $30 per week, so that is $30x$. Since she already has $90, now it is $30x + 90$. She wants to have *at least* 300, so $30x + 90 > 300$.

7. (C) First, formulate a question you can translate into an equation: what percent of the total number of toys is the number of blocks?

Let A equal the percent you are looking for. Now the question translates to $\dfrac{A}{100} \times (x + y + z) = z$. Multiply both sides by 100 to get $A(x + y + z) = 100z$. Divide both sides by $(x + y + z)$ to get $A = \dfrac{100z}{x + y + z}$.

8. (B) The driver gets paid x regardless. Then the driver also makes y per hour. If the number of hours is z, then the driver gets yz plus x. The answer is $x + yz$.

9. (C) Let t = the number of teachers needed. Set up a proportion. The needed ratio is 12:1, so $\dfrac{364}{t} \leq \dfrac{12}{1}$. You need to use the *less than or equal to* symbol to be sure that there are no more than 12 students per teacher.

10. (D) Translate each expression. "Twelve less than a certain number" can be written as $x - 12$. Then you will use the *greater than* symbol. "Ten more than another number" can be written as $y + 10$. Put it all together and you get $x - 12 > y + 10$.

CHAPTER 21

Geometry

PERIMETER

Perimeter is the measure of length around the exterior of a shape. For example, to find the perimeter of a rectangle, add up the lengths of all four sides.

If you need to find the perimeter of an irregular shape, you may need to subtract to find missing values. Try an example:

What is the perimeter of the shape below?

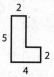

A) 11
B) 13
C) 18
D) 20

The correct answer is **C**. As you can see, two of the lengths are not marked. You will need to find them by subtracting from the values of parallel sides. The vertical piece on the right side plus the vertical piece with length 2 on the right side must equal the 5 on the left side. The missing value must equal 3. The horizontal piece plus the horizontal piece at the top with length 2 must add up to the 4 at the bottom. The missing value must equal 2. The perimeter is $5 + 2 + 3 + 2 + 2 + 4 = 18$.

CIRCUMFERENCE

The perimeter of a circle is called its circumference. Circumference can be found by using the formula $C = 2\pi r$ or $C = \pi d$, where r is the radius of the circle and d is the diameter. If you need to estimate the value of π for a question, use 3.14 (or just 3 for a rough estimation).

What is the circumference of a circle with a radius of 3 cm?

A) 6 cm
B) 3π cm
C) 6π cm
D) 9π cm

The correct answer is **C**. Use the formula $C = 2\pi r$. Since $r = 3$ cm, $2r = 6$ cm and the circumference is 6π cm.

AREA

Area is the amount of two-dimensional space taken up by an object. It is measured in units squared (square inches, square yards, square miles, and so on). The table below shows some common shapes and the formula for finding their area.

Square	□	$A = s^2$
Rectangle	▭	$A = l \times w$
Parallelogram	▱	$A = b \times h$
Trapezoid	⏢	$A = \frac{1}{2}(b_1 + b_2) \times h$
Triangle	△	$A = \frac{1}{2}b \times h$
Circle	○	$A = \pi r^2$

For parallelograms, trapezoids, and triangles, be sure you measure the height from the highest point straight down to the base—do not use the length of the slanted side as the height! You may notice that many of these formulas are related. The areas of a square, rectangle, and parallelogram are all really the same: base × height. A triangle is like a rectangle that has been cut in half, and the area formula is just that: $\frac{1}{2}b \times h$. Let's try a practice question involving area:

What is the area of the figure below?

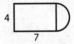

A) 28
B) $28 + 2\pi$
C) $28 + 4\pi$
D) $28 + 8\pi$

The correct answer is **B**. To find the area of the rectangle, simply multiply $4 \times 7 = 28$. To find the area of the semicircle, use the formula for area of a circle, and then divide the result in half. The diameter of the circle is the same as the width of the rectangle, 4. That means the radius of the circle is 2. $A = \pi r^2$, so $A = \pi 2^2 = 4\pi$. Now divide that in half to get the area of the semicircle. $A = 2\pi$. Add that to the area of the rectangle to get $28 + 2\pi$.

Surface Area

Surface area is the sum of the exterior areas of a three-dimensional object. A square in three dimensions is a six-sided cube, so the surface area would be six times the area of one side:

$$A = 6 \times s^2$$

A rectangle is more complicated as a three-dimensional box, since all three dimensions may be different lengths. The principle remains the same, however: Find the area of each face and add them up.

REVIEW QUESTIONS

1. A circular garden has a diameter of 140 yards. What is the area of the garden?

   A) 15,386 yards^2
   B) 21,980 yards^2
   C) 43,960 yards^2
   D) 61,544 yards^2

2. A swimming pool is 35 feet long and 12 feet wide. What is the perimeter of the pool?

   A) 37 feet
   B) 47 feet
   C) 94 feet
   D) 188 feet

3. The area of a square patio is 289 square feet. If the owner wants to put a border around the patio, what length of border will be needed?

   A) 17 feet
   B) 34 feet
   C) 51 feet
   D) 68 feet

4. Rectangle 1 has a length of l and a width of w. Rectangle 2 has a length of l and a width of $2w$. Which of the following statements is true? Select all that apply.

   A) The area of Rectangle 1 is twice the area of Rectangle 2.
   B) The area of Rectangle 1 is half the area of Rectangle 2.
   C) The perimeter of Rectangle 1 is 2 less than the perimeter of Rectangle 2.
   D) The perimeter of Rectangle 1 is less than the perimeter of Rectangle 2.

5. The triangle below is an equilateral triangle with a perimeter of 9. What is the length of side *BC*?

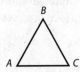

A) 18
B) 9
C) 6
D) 3

6. A courtyard measuring 7 yards by 9 yards will be tiled. How many 12-inch square tiles will be required to cover the courtyard?

A) 21
B) 63
C) 189
D) 756

7. What is the area of a circle with a diameter of 8?

A) 4π
B) 8π
C) 16π
D) 64π

8. A bicycle wheel has a radius of 21 cm. What is the distance covered by the wheel in 10 revolutions?

A) 65.94 cm
B) 131.88 cm
C) 659.41 cm
D) 1,318.80 cm

9. The area of triangle A is 4. The height of triangle B is twice that of triangle A, and the length of the base of triangle B is the same as that of triangle A. What is the area of triangle B?

A) 4
B) 8
C) 16
D) 32

10. What is the area of the figure below?

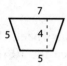

A) 24
B) 25
C) 30
D) 35

ANSWER KEY

1. A   **5.** D   **9.** B
2. C   **6.** C   **10.** A
3. D   **7.** C
4. B and D   **8.** D

ANSWERS AND EXPLANATIONS

1. (A) The formula for area of a circle is $A = \pi r^2$. If the diameter is 140 yards, then the radius is 70 yards. So $A = \pi 70^2 = 4,900\pi$. Since the answer choices are far apart from each other, you can estimate $\pi = 3$ and $4,900 \times 3 = 14,700$. Since π is a bit larger than 3, the real answer will be a bit larger than 14,700. Choice A is close and the other choices are far too large.

2. (C) The perimeter will be twice the length plus twice the width, so $(35 \times 2) + (12 \times 2) = 70 + 24 = 94$.

3. (D) To answer this question, you will need to find the perimeter of the patio. If the area is 289 and the patio is square, take the square root of 289 to find the length of each side. $\sqrt{289} = 17$. To find the perimeter, add up the lengths of the sides: $4 \times 17 = 68$.

4. (B and D) The area of Rectangle 1 is $l \times w$. The area of Rectangle 2 is $l \times 2w$ or $2(l \times w)$. Rectangle 2 is twice as big as Rectangle 1, so the area of Rectangle 1 is half that of Rectangle 2, and the perimeter of Rectangle 1 is less than the perimeter of Rectangle 2.

5. (D) An equilateral triangle has sides of equal length. If the perimeter is 9, then divide by 3 sides to get a length of 3 for each side.

6. (C) First, find the area of the courtyard. $9 \times 7 = 63$ yards^2. The tiles are 12-inch squares, so you need to convert that to yards. 36 inches = 1 yard, so 12 inches = $\frac{1}{3}$ yard. Write an equation to find the number of tiles: $t \times \frac{1}{3} = 63$. Multiply both sides by 3 to get $t = 189$.

7. (C) If the diameter is 8, then the radius is 4. Use the formula $A = \pi r^2$. $A = \pi 4^2 = 16\pi$.

8. (D) First find the circumference, the distance around the wheel. Use the formula $C = 2\pi r$. $C = 2\pi \times 21 = 42\pi$. To find the distance for 10 revolutions, multiply by 10 to get 420π. Since the answers are far apart, estimate $\pi = 3$ and $420 \times 3 = 1,260$. Look for an answer a bit larger than 1,260 cm. The best choice is D.

9. (B) Let the height of triangle A = h and the base = b. Since the area of triangle A is 4, we can say $4 = \frac{1}{2}bh$. Since the height of triangle B is twice the height of triangle A, and the length of the base is the same, the area of triangle B is $\frac{1}{2}b(2h) = bh$. If the area of A is $4 = \frac{1}{2}bh$ and the area of B is bh, then B is twice the area of A. If A = 4, then B = 8.

10. (A) The formula for the area of a trapezoid is $A = \frac{1}{2}(b_1 + b_2) \times h$. Make sure you use 4 for the height. $A = \frac{1}{2}(5 + 7) \times 4 = \frac{1}{2} \times 12 \times 4 = 6 \times 4 = 24$.

CHAPTER 22

Measurements and Conversions

Measurements and conversions questions ask you to make conversions between units of measurement in the metric system or the English system. You may also be asked to convert measurements from units in one system to units in the other. Some questions ask about the appropriate tool to be used to measure a particular quantity as well.

ENGLISH SYSTEM CONVERSIONS

The **English system** of measurement uses the following units to measure weight, volume, and length. Weight is measured in ounces, pounds, and tons. Volume is measured in ounces, cups, pints, quarts, and gallons. Length is measured in inches, feet, yards, and miles.

To convert between units in the English system, you must know the equivalent measures for each step in the measurement system. A table of equivalents is given below:

Measurement Type	Equivalents	
Weight	16 ounces	= 1 pound
	2,000 pounds	= 1 ton
Volume	8 ounces	= 1 cup
	2 cups	= 1 pint
	2 pints	= 1 quart
	4 quarts	= 1 gallon
Length	12 inches	= 1 foot
	3 feet	= 1 yard
	5,280 feet	= 1 mile

METRIC SYSTEM CONVERSIONS

The **metric system** also measures weight, volume, and length, but it uses a different set of units for measurement. The basic unit of weight measurement is the gram. The basic unit of volume measurement is the liter, and the basic unit of length measurement is the meter.

In the metric system, each unit of measurement starts with a prefix that indicates whether the measurement is smaller than the basic unit or larger than it.

Prefix	Measurement Compared to Basic Unit	Weight	Volume	Length
kilo	1,000 times	kilogram (kg)	kiloliter (kL)	kilometer (km)
hecto	100 times	hectogram (hg)	hectoliter (hL)	hectometer (hm)
deka	10 times	dekagram (dag)	dekaliter (daL)	dekameter (dam)
Basic unit	Basic unit	gram (g)	liter (L)	meter (m)
deci	1/10	decigram (dg)	deciliter (dL)	decimeter (dm)
centi	1/100	centigram (cg)	centiliter (cL)	centimeter (cm)
milli	1/1,000	milligram (mg)	milliliter (mL)	millimeter (mm)

As the table shows, each unit of measurement in the different levels of the metric system is 10 times smaller than the unit above it and 10 times larger than the unit below it. One centimeter is equal to 10 millimeters, one gram is equal to 10 decigrams, and so on.

CONVERSIONS BETWEEN SYSTEMS

To convert between measurements in the English and metric systems, you need to know the approximate equivalents between units. Some of the common equivalents are as follows:

English Measurement	Metric Equivalent
1 kilogram	Approx. 2.2 pounds
1 liter	Approx. 1 quart
2.5 centimeters	Approx. 1 inch
1 meter	Approx. 1 yard

Temperature Conversions

In the English system, temperature is measured on the Fahrenheit scale. In the metric system, temperature is measured on the Celsius scale. You will need to know how to convert temperature measurements from one scale to the other. Some common temperatures are shown in the chart below.

	Celsius	Fahrenheit
Absolute zero	−273.15	−459.67
Parity	−40	−40
Freezing point	0	32
Body temperature	37	98.6
Boiling point	100	212

To get a rough approximation of Celsius temperature from a Fahrenheit measurement, subtract 30 and then divide by 2. For an exact conversion, the formula is $C = (F - 32) \times \dfrac{5}{9}$.

Conversion Factors

A **conversion factor** is the mathematical tool used to convert from one unit of measurement to another. It is a proportion in which the denominator is equal to the numerator and is sometimes referred to as a unit multiplier. For example, the conversion factor for inches and feet is 12 inches = 1 foot. For less common conversions, the conversion factor will be given to you.

MEASUREMENT TOOLS

Measurement tools tested on the TEAS can be divided into three categories based on whether they measure weight, volume, or length. For measuring weight, **scales** are traditionally used and may have varying degrees of accuracy. For measuring volume, **pipettes** are measuring tubes or droppers used to measure small amounts of liquid with high precision, whereas **measuring cups**, **flasks**, and **beakers** provide less precise measurements for larger amounts of liquid. **Graduated cylinders** vary in size and are typically less precise than pipettes but more precise than measuring cups, flasks, and beakers.

For measuring length, **calipers** are the most precise measuring tool and take measurements using two points. **Rulers** are the next most precise tool, followed by **yardsticks** and **metersticks**. For measuring longer distances, **tape measures** may be used in varying sizes. **Odometers** measure the distances traveled by a vehicle and would be appropriate for measurements taken in miles or kilometers.

REVIEW QUESTIONS

1. A powdered chemical must be measured to the nearest $\frac{1}{4}$ of a pound.

Which of the following is the most appropriate measurement tool for this task?

A) Graduated cylinder
B) Beaker
C) Yardstick
D) Scale

2. How many pints are in 3 gallons? Write your answer in the blank:
_____

3. Which of the following is an approximate metric quantity for the volume of a glass of water?

A) 10 mL
B) 0.1 cL
C) 0.5 L
D) 1 kL

4. If a piece of wood measures 25.4 centimeters in length, which of the following is the wood's approximate length in English measurement? (Note: 1 inch ≈ 2.54 centimeters)

A) 10 inches
B) 35.4 inches
C) 64.52 inches
D) 100 inches

5. Which of the following metric units of measurement is most reasonable to measure the weight of a full tube of a cream medication?

A) Milligram (mg)
B) Gram (g)
C) Hectogram (hg)
D) Kilogram (kg)

6. Which of the following is the number of centimeters in 1.46 meters?

A) 1.46
B) 14.6
C) 146
D) 1,460

7. A builder must measure a steel rod exactly 5 inches long for a building project. Which of the following measurement tools is appropriate for this task?

A) Ruler
B) Pipette
C) Yardstick
D) Odometer

8. How many centimeters are in 20 decimeters? Write your answer in the blank: _____

9. A technician must measure exactly 6 ounces of a liquid to add to a medical preparation. It is important for the measurement to be as precise as possible. Which of the following measurement tools is most appropriate for this task?

A) Scale
B) Beaker
C) Caliper
D) Graduated cylinder

10. If a container holds about 4 liters, which of the following is the container's approximate volume in English measurement? (Note: 1 liter ≈ 1 quart)

A) 2 pints
B) 4 pints
C) 1 gallon
D) 4 gallons

ANSWER KEY

1. D **5.** B **9.** D
2. 24 **6.** C **10.** C
3. C **7.** A
4. A **8.** 200

ANSWERS AND EXPLANATIONS

1. (D) A scale is the appropriate measuring tool for measuring weight. Graduated cylinders and beakers are used to measure volume, while yardsticks are used to measure length.

2. (24) A gallon consists of 4 quarts, and there are 2 pints in each quart. Since $4 \times 2 = 8$, there are 8 pints in each gallon. Multiply 3 gallons by 8 pints: $3 \times 8 = 24$. There are 24 pints in 3 gallons.

3. (C) A glass of water is best approximated by a measurement of about half a liter, or 0.5 L. The measurements of 10 mL and 0.10 cL are equal and are both too small. The measurement of 1 kL too large.

4. (A) Set up a proportion to determine the missing measurement. Cross multiply to solve:

$$\frac{1 \text{ inch}}{2.54 \text{ centimeters}} = \frac{x \text{ inches}}{25.4 \text{ centimeters}}$$

$$2.54 \times x = 1 \times 25.4$$

$$2.54x = 25.4$$

$$x = \frac{25.4}{2.54}$$

$$x = 10$$

The wood measures approximately 10 inches.

5. (B) A full tube of a cream medication would most likely be measured in grams. The unit of milligrams would be too small. Hectogram and kilogram units would be too large.

6. (C) Convert the number of meters to centimeters. One meter equals 100 centimeters. Multiply $1.46 \times 100 = 146$.

7. (A) A ruler would be most suited for measuring a length in inches. A yardstick would be too large, so C is incorrect.

8. (200) Convert decimeters to centimeters. One decimeter equals 10 centimeters. Multiply $20 \times 10 = 200$. There are 200 centimeters in 20 decimeters.

9. (D) The volume of a liquid is best measured by a graduated cylinder or beaker, among the choices listed here. Graduated cylinders generally provide more precise measurements than beakers, so a graduated cylinder would be the most appropriate tool for this task.

10. (C) Set up a proportion to determine the missing measurement. Cross multiply to solve:

$$\frac{1 \text{ liter}}{1 \text{ quart}} = \frac{4 \text{ liters}}{x \text{ quarts}}$$

$$1 \times x = 1 \times 4$$

$$x = 4$$

The container's approximate volume is 4 quarts. There are 4 quarts in a gallon, so the container holds approximately 1 gallon.

CHAPTER 23

Data Interpretation

Data interpretation questions ask you to interpret data given in certain types of graphs. Other questions may ask you to distinguish between dependent and independent variables in a statement or description of an event.

READING GRAPHS

In the Reading chapters earlier in this book, we reviewed certain questions that involved using maps and resources. Data interpretation questions on the TEAS are similar to some of the Reading questions involving graphs that we saw earlier, except the questions may be more complex.

Games Won by League Teams

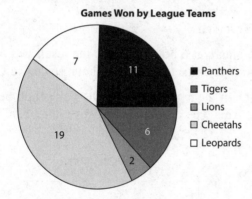

- ■ Panthers
- ■ Tigers
- ■ Lions
- ☐ Cheetahs
- ☐ Leopards

The graph above shows the distribution of 45 games won by teams in a soccer league during one season.

Games won by the Panthers represent what percentage of all games won that season? (Round the solution to the nearest tenth of a percent.)

A) 4.4%
B) 24.4%
C) 27.6%
D) 42.2%

To solve this problem, locate the section of the circle graph that shows games won by the Panthers. According to the key, the Panthers' section is in the top right quadrant. The Panthers won 11 out of 45 games during the season, or $\frac{11}{45}$. Divide 11 by 45 to determine the percentage: $11 \div 45$ is approximately 0.244. Convert this decimal to a percentage by moving the decimal point to the right two places. The Panthers won 24.4% of the games. The correct answer is **B**.

The **circle graph** shows visually how a whole is divided into parts. Here is another data interpretation example involving a **line graph**, which shows change over time:

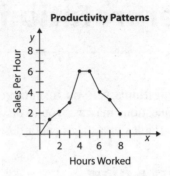

Productivity Patterns

The graph above shows the relationship between the number of hours worked by members of a sales team and the number of sales made per hour. Which of the following resulted in the highest sales per hour?

A) 2 hours worked
B) 3 hours worked
C) 6 hours worked
D) 8 hours worked

According to the graph, at 6 hours worked, the result was 4 sales per hour. At 8 hours, the number drops to 2 sales per hour, so choice **C** is correct.

Like the line graph in the example above, the **bar graph** below also shows change over time. This type of graph uses bars, rather than lines, to indicate values.

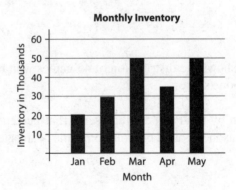

Monthly Inventory

The graph above shows the number of products held in the inventory of a warehouse over a period of five months. During which of the following months did the warehouse have more than 30,000 products in inventory?

A) January, March, and April
B) February, March, and April
C) February, March, and May
D) March, April, and May

According to the graph, the warehouse had 50,000 products in inventory during March, 35,000 during April, and 50,000 in May. Therefore, choice **D** is correct.

DEPENDENT AND INDEPENDENT VARIABLES

Some data interpretation questions ask you to identify dependent or independent variables in a given statement. The topic of dependent and independent variables is discussed in greater detail in Chapter 24. To answer Math questions regarding dependent and independent variables, you must understand the difference between the two.

Dependent and independent variables define a causal relationship between two factors. The **dependent variable** is the factor being acted upon. The **independent variable** is the factor that influences the outcome. In cause-and-effect terms, we would say that the dependent variable is the effect, and the independent variable is the cause.

Certain flowering plants have more blooms with increased sunlight.

What is the independent variable in the event described above?

In the above example, the statement explains that increased sunlight causes the plants to have more blooms. Sunlight is the independent variable in the relationship, because it is the factor that influences plants to bloom. The number of blooms is the dependent variable in the relationship, because this is the outcome that results from the influence of more sunlight.

COVARIANCE

Covariance is a measure of the joint variability of two random variables. If the value of x increases when the value of y increases, and the value of x decreases when the value of y decreases, then x and y are said to have **positive covariance**. If the value of x increases when the value of y decreases, and the value of x decreases when the value of y increases, then x and y are said to have **negative covariance**.

MEASURES OF CENTRAL TENDENCY

Measures of central tendency include mean, median, and mode. The **mean** of a data set is the average of the values. To find the mean, add up all the values and divide that sum by the number of values.

The **median** is the middle number in an ordered set of values. To find the median, put all the values in increasing order. If there are an odd number of values, the median is the value in the middle position. If there are an even number of values, find the average of the two values in the middle and the result is the median.

The **mode** of a data set is the value that occurs the most. Some data sets do not have a mode, and some may have more than one mode.

Find the mean, median, and mode of this data set: {3, 7, −2, 5, 3, 9, −6}

The mean is found by adding up the 7 values and dividing the sum by 7. $3 + 7 + -2 + 5 + 3 + 9 + -6 = 19$. The mean is $\frac{19}{7}$.

The median is found by ordering the values: −6, −2, 3, 3, 5, 7, 9. The middle value is 3, so the median = 3.

The mode is the most frequently occurring value, so the mode = 3.

RANGE

The **range** of a data set is found by subtracting the smallest value from the largest value. For the data set we used above, {3, 7, −2, 5, 3, 9, −6}, the range is $9 − (−6) = 15$.

DATA DISTRIBUTION

The shape of a data distribution may reveal useful information. A **symmetrical distribution** can be divided at the center and will create mirror images on the left and right of the dividing line.

A **uniform distribution** shows points spread evenly over the range of the data, but many data sets show peaks when graphed. A graph with a single peak is called **unimodal**, and if that peak is at the center and is symmetrical, that graph is a **bell-shaped graph** or a **normal distribution**. A graph with a single peak to the left of center (with fewer higher values on the right) is said to be **skewed right**. A graph with a single peak to the right of center (with fewer higher values on the left) is said to be **skewed left**. If only a small number of values are separated away from the rest, these are called **outliers**.

REVIEW QUESTIONS

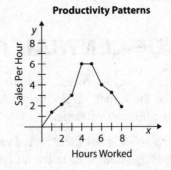

1. The graph above shows the relationship between the number of hours worked by members of a sales team and the number of sales made per hour. Based on the information given in the graph, which of the following achieved the highest number of sales per hour?

   A) A team member who worked for 2 or 3 hours
   B) A team member who worked for 3 hours
   C) A team member who worked for 4 or 5 hours
   D) A team member who worked for 6 hours

2. Most companies increase their customers with more advertising.

   Which of the following is the dependent variable in the statement above?

   A) Marketing
   B) Customers
   C) Advertising
   D) Products

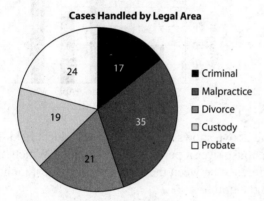

Cases Handled by Legal Area

- Criminal
- Malpractice
- Divorce
- Custody
- Probate

3. The graph above shows the distribution of 116 cases handled by a law firm in certain legal areas over a period of one year.

   Custody cases represent what percentage of all cases handled by the firm that year? (Round the solution to the nearest tenth of a percent.)

   A) 16.4%
   B) 18.1%
   C) 21.0%
   D) 30.1%

4. A scientist is presenting a report on the results of a survey that shows the number of people taking different medications to treat the same illness. Which of the following graphs should the scientist use to visually emphasize the percentage of patients taking each medication?

   A) Bar graph
   B) Line graph
   C) Circle graph
   D) Table

5. The chart shows the number of miles Paul drove each day last week.

Monday	15
Tuesday	17
Wednesday	15
Thursday	16
Friday	19
Saturday	43
Sunday	5

Put the following elements of the data set in order from least to greatest: the range, the median, and the mode.

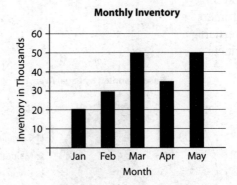

6. The graph above shows the number of products held in the inventory of a warehouse over a period of five months. Which of the following is the difference between the largest and smallest monthly inventories shown in the graph?

A) 15,000
B) 20,000
C) 27,000
D) 30,000

7. Stock prices usually decrease when investors panic.

Which of the following is the independent variable in the event described above?

A) Investor panic
B) Stock prices
C) Market fluctuations
D) News reports

Units Shipped by Vendor

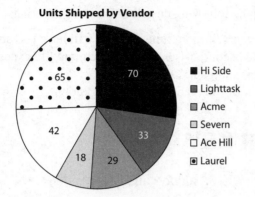

- ■ Hi Side
- ■ Lighttask
- ■ Acme
- ☐ Severn
- ☐ Ace Hill
- ◉ Laurel

8. The graph above shows the distribution of 257 units shipped by particular vendors to a company over a six-month period.

The units shipped by Severn represent what percentage of all units shipped by vendors during that period? (Round the solution to the nearest tenth of a percent.)

A) 5.2%
B) 6.3%
C) 7.0%
D) 27.2%

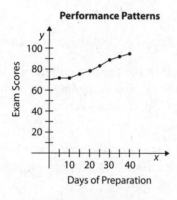

9. The graph above shows the relationship between the number of days of preparation by students studying for an exam and the exam scores received. Based on the information given in the graph, which of the following conclusions can be drawn?

A) Students needed at least 5 days of preparation to score a 70 or higher.
B) There was no score difference recorded between 5 and 10 days of preparation.
C) The highest scores were achieved by those who had 30 days of preparation.
D) Students who scored over 90 spent at least 20 days preparing for the exam.

10. Which of the following describes negative covariance?

    A) Give yourself more time and you will have less stress.
    B) People become wiser as they have more life experiences.
    C) No pain, no gain.
    D) The more you read, the more you know.

ANSWER KEY

1. C
2. B
3. A
4. C

5. mode < median < range
6. D
7. A
8. C

9. B
10. A

ANSWERS AND EXPLANATIONS

1. (C) The line graph shows that the highest number of sales per hour were achieved at 4 and 5 hours worked.

2. (B) In this statement, *customers* is the dependent variable. The number of customers is influenced by the level of *advertising,* which is the independent variable.

3. (A) The firm handled 19 custody cases during the year, or $\frac{19}{116}$.

Divide 19 by 116 to determine the percentage: $19 \div 116$ is approximately 0.164. Convert this decimal to a percentage by moving the decimal point to the right two places. Custody cases represent 16.4% of all cases handled by the firm.

4. (C) A circle graph shows visually how a whole is divided into parts. It would be the best choice to use to visually emphasize the percentage of patients taking each medication.

5. (mode < median < range) Find the median, mode, and range. Put the values in increasing order: 5, 15, 15, 16, 17, 19, 43. There are 7 values, so the median is the middle value, 16. The mode is 15. The range is $43 - 15 = 28$. Ordering those values gives you mode < median < range.

6. (D) The largest monthly inventory is 50,000 products, held in March and May. The smallest monthly inventory is 20,000 products, held in January. To find the difference between these two, use subtraction: $50,000 - 20,000 = 30,000$.

7. (A) In this statement, the cause is panic of investors, and the effect is the decrease in stock prices. *Investor panic* is the independent variable, because it influences the outcome of stock price decline.

8. (C) According to the graph, Severn shipped 18 units during the six-month period. This amounts to $\frac{18}{257}$ of the total units shipped. Divide 18 by 257 to determine the percentage: $18 \div 257 = 0.07$. Convert this decimal to a percentage by moving the decimal point to the right two places. The units shipped by Severn represent 7% of all units shipped.

9. (B) Looking at the graph, we can see that students who prepared for 5 days scored just over 70 on the exam. Students who prepared for 10 days scored the same. Therefore, there was no difference recorded between 5 and 10 days of preparation, as choice B states. Choice A is incorrect because students who spent no days preparing scored a 70 on the exam.

10. (A) Negative covariance occurs when one variable increases as the other decreases. This is the case in choice A. As time increases, stress decreases.

PART III

SCIENCE

The **TEAS Science section** tests your scientific knowledge and skills in three areas: scientific reasoning, human anatomy and physiology, and life and physical sciences. In this part, we'll review scientific concepts essential for success on the test, along with key formulas you'll need to solve problems involving calculations.

CHAPTER 24

Scientific Reasoning

Questions concerning **scientific reasoning** test your understanding of the steps and tools in the process of developing scientific knowledge. You will need to demonstrate understanding of how experiments are designed and be able to critique them. These questions also address concepts such as: deductive and inductive reasoning, dependent and independent variables, experimental and control groups, and direct and inverse correlations.

DESIGNING AN EXPERIMENT

There are many things to consider when designing an experiment. Scientists use a plan called the **scientific method**, which was developed over time by many scientists as they performed experiments and discussed their results with one another. The scientific method is not specific to a certain type of experiment and is used in all different areas of science. It allows experiments to be repeated to confirm results and allows those results to be communicated easily and uniformly.

Steps in the Scientific Method

There are six steps in the scientific method, and they are always conducted in the same order, as follows:

Step 1	Make an observation and identify the **problem** to be studied.
Step 2	Ask a **question** or questions about the problem.
Step 3	Formulate a **hypothesis** that attempts to answer one of the questions raised about the problem.
Step 4	Gather data and/or conduct an **experiment** to test the hypothesis.
Step 5	**Analyze** the data gathered.
Step 6	Draw a **conclusion** regarding whether or not the hypothesis is supported by the data.

As a scientist works through the first few steps of the process to come up with a hypothesis, he or she must pay attention to the type of logical reasoning used to form the hypothesis. There are two basic types of logical reasoning, inductive and deductive, and both can lead to faulty assumptions if the scientist is not careful.

Inductive Versus Deductive Reasoning

Scientific progress proceeds based on logical reasoning. **Inductive reasoning** involves drawing general conclusions based on observation of specific events. If a scientist observes swans on a lake, and all of the swans that he sees are white, the scientist might conclude that *all swans are white*.

Inductive reasoning is based on observation, but it has its flaws. Suppose black swans do exist somewhere, but the scientist has never seen them. It would be incorrect for the scientist to conclude definitively that all swans are white because it is impossible for him to research all swans on the planet to verify this conclusion.

Deductive reasoning involves drawing a specific conclusion based on a general premise. A scientist might start out with the general premise that all accountants are good with numbers. She might then meet Omar, who is an accountant. The scientist would conclude that Omar is good with numbers.

When using deductive reasoning, the conclusion can only be true if the general premise is also true. If a scientist starts out with a false premise, the conclusion will be false. Here is an example:

All men are over six feet tall. Jerome is a man. Therefore, Jerome is over six feet tall.

In the argument above, the conclusion is false because the general premise is false. Some men are less than six feet tall.

Dependent and Independent Variables

Science experiments are often designed in terms of dependent and independent variables. The **dependent variable** is the outcome, or effect, being studied. The **independent variable** is the causal factor being studied.

It may help to think of the two types of variables in terms of the following diagram:

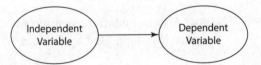

The independent variable acts on the dependent variable to produce a certain outcome. We say the dependent variable is *dependent* because it is influenced by the action of the independent variable. The independent variable, on the other hand, is free to act and is not influenced by another source, at least in terms of the design of the study.

The study described in the example below gives an example of independent and dependent variables in an experiment.

Scientists wish to investigate whether the growth of a certain plant is affected by a fertilizer. One group of ten plants is grown with no fertilizer. A second group of ten plants is grown with fertilizer administered at regular intervals with each watering. At the end of the study, the fertilized plants are 10 centimeters taller, on average, than the plants that received no fertilizer.

In this experiment, fertilizer is the independent variable, and plant growth is the dependent variable. The scientists are testing whether the fertilizer has an effect on plant growth.

Fertilizer	Plant growth
Independent variable	**Dependent variable**

We can conceptualize the relationship between fertilizer and plant growth visually as shown:

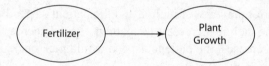

Experimental and Control Groups

Experiments are often designed with two types of test groups: experimental groups and control groups. **Experimental groups** are the test groups that receive a particular factor being tested, such as a medication or fertilizer, as in the example above. Experimental groups may also be called **treatment groups.** They are receiving the treatment being tested.

Control groups are groups that do not receive the treatment or factor being tested. Control groups may receive no factors, such as in the example above, where one group received no fertilizer. Control groups may also be given a "false" factor, known as a **placebo.** In pharmaceutical experiments, for example, placebos can take the form of pills that are made to resemble a certain medication being tested—but the placebo actually contains none of the medication itself.

CRITIQUING AN EXPERIMENT

Once an experiment has been performed, scientists must analyze the results and form conclusions. In doing this, they must be careful to make conclusions that are supported by **empirical evidence**, data that was gathered through scientific experimentation. Conclusions should never be drawn based on opinions or **bias** (favoring one idea over another).

When analyzing data, scientists often look for cause-and-effect relationships, and the first step in that process is to look for factors that appear to be correlated. There are two ways to describe these relationships: direct correlations and inverse correlations.

Direct and Inverse Correlations

When we say that there is a correlation between two factors, this means that the factors have a relationship. A **direct correlation** shows that as one factor increases, the other factor also increases. An **inverse correlation**, by contrast, shows that as one factor increases, the other decreases:

The higher the temperature rose, the more quickly the substance melted.

In the scenario above, temperature and melting rate are directly correlated. As temperature increases, the rate of melting also increases. As temperature decreases, the rate of melting slows down.

Here is an example of inverse correlation:

As the incline on the treadmill increased, the patient's speed slowed down.

In this scenario, the level of incline and the patient's speed are inversely correlated. As the incline increases, the patient's speed decreases. Presumably as the incline decreases, the patient's speed would pick back up.

Direct correlations are also known as **positive correlations**. These terms are used interchangeably. Inverse correlations can be referred to as **negative correlations** or as **indirect correlations**. Inverse, negative, and indirect correlation all mean the same thing.

In addition, correlations can sometimes be referred to as **variations**. A direct variation is the same as a direct correlation or a positive correlation. An inverse variation is the same as an inverse correlation, a negative correlation, or an indirect correlation.

Term	Means the Same as
Positive correlation	
Direct variation	Direct correlation
Positive variation	
Negative correlation	
Indirect correlation	
Inverse variation	Inverse correlation
Negative variation	
Indirect variation	

Reading Graphs of Experimental Results

Correlations can be graphed to show the results of an experiment. The line of a line graph with a direct or positive correlation will have a positive slope:

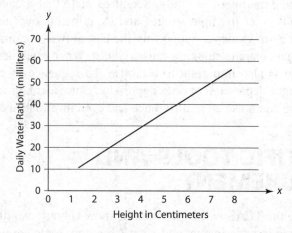

The graph above shows a line slanting upward to the right, which indicates a **positive slope**. As the daily water ration increases, the height also increases. The results of this graph show that height and daily water intake are *directly correlated*. Another way to say this is that height *varies directly* with daily water intake.

The line graph below shows an inverse correlation, or an inverse variation, which is represented by a line with a negative slope. This time, as the daily water ration increases, the height decreases.

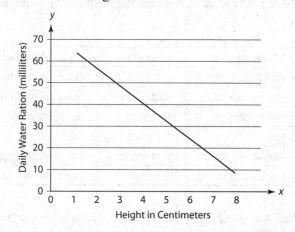

The line slanting downward to the right shows a **negative slope.** Based on the results shown in this graph, it can be concluded that height and daily water intake are *inversely correlated.* We might also say that height *varies indirectly* with the daily water intake.

Causal Relationships and Sequencing

It is important to note that correlations do not always prove causation. To conclude that one thing caused another thing to occur is difficult and takes more than one experiment or study. Scientists state that a causal relationship exists only after multiple studies and experiments over time produce a preponderance of evidence supporting the causality. For example, studies have shown that cigarette smoking causes cancer. When establishing a causal relationship, it is also important to establish the sequence of events. Does alcoholism cause depression or does depression cause alcoholism? Knowing the sequencing can make a big difference and even invalidate a conclusion.

SCIENTIFIC TOOLS AND MEASUREMENT

Another thing the TEAS will expect you to know is how scientific measurements are made in experiments and what laboratory tools are used to make them. Accuracy in measurement is vital in an experiment, and knowing the proper tool to use is equally important.

Scientists use the SI (Système Internationale) system, or **metric system**, to measure the mass, volume, and length of objects. The metric system has base units and adds prefixes to describe increased or decreased levels of those units. For example, the base *gram* is modified with the prefix *kilo* to form the term *kilogram*, or 1,000 grams. Any measurement with the prefix *kilo* will have 1,000 of the base unit. Here are the most common prefixes you will need to know:

Prefix	Meaning	Example	Example Meaning
milli	one thousandth	milliliter	one thousandth of a liter
centi	one hundredth	centimeter	one hundredth of a meter
deci	one tenth	decigram	one tenth of a gram
deka	ten	dekaliter	ten liters
hecto	one hundred	hectometer	one hundred meters
kilo	one thousand	kilogram	one thousand grams

The TEAS will test your understanding of the appropriate unit of measure to use when measuring an item. For example, you would not use kilograms to measure the mass of a paper clip. The most appropriate scale to use would be grams. To measure the length of a pencil, centimeters is more appropriate than meters.

You will also need to know which tool is appropriate to measure an item's mass, volume, or length. Here are some common scientific tools and what they can be used to measure:

Tool	Measures
thermometer	temperature
graduated cylinder	volume of liquid
volumetric pipette	small volume of liquid
meter stick	length
triple beam balance	compares mass of an object to a known mass
caliper	thickness
spring scale	force
stopwatch	time

REVIEW QUESTIONS

1. Which of the following tools would be most appropriate to measure the mass of a human liver?

   A) Balance scale
   B) Meter stick
   C) Spring scale
   D) Barometer

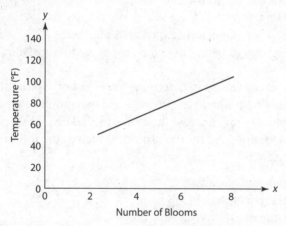

2. A scientist concluded, based on the graph above, that increasing the temperature results in an increasing number of blooms on a given flower. Which of the following correctly identifies one problem with this conclusion?

   A) The scientist is biased because he or she prefers flowers with multiple blooms.
   B) The scientist failed to include a control group in the experiment.
   C) The scientist assumed that the correlation observed does not apply to other types of plants.
   D) The scientist failed to identify a point at which increasingly higher temperatures become a barrier to bloom formation.

3. Put the steps in the scientific method in order from first (1) to last (5).

_____ Conduct an experiment
_____ Draw a conclusion
_____ Form a hypothesis
_____ Analyze the data
_____ Identify a problem

4. Which of the following provides an example of inductive reasoning?

A) All of the singers in the choir are talented. Elana is in the choir. Therefore, Elana is talented.
B) All of the gorillas observed in the zoo have brown hair. Therefore, all gorillas have brown hair.
C) All surgeons are detail oriented. Jorge is a surgeon. Therefore, Jorge is detail oriented.
D) All libraries are quiet. The MacArthur Reading Room is a library. Therefore, the MacArthur Reading Room is quiet.

5. Scientists conduct an experiment to assess the effect of a certain substance, Substance A, on bacterial cell division. One group of bacteria is exposed to Substance A at regular intervals over a period of 10 days. A second group of bacteria receives no exposure to Substance A. Which of the following is the dependent variable in this study?

A) Bacterial cell division
B) Substance A
C) The group of bacteria exposed to Substance A
D) The group of bacteria with no exposure to Substance A

6. A study is conducted to determine the effect of aspirin on heart attack risk. Study participants are divided into two groups. Participants in the first group are given a low dose of aspirin daily, while participants in the second group receive no aspirin. Which of the following describes the first group?

A) Dependent variable
B) Independent variable
C) Treatment group
D) Control group

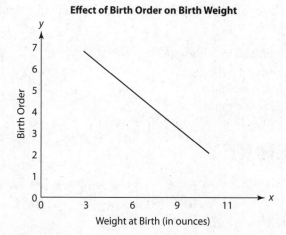

Effect of Birth Order on Birth Weight

7. Based on the graph above, which of the following statements accurately describes the relationship between birth order and weight at birth?

   A) Birth order varies directly with weight at birth.
   B) Birth order varies indirectly with weight at birth.
   C) Birth order is directly correlated with weight at birth.
   D) Birth order is positively correlated with weight at birth.

8. In a pregnancy study, women in Group 1 were given a low dose of medication X daily. Women in Group 2 did not receive medication X. The pregnancy rate for the medication X users was 60%, and the pregnancy rate for the nonusers was 40%.

   Which of the following is a reasonable hypothesis related to this experiment?

   A) Women in Group 2 have higher pregnancy rates than women in Group 1.
   B) Women in Group 1 have higher pregnancy rates than women in Group 2.
   C) Therapy with medication X reduces labor time.
   D) Therapy with medication X improves pregnancy rates.

9. Which of the following is the most appropriate unit to measure the length of a standard basketball court?

   A) Yards
   B) Millimeters
   C) Kilometers
   D) Liters

10. The final step in the scientific method is reflected by which of the following?

A) Formulate a hypothesis
B) Conduct an experiment
C) Draw a conclusion
D) Analyze the evidence

ANSWER KEY

1. A   **5.** A   **9.** A
2. D   **6.** C   **10.** C
3. 3, 5, 2, 4, 1   **7.** B
4. B   **8.** D

ANSWERS AND EXPLANATIONS

1. (A) The most appropriate tool to measure the mass of a human liver is a balance scale.

2. (D) The scientist concluded that continuing to increase the temperature would continue to increase the number of blooms. The data only shows the number of blooms increasing over a certain range of temperature, so the scientist's conclusion is not supported.

3. (3, 5, 2, 4, 1) The correct order of steps in the scientific method is as follows: identify a problem, ask questions about the problem, form a hypothesis, gather data or conduct an experiment, analyze the data, and draw a conclusion.

4. (B) The argument in choice B is an example of inductive reasoning. It starts with a statement regarding specific observations: *All of the gorillas observed in the zoo have brown hair.* It then draws a general conclusion: *Therefore, all gorillas have brown hair.* Only certain gorillas have been observed—the ones in the zoo—but the conclusion refers to all gorillas in general. Choices A, C, and D are all examples of deductive reasoning.

5. (A) In this experiment, bacterial cell division is the dependent variable under study. Substance A is the independent variable. The scientists are assessing the effect that Substance A has on bacterial cell division, so Substance A is the "cause" in this instance. Bacterial cell division is the "outcome" or "effect."

6. (C) The first group is the treatment group, or experimental group. Participants in the first group receive a dose of aspirin, which is the independent variable under study. The second group is the control group, because participants in this group do not receive the factor under study.

7. (B) The graph shows that as the position in the birth order increases, the birth weight decreases. Therefore, the two factors are inversely correlated. Another way to say this would be to say that they show indirect variation, or that birth order varies indirectly with birth weight.

8. (D) The study tested the effect of medication X on pregnancy rates in women. A reasonable hypothesis related to this study would be that *therapy with medication X improves pregnancy rates.* Choices A and B are incorrect, because the study focused on how medication X affected pregnancy rates specifically. Choice C is incorrect, because the study did not address labor time.

9. (A) The most appropriate unit to measure the length of a standard basketball court is in yards. Millimeters and kilometers also measure length, but the scale of a basketball court is too large for millimeters and too small for kilometers.

10. (C) The final step in the scientific method is to draw a conclusion. Scientists must analyze the evidence before drawing a conclusion, and they must conduct an experiment before analyzing the evidence, so choices D and B are incorrect.

Anatomy and Physiology

A large portion of the science test consists of questions about anatomy and physiology, so you will need to be familiar with the structures and functions of the ten major body systems, many of which work together to perform certain tasks. You may also be tested on specific vocabulary terms related to the understanding of anatomy.

Relevant Anatomical Terms

The following terms are commonly used when discussing anatomy:

- **anterior:** In the front or in front of
- **posterior:** In the back or in back of
- **ventral:** Refers to the front of the body
- **dorsal:** Refers to the back of the body
- **medial:** Closer to the center line of the body
- **lateral:** Farther from the center line of the body
- **proximal:** Closer to the origin of a limb or attachment point
- **distal:** Farther from the origin of a limb or attachment point
- **superior:** Above or higher up
- **inferior:** Below or lower down
- **sagittal:** The plane that divides the body vertically from right to left
- **transverse:** The plane that divides the body horizontally from top to bottom
- **coronal (also called frontal):** The plane that divides the body vertically from front to back

CHAPTER 25

The Skeletal System

The **skeletal system** serves several important functions in the body. It provides support and structure for movement, protects vital organs, produces blood cells, and stores and regulates certain minerals. The skeletal system works closely with the neuromuscular system to allow us to move our bodies.

STRUCTURE

Bones are **dynamic** tissues that are made and broken down continuously. Bones are nearly as strong as steel, which allows them to act as the armor for the soft organs of the body. The body contains 206 bones. These bones can be classified into two groups. The **axial skeleton** consists of the skeleton's center and includes the skull, the vertebral column, and the rib cage. The **appendicular skeleton** consists of the pelvic and shoulder girdles and the **appendages** (limbs).

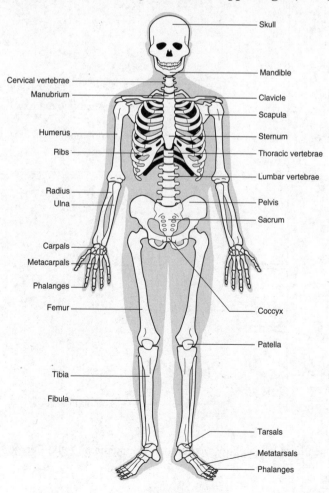

Skull
Mandible
Cervical vertebrae
Manubrium
Clavicle
Scapula
Humerus
Sternum
Ribs
Thoracic vertebrae
Lumbar vertebrae
Radius
Ulna
Pelvis
Sacrum
Carpals
Metacarpals
Phalanges
Femur
Coccyx
Patella
Tibia
Fibula
Tarsals
Metatarsals
Phalanges

The figure above shows the **anterior**, or frontal, view of the skeleton. The **posterior** view is the back of the skeleton.

There are four types of bones:

- **Long bones** have hollow shafts that contain a spongy tissue called **marrow**.
- **Short bones** are wider than they are long.
- **Flat bones** are not hollow, but they do contain marrow.
- **Irregular bones** are those with nonsymmetrical shapes.

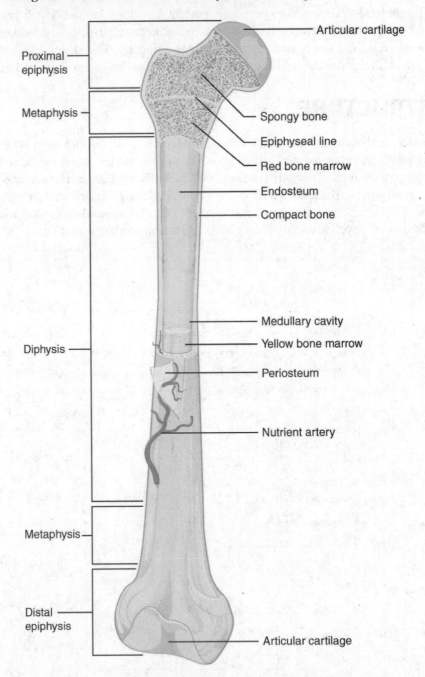

Author: OpenStax College. https://commons.wikimedia.org/wiki/File:603_Anatomy_of_Long_Bone.jpg.

SUPPORT AND MOVEMENT

The skeletal system provides a framework of support for all the organ systems of the body and allows the body to move and function. Some bones are fused together, such as the plates that form the skull. Most bones, however, are joined to other bones by strong fibrous bands called **ligaments**. Ligaments are made up of dense bundles composed of collagenous fibers and spindle-shaped cells called **fibrocytes**. There are two major types of ligaments: **white ligaments**, which have a lot of collagenous fibers and are inelastic, and **yellow ligaments**, which have a lot of elastic fibers and allow elastic movement.

Ligaments connect and hold bones or cartilages together at the joints. The ends of long bones are padded with **cartilage**, which is a smooth elastic tissue that protects the ends of the bones by not allowing them to rub directly together. Cartilage also acts as a structural component of the ear, nose, rib cage, intervertebral discs, bronchial tubes, and many other parts of the body. Most of the major joints also have a fluid-filled sac at the end of each bone to provide a cushion between the bones and the muscles and tendons around a joint. This sac, called a **bursa**, is lined by **synovial tissue** and contains a

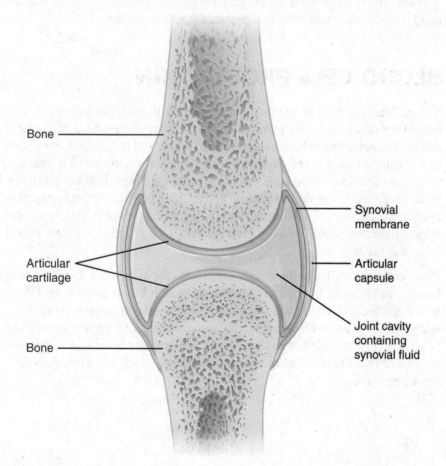

Author: OpenStax College. https://commons.wikimedia.org/wiki/File:907_Synovial _Joints.jpg.

lubricating membrane called the synovial membrane. This structure reduces friction between bones and allows the joint to move freely. Other ligaments attach around or across the ends of bones like bands. They may allow movement or may restrict movement depending on their elasticity.

Another important function of the skeletal system is the interaction between the bones and the muscles. As the muscles contract, **tendons** pull on the bones, thus moving certain parts of the body. Tendons, like ligaments, are also made of inelastic fibrous collagenous tissue. A tendon is connected to muscle fibers at one end and to components of the bone at the other end. These connections are very strong and can withstand tension from pulling and twisting. In fact, tendons have one of the highest tensile strengths of any of the soft tissues.

PROTECTION

The axial skeleton not only provides the framework for vital organs, but it also protects these same organs from injury. The thoracic cage surrounds the heart and lungs and protects them. The heart and lungs are protected by the sternum. The skull protects the brain. The vertebral column, or spine, is made up of 33 individual vertebrae that protect the spinal column.

BLOOD CELL PRODUCTION

The skeletal system has another main function in addition to support and protection: new blood cells are produced inside some bones. Almost all bones contain bone marrow, which has two types: yellow and red. Yellow bone marrow is mainly found in the cavities of long bones. It is composed of inactive cells that can release blood cells in emergency situations. Red bone marrow is mainly found in the skull, shoulder blades, long bones, and flat bones. It is composed of active cells that continuously divide and multiply to develop and release blood cells. Red bone marrow produces red blood cells, white blood cells, and platelets.

Bone cells are called **osteocytes**, and there are two main types: **osteoblasts**, which make bone, and **osteoclasts**, which break down bone. Bone is synthesized within tubular structures called **osteon**, which is made of hydroxyapatite embedded in a matrix of collagen. Each osteon consists of concentric layers called **lamellae**, which are compact bone tissue that surround a central canal called the **haversian canal**, which contains the bone's blood supplies.

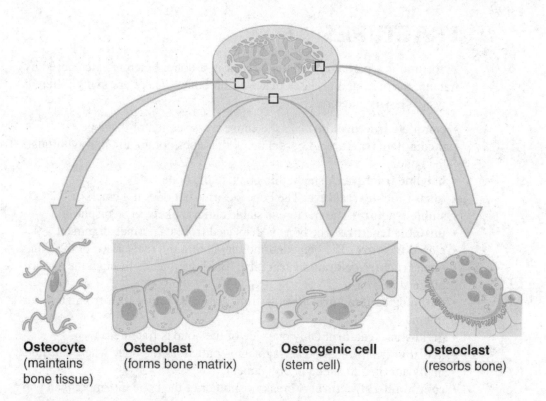

Osteocyte (maintains bone tissue)

Osteoblast (forms bone matrix)

Osteogenic cell (stem cell)

Osteoclast (resorbs bone)

Author: OpenStax College. https://commons.wikimedia.org/wiki/File:604_Bone_cells .jpg.

MINERAL STORAGE AND REGULATION

There is one more function of the skeletal system that you should be aware of: storage and release of minerals. Bones act as reservoirs for several important minerals, especially calcium and phosphorus. The skeletal system helps maintain homeostasis in the body by regulating mineral levels in the blood. For example, when calcium levels in the blood fall, the bones release some of their stored calcium to maintain an adequate level of calcium in the blood for the muscles to function.

FRACTURES

A fracture is a partial or complete break in a bone. Fractures are caused by trauma, overuse, and diseases that weaken bones. There are many different ways to classify fractures:

- **complete fracture:** Involves the entire cross section of the bone.
- **incomplete fracture:** A partial break that does not go all the way through the bone.
- **hairline fracture:** A small, thin crack in the bone.
- **torus (buckle) fracture:** The bone deforms but does not crack.
- **stable fracture:** The fracture is stable and not likely to be displaced.
- **unstable fracture:** The bone is displaced from its normal alignment.
- **closed fracture:** The bone does not break through the surface of the skin.
- **open fracture/compound fracture:** The bone breaks through the surface of the skin.
- **pathological fracture:** Results from a disease rather than from stress or trauma.
- **greenstick fracture:** Only one side of the bone is fractured.
- **avulsion fracture:** A bone fragment is pulled off the bone where it is normally attached to a tendon or ligament.
- **comminuted fracture:** A break or splinter of the bone into more than two fragments.
- **intra-articular fracture:** The break crosses into the surface of a joint, causing damage to the cartilage.
- **transverse fracture:** The fracture goes straight across the bone.
- **longitudinal fracture:** The fracture goes along the length of the bone.
- **oblique fracture:** The fracture goes at an angle across the bone.
- **spiral fracture:** The fracture goes in a twisted pattern around the bone.
- **impacted fracture:** One fragment of the fractured bone is wedged into another fragment.
- **compression (crush) fracture:** The fractured bone collapses; most common in spongy bone.
- **depressed fracture:** Bone fragments are pushed in beyond the surrounding skin.

Bones can also become dislocated. In a **complete dislocation**, the joints are completely separated. In a **subluxation**, the joints are only partially separated.

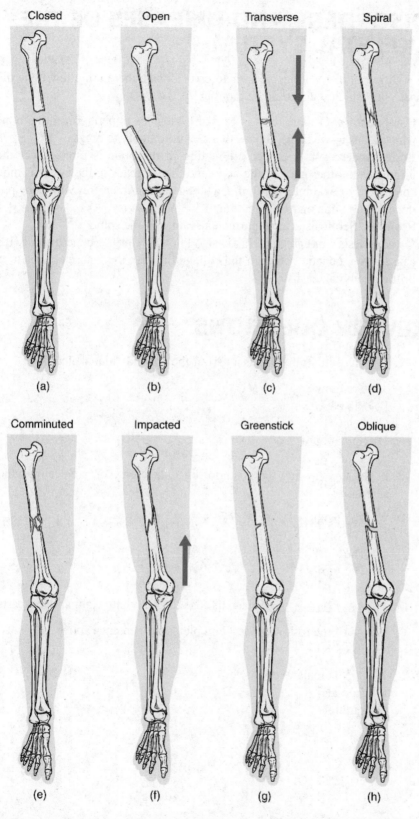

Closed (a)   Open (b)   Transverse (c)   Spiral (d)

Comminuted (e)   Impacted (f)   Greenstick (g)   Oblique (h)

Author: OpenStax College. https://commons.wikimedia.org/wiki/File:612_Types_of _Fractures.jpg.

DISORDERS AND DISEASES OF THE SKELETAL SYSTEM

In addition to dislocations and fractures of bones, there are a few bone diseases with which you should be familiar.

- **Osteoporosis**: Osteoporosis is caused by loss of minerals from the bone, which leads to weakened bones that are more likely to break.
- **Bone cancer:** While cancer originating in the bone is rare, cancer that originates in other parts of the body and then spreads to the bones is more common. For example, **myeloma**, a blood cancer, interferes with bone production and bone marrow function.
- **Scoliosis**: Scoliosis is an abnormal curvature of the spine.
- **Osteogenesis imperfecta**: This is also known as brittle bone disease. It is caused by a genetic defect in the collagen matrix that causes bones to be brittle and break easily.

REVIEW QUESTIONS

1. Which of the following is a part of the appendicular skeleton?

   A) Cranium
   B) Rib cage
   C) Legs
   D) Spinal cord

2. If you are viewing the posterior of a skeleton, you are seeing which side of it?

   A) The front
   B) The back
   C) The side
   D) The top

3. The _____ plane divides the body into right and left parts.

   Which of the following best completes the sentence above?

   A) axial
   B) appendicular
   C) frontal
   D) sagittal

4. Which of the following are functions of the skeletal system? Select all that apply.

   A) To protect internal organs
   B) To regulate levels of calcium in the blood
   C) To add carbon dioxide to the blood
   D) To produce blood cells

5. Bones are attached to other bones by

   A) ligaments
   B) tendons
   C) myosin
   D) flexors

ANSWER KEY

1. C
2. B
3. D
4. A, B, and D
5. A

ANSWERS AND EXPLANATIONS

1. (C) The appendicular portion of the body includes the limbs, which are the legs and arms. The cranium, rib cage, and spinal cord are all part of the axial portion of the body.

2. (B) If you are viewing the posterior of a skeleton, then you are looking at the back of it. The term *anterior* describes the front of the skeleton.

3. (D) The sagittal plane divides the body into right and left parts. The axial portion of the body consists of the head, neck, and torso. The appendicular portion consists of the limbs. The frontal plane divides the body into anterior and posterior parts.

4. (A, B, and D) Adding carbon dioxide to the blood is not a function of the skeletal system. The skeletal system provides support and protection for internal organs, produces blood cells, regulates blood calcium levels, and helps with the movement of the body.

5. (A) Ligaments attach one bone to another. Tendons attach muscles to bone.

CHAPTER 26

The Neuromuscular System

The **neuromuscular system** includes all the muscles in the human body and the nerve system that serve them. The neuromuscular system is responsible for coordinating all movement in the body, such as walking, chewing, and circulating blood. It also controls posture and breathing.

MOVEMENT: THE MUSCULAR SYSTEM

Muscles work with the skeletal system for movement and to provide support and protection for the body. Muscles are made up of bundles of **myofibrils** made of **sarcomere units**. Each sarcomere unit contains long protein filaments: **actin** (thin) and **myosin** (thick). These filaments slide past each other to contract or relax the muscle. There are three types of muscle: smooth, skeletal, and cardiac.

Smooth muscle, also known as **visceral muscle**, is found in the walls of internal organs, such as the stomach, intestines, bladder, uterus, and blood vessels. These muscles contract to help move substances through the organs. Their functions are also controlled by the nervous system and are involuntary. Smooth muscle cells each have one nucleus and contain actin and myosin but are not organized into sarcomere units.

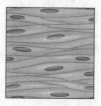

Smooth
muscle

Author: OpenStax College. Portion of full illustration at:
https://commons.wikimedia.org/wiki/File:419_420_421_Table_04_01_updated.jpg.

Skeletal muscle is attached to bone by tendons and provides movement to the body when the muscles pull on the bones. The movement of these muscles is voluntary, meaning that you are able to control them. Each skeletal muscle is made up of thousands of cylindrical **muscle fibers**. These muscle fibers have more than one nucleus and multiple mitochondria to better meet energy needs. They are composed of myofibrils (made of actin and myosin) that repeat in sarcomere units. These alternating light and dark bands form a pattern or striations, so we also call this type of muscle **striated muscle**.

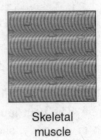

Skeletal
muscle

Author: OpenStax College. Portion of full illustration at: https://commons.wikimedia.org/wiki/File:419_420_421_Table_04_01_updated.jpg.

Skeletal muscles function with two opposing skeletal muscles working together to move bones. A **flexor** contracts to bring two bones closer together, and an **extensor** contracts to straighten the two bones. When the extensor contracts to straighten the two bones, the flexor relaxes. When a flexor contracts, the extensor relaxes.

The **origin** of a muscle is the location on the immobile bone where the muscle is connected. The **attachment** of the muscle to the mobile bone is called the **insertion**. Muscle groups are identified by several different characteristics, such as size, location, number of origins and insertions, and functions of the muscles.

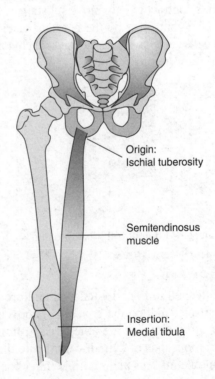

Origin:
Ischial tuberosity

Semitendinosus
muscle

Insertion:
Medial tibula

Cardiac muscle makes up the walls of the heart. Cardiac muscle contracts the heart to pump blood from the heart to the entire body. These muscles are controlled by the nervous system, and their functions are involuntary. Like skeletal muscle tissue, cardiac muscle tissue is striated.

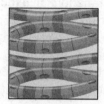

Cardiac
muscle

Author: OpenStax College. Portion of full illustration at: https://commons.wikimedia.org/wiki/File:419_420_421_Table_04_01_updated.jpg.

COORDINATION: THE NERVOUS SYSTEM

The **nervous system** coordinates the tasks of all the systems of the body. It consists of the brain, spinal cord, and nerves. It regulates the body by responding to different **stimuli**, changes that occur both inside and outside of the body. It is also the source of all mental activity, such as learning and thought.

The nervous system is divided into two main subparts: the **central nervous system (CNS)** and the **peripheral nervous system (PNS)**. The CNS contains the brain and spinal cord, which read information and decide on a correct response. The PNS consists of nerves that transmit messages to and from the CNS. The peripheral nervous system can be divided even further into the **somatic** and **autonomic** systems. The somatic system responds to outside changes, while the autonomic system regulates internal changes. The somatic system is under voluntary control and directs the skeletal muscles. The autonomic system is involuntary and is divided into the **sympathetic division** and the **parasympathetic division**. The sympathetic division directs the "fight or flight" responses, while the parasympathetic division directs "rest and digest" or "feed and breed" responses by slowing down muscle and gland activity. The nervous system also carries out reflex actions.

Neurons

Both the PNS and the CNS contain two types of **neurons**, special cells that receive and transmit chemical signals to the brain. **Afferent** or **sensory neurons** convey information from receptors in the body to the CNS. **Efferent** or **motor neurons** then bring information from the CNS back to the appropriate effectors in the body. Most of the larger nerves consist of both afferent and efferent nerve fibers.

The basic structural and functional units of the nervous system are cells called neurons. The neuron, pictured below, consists of a main cell body or **soma**, the center of which is the nucleus. Stemming off the cell body are **dendrites**, which receive neural impulses and convey them to the cell body. After receiving this information, an **axon** will transmit the message to another neuron. In some neurons, the axon is covered by a **myelin sheath**, which acts as an insulator to allow for electrical impulses to transmit into the cell. The ends of the axons are **synaptic terminals** where the electrical impulses are converted into chemical messages in the form of **neurotransmitters**. Neurons do not come into contact with one another. There is a gap between the synaptic terminals of one neuron and the dendrites of another that we call a **synapse**.

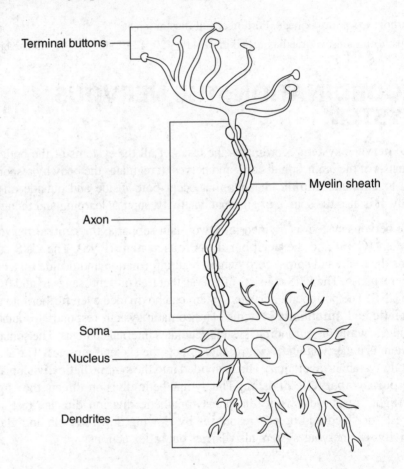

Neurons are different from nerves. A nerve is a bundle of axons wrapped in a tough connective tissue that provides a structured path for electrochemical nerve impulses to be transmitted throughout the body. Nerves are only found in the PNS.

To form a nerve, axons are bundled together into a group called a fascicle, which is wrapped in a layer of connective tissue called the **perineurium**. A strong dense outer covering of irregular connective tissue called the **epineurium** protects the nerve.

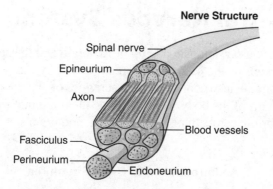

Nerve Structure

Spinal nerve

Epineurium

Axon

Blood vessels

Fasciculus

Perineurium

Endoneurium

Based on an illustration by the U.S. government: https://commons.wikimedia.org/wiki/File:Illu_nerve_structure.jpg.

Resting and Acting Potential

When a neuron is not conducting a signal, it is said to have **resting potential**. Resting potential results from an imbalance of ions on either side of the cell membrane. There are more positive ions than negative ions on the outside of the neuron's cell membrane. Inside the cell, there are more negative ions than positive ions.

To transmit a message, the resting potential must be disrupted by and changed to an **action potential**. The neuron depolarizes so that the outside of the cell membrane has more negative ions than positive ions and the inside of the cell has more positive ions than negative ions. When a neuron receives a signal, the impulse travels through the dendrite into the body of the cell and then flows along the axon. Then the concentration of ions returns to the state of resting potential. If another signal arrives while the neuron is in action potential, the neuron cannot transmit the impulse until after the neuron returns to resting potential. This period when the neuron cannot process a second signal is called the **refractory period**.

Once an impulse has traveled across one neuron, chemical messengers called **neurotransmitters** carry the impulse across the synapse between neurons to the dendrites of another neuron, which can then enter action potential and pass along the signal. After the neurotransmitters cross the synapse, they are destroyed so that the first neuron can return to resting potential. Not all neurotransmitters stimulate neurons. Some actually inhibit a neuron from firing by raising the action potential necessary.

Some neurons, such as large muscle command neurons, can conduct impulses faster than others. The average speed for a neuron to conduct a signal is about 100 miles per hour. The fastest can transmit at nearly 270 miles per hour! The axons of these large neurons are wrapped in a myelin sheath that has gaps called **nodes of Ranvier**. When an impulse moves from the cell body of the neuron across the axon, it can jump across the nodes of Ranvier and travel faster. This allows our muscles to react faster.

The Central Nervous System

The central nervous system is made up of the brain and the spinal cord. The brain processes all of the sensory information sent by the body, as well as conscious thought. It also coordinates the activities of all the skeletal muscles and organ systems of the body. We can divide the brain into four main structures: the cerebrum, cerebellum, diencephalon, and brain stem.

An Introduction to Brain Structures

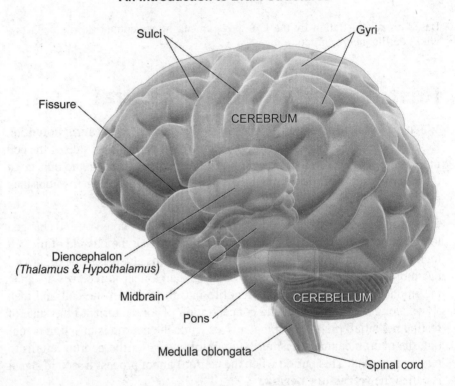

Author: BruceBlaus. https://commons.wikimedia.org/wiki/File:Blausen_0115 _BrainStructures.png.

The **cerebrum** has many diverse functions, including initiating and coordinating movement, processing sensory input, controlling memory and emotion, and governing learning, reasoning, and problem solving.

The cerebrum can be divided into two hemispheres: the left side is in charge of language and analytical thinking, while the right side is in charge of spatial and pattern recognition. These hemispheres are joined by the corpus callosum, which integrates the functions of the two hemispheres. The outer tissue of the cerebellum is called the **cerebral cortex**.

The cerebrum can be further divided into four lobes: the frontal, parietal, occipital, and temporal. The **frontal lobe** is located at the upper front of the brain. It controls higher-level thinking and behavior, such as planning, judgment and decision making, and attention and impulse control. The **parietal lobe** is located behind the frontal lobe. It processes sensory information. The **occipital lobe** is located at the back of the brain. It processes visual input from the eyes. The **temporal lobe** is located at the lower front of the brain. It controls language, visual memory, and emotion.

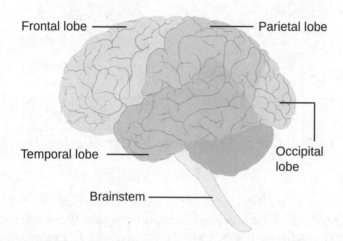

Author: Cancer Research UK. https://commons.wikimedia.org/wiki/File:Diagram
_showing_the_lobes_of_the_brain_CRUK_308.svg.

The **cerebellum** is located at the base of the brain, behind the brain stem. Like the cerebrum, it can be divided into two hemispheres. About half of the neurons in the brain are contained in the cerebellum. The cerebellum controls sensorimotor coordination, balance, posture, complex muscle movements, and speech.

The **diencephalon** is located at the posterior of the forebrain, between the brain stem and the cerebral cortex. It is composed of four parts: the thalamus, hypothalamus, epithalamus, and subthalamus. The **thalamus** routes incoming sensory information to the appropriate parts of the cerebrum. It also regulates motor function and controls the sleep cycle. The **hypothalamus** works with the endocrine system to control many autonomic functions through the release of hormones. It also maintains homeostasis, including body temperature and blood pressure. The pituitary gland is located in the hypothalamus. The **epithalamus** controls the sense of smell and helps regulate the sleep and wake cycle. The pineal gland is located in the epithalamus. The **subthalamus** is interconnected with the cerebrum and is largely responsible for movement.

The **brain stem** connects the brain to the spinal cord. It is composed of the midbrain, pons, and medulla oblongata (or medulla).

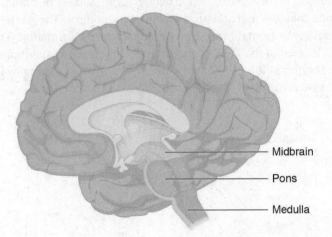

Midbrain

Pons

Medulla

Author: OpenStax College. https://commons.wikimedia.org/wiki/File:1311_Brain_Stem.jpg.

The **midbrain** is involved in motor movement, especially of the eye, and in visual and auditory processing. The **pons** connects the cerebral cortex to the medulla oblongata. It aids with many autonomic and sensory functions, including regulating sleep, respiratory processes, and fine motor control. The **medulla oblongata** transmits signals between the spinal cord and the brain. It controls autonomic activities such as circulation and respiration.

DISORDERS AND DISEASES OF THE NEUROMUSCULAR SYSTEM

There are many diseases of the nervous system, so let's categorize them into types:

- myopathies: These are problems with the muscles, the most well-known of which is **muscular dystrophy**.
- neuropathies: These are problems with the nerves, such as **Parkinson's disease**, **Charcot-Marie-Tooth disease**, and **motor neuron disease**.
- neuromuscular autoimmune conditions: These are neuromuscular system problems that also involve the immune system, such as **multiple sclerosis** or **myasthenia gravis**.
- dementia: This is a group of conditions characterized by impairment of more than one brain function. The most well-known type is **Alzheimer's disease**.
- **cerebral palsy**: This is a group of disorders that affect muscle movement and coordination.

REVIEW QUESTIONS

1. What is the main function of the nervous system?

   A) It regulates the body's movement.
   B) It maintains homeostasis in the body.
   C) It breaks down the food we eat through digestion.
   D) It coordinates the body's responses to different stimuli.

2. Which human muscle types are classified as involuntary? Select all that apply.

   A) Skeletal
   B) Smooth
   C) Cardiac

3. Which part of the brain is responsible for coordinating movement and balance?

   A) Spinal cord
   B) Cerebellum
   C) Brain stem
   D) Cerebrum

4. Which of the following controls the "fight or flight" response?

   A) Central nervous system
   B) Somatic nervous system
   C) Autonomic nervous system
   D) Enteric nervous system

5. Which of the following is a function of the central nervous system?

   A) Controlling the gastrointestinal system
   B) Controlling skeletal muscles
   C) Regulating blood pressure
   D) Storing information

ANSWER KEY

1. D	**3.** B	**5.** D
2. B and C	**4.** C	

ANSWERS AND EXPLANATIONS

1. (D) The main function of the nervous system is to coordinate the body's responses to different stimuli. The nervous system acts a regulator for the body by responding to stimuli through receptors.

2. (B and C) Skeletal muscles are classified as voluntary because we can consciously control them. Smooth and cardiac muscles are involuntary because we do not consciously control them.

3. (B) The cerebellum coordinates movement and balance.

4. (C) The sympathetic division of the autonomic nervous system is responsible for the "fight or flight" response. The autonomic nervous system is a subsystem of the peripheral nervous system, not the central nervous system.

5. (D) Information is stored by the brain, which is a part of the central nervous system.

CHAPTER 27

The Endocrine System

Working closely with the neuromuscular system to maintain balance in the body, the **endocrine system** helps to regulate the various endocrine glands and hormone production. The hypothalamus in the brain is the main link between the endocrine and nervous systems. Unlike the nervous system, which uses both electrical and chemical signals, the endocrine system uses only chemical signals. **Endocrine glands** are organs that secrete chemicals called **hormones**. The hormones are then transported throughout the body primarily through the bloodstream using the circulatory system. Once the hormones reach their destination, they bind to receptors on the **target cells**—the particular cells they are meant to act upon. The hormones produce a particular reaction in the target cells, depending on the function of those hormones. This process requires more time than the firing of a neuron, though the exact amount of time varies among the different hormones.

REGULATING HORMONES

The endocrine system is responsible for regulating hormones, which are transmitted to maintain homeostasis in the body. If the gland producing the hormone receives feedback from a system, the gland can respond appropriately by increasing or decreasing the production of that hormone. Some hormones have opposite partners—one hormone increases a function while a different hormone decreases a function. These are called **counterregulatory hormones**. For example, if the level of glucose in the blood gets too high, the hormone insulin is released to lower blood sugar. If the level of glucose in the blood gets too low, the hormone glucagon is released to raise it back up to homeostasis.

Hormones can be classified into three groups: peptide hormones, amino acid–derived hormones, and lipid-derived hormones.

- **Peptide hormones** are short chains of amino acids or small proteins. They are water soluble and cannot pass through a cell membrane, so their receptors are on the outside of cell membranes. Peptide hormones include oxytocin, antidiuretic hormone, growth hormone, follicle-stimulating hormone, and insulin.
- **Amino acid–derived hormones** are small molecules derived from the amino acids tryptophan and tyrosine. They are also water soluble and cannot pass through a cell membrane, so their receptors are on the outside of cell membranes. Amino acid–derived hormones include melatonin, thyroxine, epinephrine, and norepinephrine.

- **Lipid-derived hormones** (primarily steroid hormones) are derived from cholesterol and are usually ketones or alcohols. Lipid molecules are insoluble in water and can diffuse across a cell membrane, since the cell membrane also contains lipids. Once they enter the cell, they bind to a cytoplasmic receptor and move into the nucleus, where they interact with DNA to activate certain genes. This process typically takes longer than the action of peptide or amino acid–derived hormones, but the effects of lipid-derived hormones last longer. Lipid-derived hormones include estradiol, testosterone, aldosterone, and cortisol.

REGULATING ENDOCRINE GLANDS

The endocrine system is also responsible for regulating the endocrine glands. There are several different endocrine glands located throughout the body.

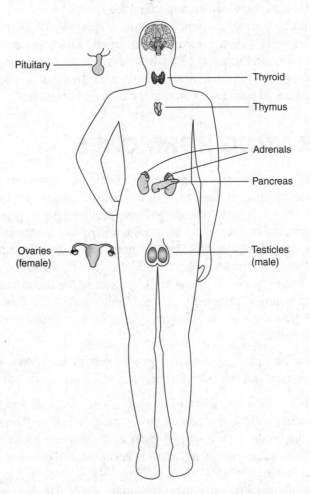

- The **pituitary gland** is controlled by the **hypothalamus** in the brain and is responsible for much of the system's regulatory function. In fact, the pituitary gland controls the functions of many other endocrine glands. One particularly important hormone it produces is growth hormone. It also produces several hormones involved in reproduction and development.

- The **pineal gland** is responsible for the hormone melatonin, which influences the sleep cycle.
- The **thyroid gland**, located in the neck, produces hormones for regular growth and metabolic rate.
- The **parathyroid gland** is attached to the thyroid gland. It produces a hormone that regulates levels of calcium and phosphate in the bones and blood.
- The **adrenal glands**, located on the kidneys, regulate metabolism and help the body deal with stress. They produce the hormone epinephrine, which is responsible for the "fight or flight" response.
- The **pancreatic gland** secretes digestive enzymes that help break down food in the body. It also produces two hormones that regulate blood sugar: insulin and glucagon.
- The **gonads** produce sex hormones in the body. They consist of the ovaries for women and the testes for men.

This chart shows the endocrine glands, their major hormones, and the functions of those hormones.

Gland	Hormone	Function
Anterior pituitary gland	Growth hormone (GH)	Promotes growth in muscles, bone, and cartilage
Anterior pituitary gland	Thyroid-stimulating hormone (TSH)	Stimulates the release of thyroid hormone
Anterior pituitary gland	Adrenocorticotropic hormone (ACTH)	Stimulates release of hormones by the adrenal cortex
Anterior pituitary gland	Endorphins	Activate the body's opiate receptors, which reduces the perception of pain
Anterior pituitary gland	Follicle-stimulating hormone (FSH)	In women, stimulates the secretion of estrogen and helps in egg production. In men, FSH is involved in sperm production.
Anterior pituitary gland	Prolactin (PRL)	Promotes milk production
Anterior pituitary gland	Luteinizing hormone (LH)	In women, stimulates estrogen and progesterone production and causes ovulation. In men, LH is involved in secreting testosterone.
Posterior pituitary gland	Antidiuretic hormone (ADH)	Stimulates water reabsorption by the kidneys and decreases urine volume
Posterior pituitary gland	Oxytocin (OT)	Stimulates uterine contractions during labor; stimulates milk ejection
Thyroid	Thyroxine (T_4) Triiodothyronine (T_3)	Stimulates basal metabolic rate
Thyroid	Calcitonin	Reduces blood calcium levels

Gland	Hormone	Function
Parathyroid	Parathyroid hormone (PTH)	Increases blood calcium levels
Adrenal (cortex)	Aldosterone	Increases blood sodium levels
Adrenal (cortex)	Cortisol Cortisone Corticosterone	Increases blood glucose levels
Adrenal (medulla)	Epinephrine Norepinephrine	Stimulates "fight or flight" response
Pineal	Melatonin	Influences patterns such as sleep, fertility, and aging
Thymus	Thymopoietin	Stimulates maturation of certain white blood cells (T-cells)
Thymus	Thymosin	Stimulates maturation of certain white blood cells (T-cells)
Pancreas	Insulin	Increases blood glucose levels
Pancreas	Glucagon	Decreases blood glucose levels
Ovaries	Estrogen	Stimulates development of female secondary sex characteristics, follicle development, and pregnancy
Ovaries	Progesterone	Prepares body for childbirth
Testes	Testosterone	Stimulates development of male secondary sex characteristics and sperm production

DISORDERS AND DISEASES OF THE ENDOCRINE SYSTEM

There are many endocrine system disorders since there are so many different endocrine glands. You should be familiar with some of the most common disorders.

- **Diabetes**: Diabetes results when the pancreas does not produce enough insulin. As a result, glucose remains in the blood instead of being transported to the cells. Type 1 diabetes, also known as juvenile diabetes, is a chronic condition in which the pancreas produces little or no insulin. Type 2 diabetes, also known as adult-onset diabetes, is a condition in which the body does not respond to insulin as well as it should and over time the pancreas may reduce or stop producing insulin.
- Thyroid disorders: These include **hypothyroidism** (low thyroid hormone levels), **hyperthyroidism** (high thyroid hormone levels), **Graves' disease** (a type of hyperthyroidism resulting in excessive thyroid hormone

production), **Hashimoto's thyroiditis** (an autoimmune disease resulting in hypothyroidism), and thyroid cancer.

- **Polycystic ovary syndrome** (PCOS): PCOS causes enlarged ovaries that contain small cysts that interfere with fertility and the menstrual cycle.
- Pituitary disorders: These include **diabetes insipidus**, **acromegaly**, and **gigantism**.
- **Addison's disease**: Addison's disease is caused by decreased production of cortisol and aldosterone due to adrenal gland damage.
- **Cushing's syndrome**: Cushing's syndrome is caused by the adrenal glands producing abnormally high levels of cortisol.

REVIEW QUESTIONS

1. Which of the following are chemical messengers produced by the endocrine glands?

   A) Hormones
   B) Sperm cells
   C) White blood cells
   D) Antigens

2. Much of the endocrine system's activity is controlled by the _____.

   A) pineal gland
   B) aorta
   C) spinal cord
   D) hypothalamus

3. Which of the following controls daily rhythm cycles?

   A) Adrenal gland
   B) Parathyroid
   C) Pineal gland
   D) Pancreas

4. Which of the following regulates the levels of calcium in the blood?

   A) Parathyroid hormone
   B) Estrogen
   C) Oxytocin
   D) Melatonin

5. The _____ gland is located on the kidney.

   A) thyroid
   B) adrenal
   C) pineal
   D) pituitary

ANSWER KEY

1. A	**3.** C	**5.** B
2. D	**4.** A	

ANSWERS AND EXPLANATIONS

1. (A) Hormones are the chemical messengers produced by the endocrine glands. Hormones are used to regulate many body functions.

2. (D) The hypothalamus controls much of the endocrine system's functions, including maintaining fluid balance, regulating body temperature, influencing sexual behavior, and acting as the link between the nervous and endocrine systems.

3. (C) The pineal gland controls day/night rhythms.

4. (A) Parathyroid hormone regulates the level of calcium in the blood.

5. (B) The adrenal gland is located on the kidney. The root word *renal* refers to the kidney.

CHAPTER 28

The Cardiovascular System

The **cardiovascular system**, or **circulatory system**, transports blood pumped from the heart throughout the entire body. The cardiovascular system works closely with several other body systems:

- Respiratory system: The cardiovascular system carries oxygen and eliminates carbon dioxide; assists with regulating blood pH.
- Genitourinary system: The cardiovascular system filters blood; removes nitrogenous waste; regulates blood volume; regulates blood pressure; regulates blood pH.
- Digestive system: The cardiovascular system picks up nutrients and distributes them throughout the body.

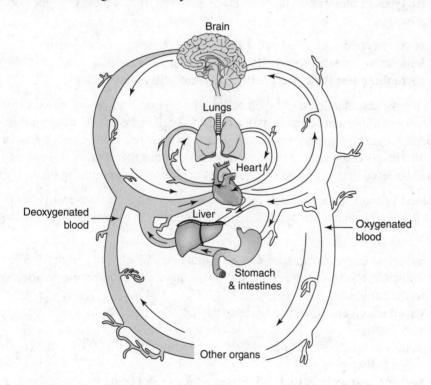

TRANSPORT: BLOOD

Blood is a connective tissue that is carried through various **blood vessels** and transports vital nutrients, oxygen, water, ions, and hormones to help maintain the body's homeostasis. Blood removes carbon dioxide and waste from the cells and carries it to the appropriate areas for elimination. Blood also fights infection and regulates temperature.

Blood is mostly liquid and is composed of blood cells and blood plasma. **Blood plasma** makes up approximately 55% of blood volume. Plasma is primarily made up of water, and the amount of water can be adjusted with the help of the kidneys in order to adjust the volume of blood in the body, which adjusts blood pressure. More water equals more blood volume and thus higher blood pressure. Less water equals less blood volume and thus lower blood pressure. The function of plasma is to take nutrients, proteins, and hormones to the parts of the body that need them, and to remove waste products from the body.

Approximately 45% of blood volume is composed of **blood cells**. There are three types of blood cells, all of which are derived from stem cells in the bone marrow:

- **erythrocytes:** Red blood cells, which carry oxygen to the tissues
- **leukocytes:** White blood cells, which fight infections
- **thrombocytes:** Platelets, smaller cells that help blood to clot

The most abundant type of blood cells is the erythrocytes, or red blood cells. The most important component of a red blood cell is the protein **hemoglobin**. Hemoglobin transports oxygen and gives blood its red color. Leukocytes, or white blood cells, have important functions within the immune system and will be discussed in greater detail in the chapter on the immune system.

Blood is transported through blood vessels, and there are several types of blood vessels that work in conjunction with the heart to provide blood to the body:

- **arteries:** Large, thick, elastic vessels that carry blood away from the heart
- **arterioles:** Smaller vessels that narrow as they carry blood from the arteries to the capillaries
- **capillaries:** The smallest vessels that serve as the site of gas exchange within tissues
- **venules:** Small vessels that widen as they bring the blood from the capillaries to the veins
- **veins:** Large vessels (not as thick as arteries) that bring the blood back to the heart

These vessels form a network that carries the blood pumped from the heart to the body's tissues and then back to the heart again. We call this system the circulatory system.

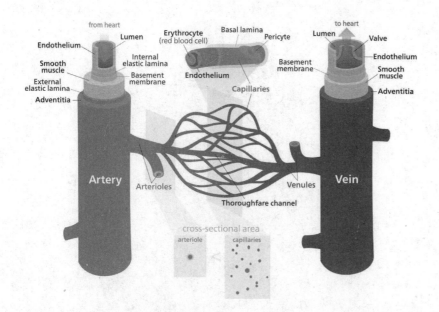

Author: Kelvinsong. Modified by Begoon. https://en.wikipedia.org/wiki/Blood_vessel.

CIRCULATION: THE HEART

The heart is the major organ relevant to the circulatory system. It consists of four chambers and two circulatory systems. **Pulmonary circulation** is the flow of blood between the heart and lungs. In pulmonary circulation, oxygen-poor blood coming from the body enters the **right atrium** of the heart through two large veins, the **inferior** and **superior vena cava**. This deoxygenated blood is high in carbon dioxide and is purplish in color. After entering through the right atrium, it is pumped by the **right ventricle** out through the **pulmonary artery** to the lungs to receive oxygen. The pulmonary artery splits to send a branch to each lung. In the lungs, the blood exchanges carbon dioxide for oxygen. The oxygenated blood leaves the lungs through **pulmonary veins** and returns to the heart, where it enters the **left atrium** and then the **left ventricle** and is then sent back out to the body through the **aorta**. The process of delivering oxygen-rich blood to the rest of the body is called **systemic circulation**.

The left and right sides of the heart are separated by a membrane called the **septum**, which keeps the flow of oxygenated and deoxygenated blood separate. The heart also has four one-way valves between chambers to keep the blood from backflowing.

- **Mitral valve**: Between the left atrium and left ventricle
- **Tricuspid valve**: Between the right atrium and right ventricle
- **Aortic valve**: Between the left ventricle and aorta
- **Pulmonic or pulmonary valve**: Between the right ventricle and pulmonary artery

The heart has its own system of blood vessels that specifically circulates blood for its own function. This system is called the **coronary system**.

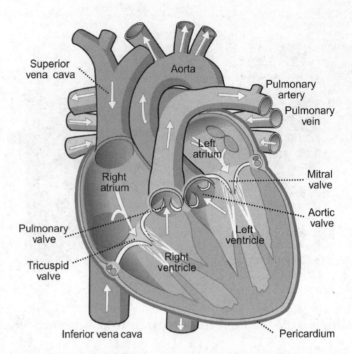

Author: Wapcaplet. https://commons.wikimedia.org/wiki/File:Diagram_of_the _human_heart_(cropped).svg.

The **cardiac cycle** is the process of one heartbeat: the heart contracts and blood is forced out; then it relaxes and the heart fills with blood. The stage of contraction is called **systole**, and the stage of relaxation is called **diastole**.

DISORDERS AND DISEASES OF THE CARDIOVASCULAR SYSTEM

The most common disorders of the cardiovascular system include:

- **coronary artery disease (CAD):** CAD is characterized by atherosclerosis, a hardening and narrowing of the coronary arteries, which produces blood vessel blockages. Atherosclerosis is usually the cause of heart attack, stroke, and peripheral vascular disease.
- **hypertension:** High blood pressure.
- **hypotension:** Low blood pressure.
- **arrhythmia:** An arrhythmia is any change in the normal sequence of the heartbeat, whether too fast, too slow, or irregular. When the heart doesn't beat normally, it can't pump blood effectively.
- **myocardial infarction:** A heart attack.
- **heart failure:** Heart failure occurs when the heart's ability to pump blood is weak and the blood moves slower. This causes the pressure in the heart to increase, and the heart cannot supply enough oxygen to the cells.
- **congenital heart defect:** These defects, such as a leaky heart valve or a hole in the heart, are the result of abnormalities in fetal development.

• **Cardiomyopathy:** Cardiomyopathy, also known as heart muscle disease, is a progressive disease that causes the heart to become abnormally enlarged, thickened, and/or stiffened, which inhibits the heart's ability to pump blood effectively.

REVIEW QUESTIONS

1. The right atrium in the heart receives what kind of blood?

A) Oxygen-rich blood from the left ventricle
B) Oxygen-poor blood from the tissues
C) Oxygen-rich blood from the right ventricle
D) Oxygen-poor blood from the left atrium

2. Which blood vessel carries oxygenated blood from the lungs to the heart?

A) Pulmonary artery
B) Pulmonary vein
C) Carotid artery
D) Subclavian vein

3. An arrhythmia is most likely to result in _____.

A) an irregular heart beat
B) low blood pressure
C) high blood pressure
D) blocked arteries

4. Where are materials exchanged between the blood and the tissues?

A) Bronchioles
B) Leukocytes
C) Capillaries
D) Alveoli

5. Which of the following statements are true about the circulatory system? Select all that apply.

A) Capillaries connect venules and bronchi.
B) Arteries generally have thicker walls than do veins.
C) The left side of the heart sends deoxygenated blood to the lungs.
D) Veins can prevent blood from backflowing.

ANSWER KEY

1. B

2. B

3. A

4. C

5. B and D

ANSWERS AND EXPLANATIONS

1. (B) The right atrium receives oxygen-poor blood from the tissues. It is the first of the four chambers to receive blood from the body. After the blood leaves the right atrium, it travels to the right ventricle and to the lungs and so on, until it leaves the heart through systemic circulation and travels through the body.

2. (B) The pulmonary vein carries oxygenated blood from the lungs to the left atrium.

3. (A) An arrhythmia is an irregular change in heartbeat.

4. (C) Capillaries allow oxygen, nutrients, and waste to be exchanged between the blood and the tissues.

5. (B and D) Veins have valves that prevent blood from backflowing, and veins generally have thinner walls than do arteries.

CHAPTER 29

The Respiratory System

The **respiratory system** works closely with the cardiovascular system. In the last chapter, we looked at how blood flows between the heart and the lungs to assist with the exchange of oxygen and carbon dioxide. The respiratory system brings oxygen from the air into the lungs and releases carbon dioxide from the lungs.

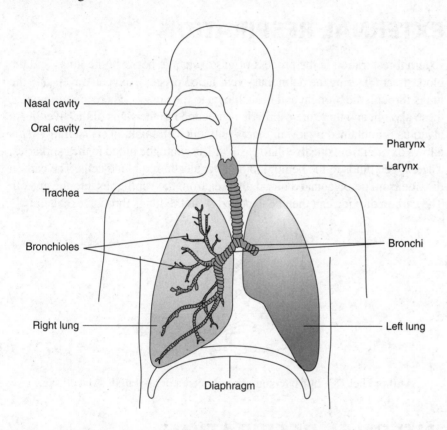

PULMONARY VENTILATION

Pulmonary ventilation is the movement of air into and out of the lungs. **Inspiration** is the process of air coming in, while **expiration** involves air flowing out. The ventilation process begins with air entering the body through the nose or mouth and then traveling through the **pharynx**, which is an area at the back of the throat behind the mouth and nasal cavity. Next, the air flows down the windpipe, or **trachea**, and divides into two **bronchi**, with one going into each lung. Each bronchus breaks down into smaller and smaller **bronchioles** within the lungs, forming a bronchial tree. Bronchioles terminate in alveoli, which are like tiny air sacs. This is where oxygen and carbon dioxide are exchanged between the respiratory system and the cardiovascular system. The **upper respiratory system** consists of the nose and **nares** (nostrils), the pharynx, and the larynx. The **lower respiratory system** consists of the trachea, bronchi, bronchioles, lungs, and alveoli.

The neuromuscular system aids in the pulmonary ventilation process. The movement of air into the lungs is the result of the diaphragm muscle that runs beneath the lungs moving downward and creating a vacuum. This causes air to flow into the lungs to fill the space and expand the lungs. The air is pushed back out by the diaphragm moving upward. The skeletal system is also involved since the ribs protect the lungs.

EXTERNAL RESPIRATION

External respiration is the process of gas exchange between the lungs and the bloodstream. During the pulmonary ventilation process, oxygen travels into the lungs through the bronchi and bronchioles to the alveoli. There are millions of these **alveoli**, and there are capillaries embedded in the walls of the alveoli. An alveolus is contained by a wall that is only one cell thick, like a capillary. This allows oxygen from the alveoli to easily diffuse into the blood in the capillaries. The oxygen binds to the hemoglobin molecules in red blood cells. The carbon dioxide from deoxygenated blood diffuses from the capillaries into the alveoli. The carbon dioxide can then be expelled from the lungs through exhalation.

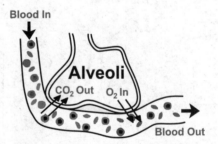

Author: helix84. https://commons.wikimedia.org/wiki/File:Alveoli.svg.

INTERNAL RESPIRATION

Internal respiration is the process of gas exchange between the bloodstream and the tissues of the body. After the lungs have absorbed oxygen from the air and diffused the oxygen into the pulmonary capillaries, the red blood cells in the capillaries carry the oxygen through the vasculature all over the body. When the oxygenated blood reaches the capillaries of body tissues, the red blood cells release the oxygen to diffuse through the capillary walls into the tissues. At the same time, carbon dioxide from the body tissues diffuses through the capillary walls into the bloodstream, where it can be carried back to the lungs to be expelled from the body.

OTHER FUNCTIONS OF THE RESPIRATORY SYSTEM

There are a few other important functions of the respiratory system with which you should be familiar.

- Cellular respiration: The respiratory system works with the cardiovascular system and digestive system to perform **cellular respiration**. Cellular respiration is the process that provides nutrients to cells for energy production and removes carbon dioxide wastes from the cells.
- Regulating pH: Carbon dioxide levels play an important role in maintaining the acid-base balance of the body, known as pH balance.
- Vocal communication: The pharynx has two passageways, the esophagus and the larynx. The **larynx** is made of cartilage and vocal cords that produce sound when they vibrate, which is why it is also called the voice box.
- Olfaction: The respiratory system works with the neuromuscular system to perform **olfaction**, commonly known as smelling. Chemicals in the air we breathe bind to and activate nervous system receptors on the tiny hairs, or **cilia**, of the nasal passages. The neurons send a signal to the olfactory area of the cerebral cortex.
- Protection from infection: Particles in the air can damage the lungs or trigger allergic responses. In order to trap these particles, the nasal cavity has cilia and mucus, the lungs produce mucus, and the bronchi and bronchioles have cilia.

DISORDERS AND DISEASES OF THE RESPIRATORY SYSTEM

In addition to lung problems caused by viruses and cancer, there are some diseases and disorders with which you should be familiar.

- **Pneumonia**: An infection that inflames the air sacs in one or both lungs.
- **Emphysema**: A lung condition characterized by the inability to expel air from the alveoli that causes shortness of breath.
- **Bronchitis/bronchiolitis**: An infection that causes inflammation of the bronchi or bronchioles.
- **Asthma**: When the bronchi become chronically inflamed, they narrow and spasm, causing asthma.
- **Chronic obstructive pulmonary disease (COPD)**: COPD is an inability to exhale normally. Emphysema and bronchitis are forms of COPD.
- **Laryngitis/pharyngitis**: An infection that causes inflammation of the larynx or pharynx.
- **Cystic fibrosis**: This is a genetic disorder that causes poor mucus clearance from the lungs, resulting in difficulty breathing and frequent infections.
- **Tuberculosis**: An infectious bacterial disease that mainly affects the lungs.

REVIEW QUESTIONS

1. Which of the following is NOT a body part involved in the respiratory system?

   A) Trachea
   B) Lungs
   C) Bronchial tree
   D) Ovaries

2. Which part of the brain controls the rate of ventilation?

   A) Hippocampus
   B) Medulla oblongata
   C) Hypothalamus
   D) Amygdala

3. The exchange of gases takes place across the _____.

   A) bronchioles
   B) pleura
   C) capillaries
   D) nasal cavity

4. The movement of air through the respiratory system depends on which of the following?

   A) Movements of the diaphragm
   B) Contractions of the muscles in the trachea
   C) Cilia within the respiratory tract pushing air in and out
   D) The pleura pushing air out of the body

5. What path does air follow when it enters the body through the nose or mouth? Put the following in order from first (1) to last (5).

   _____ Alveoli
   _____ Bronchi
   _____ Trachea
   _____ Bronchioles
   _____ Pharynx

ANSWER KEY

1. D   3. C   5. 5, 3, 2, 4, 1
2. B   4. A

ANSWERS AND EXPLANATIONS

1. (D) The ovaries are part of the female reproductive system. The trachea, lungs, and bronchial tree are all part of the respiratory system.

2. (B) The medulla oblongata is the part of the brain responsible for respiration, circulation, and other autonomic functions. It helps regulate breathing, heart and blood vessel function, and digestion.

3. (C) Capillaries have very thin walls, which allow oxygen to pass from the alveoli to the blood and carbon dioxide to pass from the blood to the alveoli.

4. (A) The movement of the diaphragm creates suction in the chest, which draws in air and expands the lungs. When the diaphragm relaxes and moves up, it pushes air out of the lungs.

5. (5, 3, 2, 4, 1) After air enters through the nose or mouth, it passes through the pharynx, then the trachea, the bronchi, the bronchioles, and then the alveoli where gas exchange takes place.

CHAPTER 30

The Digestive System

The **digestive tract**, or **gastrointestinal (GI) tract**, is about eight to nine meters long and begins with the mouth, where food enters, and ends at the anus, where waste is eliminated. In between, the GI tract is made up of various organs through which food passes and is broken down. The sequence of the GI tract includes the mouth, throat, esophagus, stomach, small intestine, and large intestine. Most digestion takes place in the small intestine.

The digestive system involves a series of processes that break down the food we eat into structures that can be delivered and then used by the cells. Food is first ingested into the mouth, chewed, and then swallowed. Next, food is digested through **mechanical digestion**, the physical breakdown of food through chewing and mixing movements in the stomach. **Chemical digestion** breaks food down further through the use of enzymes so that the nutrients can be absorbed. The **absorption** process transports the digested food through the intestine into the circulatory system. Lastly, undigested food is **eliminated** from the body.

The numbered diagram below shows the order in which food passes through different parts of the body in the process of digestion.

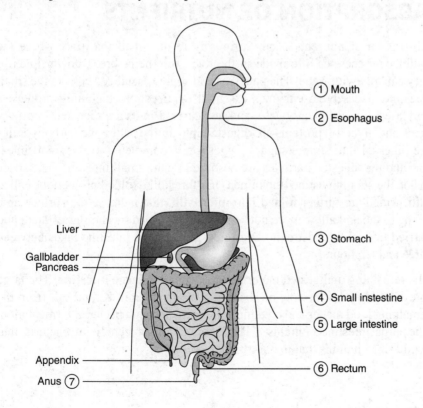

MECHANICAL AND CHEMICAL DIGESTION

The process of mechanical and chemical digestion begins in the mouth, where the salivary glands secrete **saliva** as food is chewed and broken down. Enzymes such as **lipase** and **amylase** in the saliva begin the chemical digestion of lipids and starches. The partially digested food mixed with saliva, called a **bolus**, then passes to the pharynx. Swallowing causes a tiny flap called the **epiglottis** to close off the trachea to ensure that the bolus passes into the **esophagus** and not the trachea, where it would cause choking. The esophagus is a narrow tube that connects the pharynx to the stomach. Contractions of the smooth muscles in the esophagus called **peristalsis** move the food along through the esophagus. No digestion occurs in the esophagus.

Once the bolus moves into the stomach, the **gastric sphincter** prevents the reflux of food back into the esophagus. Peristaltic contractions churn the bolus, continuing the process of mechanical digestion. The enzyme **pepsin** initiates chemical digestion of the food in the stomach. Secretions in the stomach further help the food to digest. There are three main secretions: pepsinogen, mucus, and hydrochloric acid. Digestion in the stomach lasts for several hours.

After the food is digested in the stomach, the product is called **chyme** and it passes through pyloric sphincter into the **duodenum**, the first part of the **small intestine**.

ABSORPTION OF NUTRIENTS

Absorption of nutrients occurs primarily in the small intestine, where the gallbladder secretes **bile** made in the liver. Bile helps break down lipids so they can mix with water. The pancreas and some specialized cells in the small intestine also secrete enzymes essential to digestion, including proteases, amylases, lipases, bicarbonate, and nucleases. Lipids are digested into fatty acids and glycerol, proteins are digested into amino acids, and carbohydrates are digested into simple sugars. Digestion is completed in the small intestine and the digested particles are absorbed by the small intestine. The space inside the small intestine (the lumen) has threadlike folded projections called **villi**, which are further folded into **microvilli**, that increase the surface area of the tissue and allow more nutrients to be absorbed by capillaries there and carried into the bloodstream. Digestion in the small intestine takes between three and ten hours.

The remaining undigested material passes into the **large intestine**. The large intestine performs the role of absorbing water, vitamin K, and salt from the remaining food matter and creating solid waste through bacterial fermentation. The large intestine contains a large population of beneficial bacteria that synthesize vitamins that the body needs.

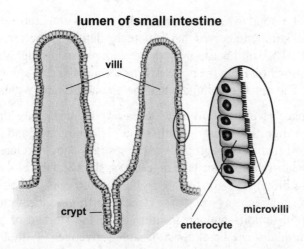

lumen of small intestine

villi

microvilli

crypt

enterocyte

Author: BallenaBlanca. https://commons.wikimedia.org/wiki/File:Villi_%26_microvilli _of_small_intestine.svg.

ELIMINATION OF WASTES

After absorbing water, vitamins, and salt, the large intestine stores the solid waste until it's time to eliminate it. There are four sections of the large intestine:

- **cecum**: This small area connects the small and large intestines. An outgrowth of the cecum is the appendix, which is a vestigial organ, although it plays a role in the lymphatic system.
- **colon**: The colon makes up the largest part of the large intestine. Its primary job is to absorb water, vitamins, and salt from the food matter and create solid waste.

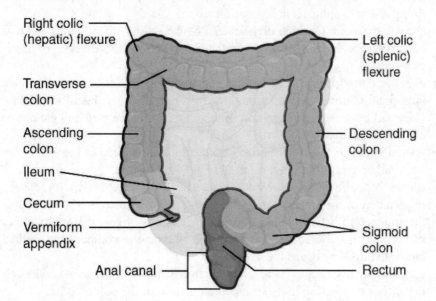

Right colic (hepatic) flexure

Left colic (splenic) flexure

Transverse colon

Ascending colon

Descending colon

Ileum

Cecum

Vermiform appendix

Sigmoid colon

Anal canal

Rectum

Author: OpenStax College. https://commons.wikimedia.org/wiki/File:2420_Large _Intestine.jpg.

- **rectum**: The solid waste from the colon passes into the rectum, which stretches to stimulate nerves that initiate the defecation reflex.
- **anal canal**: The solid waste from the rectum passes through the anal canal during elimination from the body. The anal canal has two sphincters to regulate exit. The first is involuntary and the second is under voluntary control.

Hormones play a vital role in digestion as well. They cause the secretions necessary for digestion. They stimulate muscle contraction and relaxation to move digested matter through the small intestine. They regulate the flow of water and electrolytes between the digestive system and the bloodstream, and they increase blood flow for the absorption of nutrients. Specific hormones perform other functions as well. For example, the hormone ghrelin stimulates appetite, leptin inhibits hunger, insulin causes the storage of glucose, and glucagon stimulates the breakdown of stored glycogen. Without hormones, the system could not function.

Other vital organs necessary for the digestion and absorption of food are the **pancreas**, the **liver**, and the **gallbladder**. The pancreas secretes pancreatic juice, which helps to break down fats into useful nutrients for the body. The liver produces bile, which is important in the digestion of fats. The bile is stored in the gallbladder until it is needed.

DISORDERS AND DISEASES OF THE DIGESTIVE SYSTEM

In addition to viruses and cancers, there are some digestive system disorders and diseases with which you should be familiar:

- **gastroesophageal reflux disease (GERD)**: The most common symptom of GERD is heartburn, but if GERD is not controlled properly, it can erode the lining of the esophagus and cause bleeding.
- chronic diarrhea: Chronic diarrhea can be caused by many things, such as **celiac disease**, **irritable bowel syndrome** (IBS), **Crohn's disease**, or **ulcerative colitis**.
- **chronic constipation**: Occasional constipation, like occasional diarrhea, is normal. Chronic constipation, however, is a disorder. **Fecal impaction** is caused by severe constipation in which the stool is dried and cannot be evacuated normally.
- **gastroenteritis**: Gastroenteritis is caused by an infection in the gut, either bacterial or viral. It is often referred to as "stomach flu."
- **ulcers**: A peptic ulcer is like a sore on the inside of the stomach. It is caused by damage to the mucus lining the stomach, which exposes the lining of the stomach to irritating acid. This damage is most likely caused by either bacteria in the stomach or the heavy use of over-the-counter nonsteroidal anti-inflammatory drugs (NSAIDs).
- gall bladder disorders: These include **cholelithiasis** (gallstones) and **cholecystitis**, an infection that causes inflammation of the gall bladder.

- liver disorders: These include **cirrhosis**, which is damage to the liver and its hepatic tissues, and **hepatitis**, which is an infection of the liver.
- **hemorrhoids**: Hemorrhoids are small, swollen rectal veins. They are caused by straining during bowel movements and are common during pregnancy as well.
- **diverticulosis**: A condition in which an area of the intestines becomes distended.
- **diverticulitis**: Infection or inflammation of an area of the intestine affected with diverticulosis.

REVIEW QUESTIONS

1. Which of the following performs chemical digestion?

A) Teeth
B) Duodenum
C) Tongue
D) Gastric enzymes

2. What is another name for the digestive tract?

A) Stomach tract
B) Food absorption tunnel
C) Gastrointestinal tract
D) Digestion path

3. Which of the following structures plays a role in mechanical digestion?

A) Salivary gland
B) Pancreas
C) Large intestine
D) Appendix

4. What is one function of bile?

A) Allows material to pass into the rectum
B) Helps with digestion and absorption of fats
C) Returns excess fluid back into the blood
D) Initiates chemical digestion

5. Which of the following enzymes aid in chemical digestion? Select all that apply.

A) Ghrelin
B) Chyme
C) Amylase
D) Pepsinogen

ANSWER KEY

1. D **3.** A **5.** C and D
2. C **4.** B

ANSWERS AND EXPLANATIONS

1. (D) Digestive enzymes perform the chemical breakdown of food in the stomach.

2. (C) The gastrointestinal tract is another name for the digestive tract, which extends from the mouth to the anus.

3. (A) Saliva, secreted by salivary glands in the mouth, aids in mechanical digestion by moistening the food and helping to break down starches.

4. (B) Bile aids in the digestion and absorption of fats and fat-soluble vitamins in the small intestine.

5. (C and D) The enzymes lipase and amylase begin chemical digestion in the mouth. Secretions of mucus, hydrochloric acid, and pepsinogen aid in chemical digestion in the stomach. Ghrelin is a hormone that stimulates appetite, and chyme is the mass of partially digested food that passes from the stomach into the small intestine.

CHAPTER 31

The Genitourinary System

The **genitourinary system** is composed of the kidneys, ureters, urinary bladder, and urethra. The genitourinary system has several functions: filtering the blood and producing urine to remove nitrogenous cellular waste products, regulating blood pressure, adjusting blood pH, and regulating osmotic concentrations of the blood.

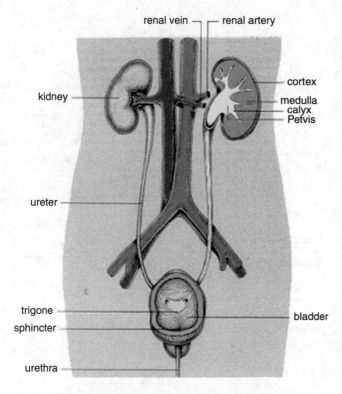

Source: http://glasgowpbl.wikispaces.com/Block+5+Scenario+3

FILTERING THE BLOOD

The **kidneys** are two bean-shaped organs located in the upper abdominal area against the back muscles, one on the left and one on the right. The left kidney is slightly lower to accommodate the liver. The kidneys work with the cardiovascular system to filter the blood. **Urea**, which is nitrogenous waste from the metabolic breakdown of proteins, is made by the liver. Urea is transported through the bloodstream to the kidneys. The blood enters each kidney through the renal artery, and the kidney filters the blood and produces **urine**, which is then stored in the **urinary bladder**, until it is discharged from the body through the **urethra** during **micturition** (urination).

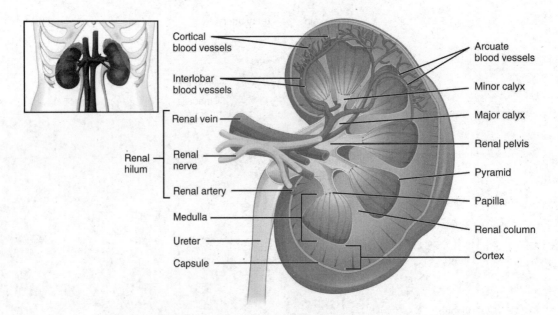

Author: OpenStax College. https://commons.wikimedia.org/wiki/File:2610_The _Kidney.jpg.

The outer layer of the kidney is called the **renal cortex**. The inner layer is called the **renal medulla** and is made up of seven **renal pyramids**. Renal pyramids appear striped because they are actually groups of parallel **nephrons**. Nephrons are the primary functional cells of the kidney, and each kidney contains about one million nephrons. A diagram of a nephron is shown on the next page.

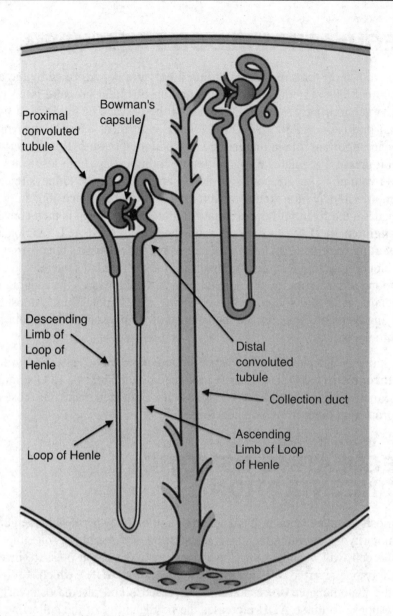

Author: Artwork by Holly Fischer. https://commons.wikimedia.org/wiki/File: Kidney_Nephron.png.

Each nephron is like a long tube. At one end, the tube is closed and folded into a cuplike sac called the **renal corpuscular capsule**, or **Bowman's capsule**. Bowman's capsule encloses a cluster of capillaries called the **glomerulus**. The glomerulus is the first stage in the filtering process. Urea and nutrients are diffused from the glomerulus into Bowman's capsule, which leads to the **proximal convoluted tubule**, then to the **loop of Henle**, then to the **distal convoluted tubule,** and finally to the **collection duct**. The collection ducts from all the nephrons in each kidney merge together and lead to a **ureter**. Each ureter leads to the **bladder**, where the urine is stored until it is excreted through the **urethra**. In males, the urethra runs through the penis. The filtered blood returns to the body through the renal vein.

REGULATING BLOOD PRESSURE

While the short-term regulation of blood pressure is performed by the auto-nomic nervous system, long-term regulation of blood pressure is provided by the genitourinary system. **Perfusion** is the passage of fluid into a tissue. Renal perfusion pressure and the kidneys' control of extracellular volume play an important role in regulating arterial blood pressure. Renal artery per-fusion pressure regulates the excretion of sodium. If sodium levels are low, blood volume is low, or potassium levels are too high, the kidneys release a hormone called **renin**. Renin converts the hormone angiotensinogen, which is made in the liver, into the hormone angiotensin I, which is then converted to **angiotensin II** by an enzyme from the lungs called ACE (angiotensin-converting enzyme). Angiotensin II causes the blood vessels to constrict, and the blood pressure increases. Angiotensin II also stimulates the release of the hormone **aldosterone** by the adrenal glands, which causes the renal tubules to retain water and sodium while excreting excess potassium. Aldosterone and angiotensin II thus restore the balance of fluids, sodium, and potassium within the body.

The kidneys also play a role in the production of red blood cells. The hormone **erythropoietin** (EPO) is primarily produced by the kidneys. EPO stimulates bone marrow cells to produce red blood cells. EPO then maintains those cells by protecting them from being destroyed.

REGULATING OSMOTIC CONCENTRATION

Osmosis is the movement of water across a selectively permeable membrane. Osmolarity is determined by the concentration of the solutions on either side of the cell wall. Another way the kidneys regulate blood pressure involves the hormone referred to as **antidiuretic hormone** (ADH), which is released by the hypothalamus in response to increased blood plasma osmolarity or in response to thirst. ADH increases the permeability of the collecting duct to allow more water to enter and stimulates reabsorption of sodium from the loop of Henle. This increases water reabsorption, which increases blood plasma volume and decreases osmolarity.

ADJUSTING BLOOD PH

The body must maintain its acid-base balance, or pH, within a fairly narrow range, and the genitourinary system plays an important role in regulating pH balance. If blood pH is not in balance, the tubular cells of the kidneys can reg-ulate the reabsorption of bicarbonate, which can increase or decrease acid secretion. The kidneys can also excrete bicarbonate by decreasing hydrogen ion secretion and lowering the rate of ammonium secretion.

DISORDERS AND DISEASES OF THE GENITOURINARY SYSTEM

In addition to cancers, the most common genitourinary system disorders and diseases include:

- **urinary tract infection** (UTI): The most common UTI is a bladder infection, but a UTI can occur anywhere in the urinary tract. UTI is more common in women.
- urolithiasis: The formation of stones within the genitourinary system includes **nephrolithiasis** (kidney stones) and **ureterolithiasis** (ureter stones).
- **glomerulonephritis**: An acute inflammation of the glomeruli within the kidney.
- **renal cysts**: These sacs of fluid that can form in the kidneys are usually harmless and are common as the body ages.
- **renal failure**: A failure of the kidneys to function properly. Without at least one functioning kidney, the body cannot survive. If a kidney cannot function properly, **dialysis** may be needed. Dialysis is an artificial process that removes excess water and filters the blood.

REVIEW QUESTIONS

1. Which of the following is **NOT** a function of the genitourinary system?

A) Producing urine
B) Regulating blood pressure
C) Neutralizing stomach acid
D) Adjusting blood pH

2. Which of the following is a function performed by the kidneys?

A) Remove metabolic waste
B) Pump blood
C) Produce sperm
D) Secrete sweat

3. A glomerulus is part of a _____.

A) sphincter
B) bladder
C) urethra
D) nephron

4. Which of the following is located inside the kidney?

A) Thymus gland
B) Calyx
C) Trigone
D) Vas deferens

5. Which of the following is a structure within the kidney that filters the blood?

A) Testes
B) Spleen
C) Nephron
D) Urethra

ANSWER KEY

1. C   3. D   5. C
2. A   4. B

ANSWERS AND EXPLANATIONS

1. (C) The genitourinary system does not neutralize stomach acid. The stomach is a part of the digestive system.

2. (A) One of the functions of the kidneys is to remove metabolic waste. The kidneys also produce urine. The heart pumps blood; the testes produce sperm; and glands in the skin secrete sweat.

3. (D) A glomerulus is a network of capillaries located at the beginning of each nephron.

4. (B) The calyx is a chamber of the kidney through which urine passes.

5. (C) Nephrons filter the blood.

CHAPTER 32

The Immune System

The **immune system** is supported by different defense mechanisms in the body that prevent harmful **pathogens** from entering or developing in the body. The immune system must differentiate between natural cells that belong in the body and foreign cells from outside the body. The system's job is to eliminate foreign cells and any abnormal natural cells. Pathogens include:

- **bacteria**: Single-cell organisms that can release toxins that damage tissues.
- **viruses**: Microscopic pathogens that have a protein coat, sometimes enclosed within a membrane, that contains either DNA or RNA. When a virus comes into contact with a host cell, it inserts its genetic material into the host cell and takes over the host's functions.
- **fungi**: Microorganisms from plants that can be pathogenic to humans. Fungal infections may be superficial (on the epidermis or hair), cutaneous (below the epidermis), subcutaneous (all layers of the skin), or systemic (the entire body).
- **parasites**: Living organisms that live on or in the host and sustain themselves at the expense of the host.
- **prions**: Misfolded proteins that can cause normal proteins in the brain to misfold.

PATHOGEN TRANSMISSION

Infections can result from many different modes of transmission. The **chain of infection** is the series of events that takes place to transmit or carry an infection. The first part of this chain is the **reservoir**, the environment in which the pathogen develops. Then the pathogen, or infectious agent, moves from its reservoir into its host via direct or indirect transmission.

Direct transmission occurs when the host has direct contact with the reservoir for the pathogen. There are two types of direct transmission:

- **person-to-person**: The host comes into direct contact with an infected person. The pathogen is transferred from the infected person to the host through touch or exchange of body fluids. This includes **bloodborne pathogens** that are transmitted to the host through contact with the blood or body fluids of an infected person. Person-to-person transmission also includes a mother transferring a pathogen to her fetus or infant.
- **droplet transmission**: The host comes into direct contact with a spray of tiny droplets ejected by an infected person coughing, sneezing, or speaking.

Indirect transmission occurs when the pathogen moves from its reservoir to the air or to a vehicle or vector, which then comes into contact with the host.

- **airborne transmission**: The host is exposed to air, or to dust in the air, that carries a pathogen.
- **vehicle transmission**: The host becomes infected by a pathogen that has been transferred from its reservoir to an inanimate object, such as a countertop or a doorknob.
- **vector transmission**: The host becomes infected by a pathogen that has been transferred from its reservoir to another living organism, such as a mosquito that bites the host.

After a person has been infected by a pathogen, the body attempts to eliminate the pathogen by creating an **immune response**. An immune response occurs when the body recognizes these pathogens and creates an action against them. Harmful molecules that are recognized and elicit an immune response are called **antigens**. In response to antigens, the body makes **antibodies**, which are protective proteins in the blood that bind to antigens and destroy them.

The immune system itself is divided into two categories: innate and adaptive (acquired). Before we discuss those categories, let's discuss white blood cells, which are vital to both categories.

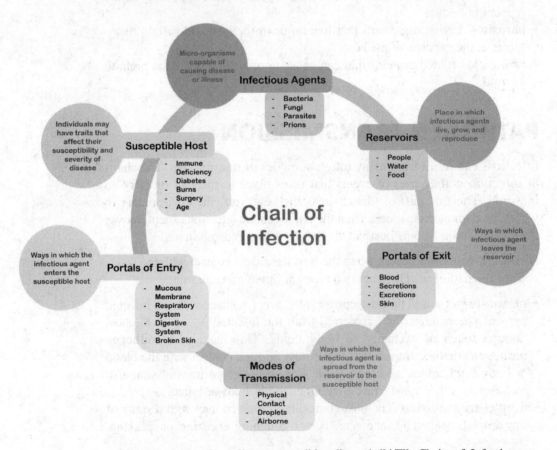

Author: Genieieiop. https://commons.wikimedia.org/wiki/File:Chain_of_Infection.png.

WHITE BLOOD CELLS

White blood cells, or **leukocytes**, play an important role in the immune system. While there is only one type of red blood cell, there are many types of white blood cells. They can be classified by structure or by cell lineage. The two structural classes are **granulocytes**, which are characterized by granules within the cells' cytoplasm, and **agranulocytes**, which have no granules. The two cell lineages are **myeloid cells**, which derive from the bone marrow, or **lymphoid cells**, which derive from the lymphatic system.

We further categorize white blood cells into five types:

- **neutrophil:** These myeloid granulocytes are found in the bloodstream and are the most abundant type of leukocyte. They mainly target bacteria and fungi.
- **eosinophil:** These myeloid granulocytes are produced in the bone marrow and reside in tissues. They combat certain infections and multicellular parasites, as well as modulate allergic inflammatory responses.
- **basophil:** These are the least common, but largest myeloid granulocyte. They reside in tissues and are responsible for inflammatory reactions, allergic responses, and helping coordinate immune responses.
- **monocyte**: These myeloid agranulocytes are found in the bloodstream and are the largest leukocyte. They can differentiate into **dendritic cells** and **macrophages**.
- **lymphocyte:** These lymphoid agranulocytes include B-cells, T-cells, and natural killer cells. We will discuss these in more detail in the Adaptive Immunity section.

INNATE IMMUNITY

Innate immunity refers to the **nonspecific** response mechanisms that begin immediately or within hours of an antigen's appearance. Innate immunity is present from birth. The innate immune response is activated by the chemical properties of the antigen. There are several of these nonspecific response mechanisms:

- **physical barriers**: Skin, mucus, hair, and cilia prevent foreign cells from entering the body.
- **chemical barriers**: Sweat, saliva, stomach acid, and lysozyme can prevent infection.
- **defensive leukocytes (white blood cells)**: White blood cells that destroy pathogens that have entered the body. These include neutrophils, eosinophils, basophils, and monocytes.
- **defensive proteins**: These include signaling proteins, complement proteins, and antibodies. **Signaling proteins**, or **cytokines**, include proteins known as **interferons**. Cells infected by viruses can secrete interferons, which signal uninfected cells that a pathogen is present so that they can shore up their defenses. This can stop the spread of a virus. Interferons are not specific to a particular virus. **Complement proteins** can defend against

bacteria by coating the germ or forming a complex around it to destroy its cell membrane.

- **inflammation**: The increased blood flow of inflammation brings in defensive leukocytes and proteins to fight infection.
- **fever**: Fever increases metabolism and stimulates immune defenses, but if a fever gets too high, it can be dangerous.

The body's first line of defense against pathogens includes the skin and various chemical secretions. If pathogens successfully enter the body, often a fever or inflammation will occur to fight off an infection. White blood cells and defensive proteins try to destroy the pathogens.

ADAPTIVE IMMUNITY

Adaptive immunity refers to an antigen-specific immune response and is more complex than innate immunity. An antigen first must be processed and recognized as foreign; then the adaptive immune system creates immune cells specifically designed to attack that antigen. Adaptive immunity also provides memory of an antigen that makes future responses to that antigen more efficient.

White blood cells play a major role in the adaptive immune system. One type of white blood cell is called a **phagocyte**. This type of white blood cell protects the body by using the cells' plasma membranes to surround particles such as pathogens or dead cells, take them inside the phagocyte cells, and then digest or destroy them. This process is called **phagocytosis**. There are several types of phagocytes, each of which is specialized. Some phagocytes present the particles they digested to other white blood cells in the immune system, including two types of **lymphocytes**: B-cells and T-cells. Both are derived from stem cells in the bone marrow.

B-cells mature in the bone marrow. They produce specific antibodies that destroy invading microbes, including viruses, bacteria, and parasites. Each pathogen brings about the response of a particular B-cell. Since there are millions of different pathogens, there are also millions of different B-cells.

T-cells mature in the thymus gland. They attack infected cells. These include several types:

- **Helper T-cells** help the B-cells and other T-cells multiply and coordinate their actions.
- **Killer T-cells** directly destroy pathogens.
- **Cytotoxic T-cells** and **natural killer (NK) cells** attack cancer cells or cells that have been infected with bacteria and viruses.

There are two main forms of adaptive immunity, humoral and cellular, both of which rely on lymphocytes.

Humoral immunity is the process of producing specific antibody proteins from B-cells that have been activated. Humoral immunity is sometimes referred to as **antibody-mediated immunity** because the B-cells are assisted by helper T-cells to differentiate into plasma B-cells and memory B-cells.

The plasma B-cells produce antibodies against a specific antigen. Memory B-cells remember the antigen and can respond to it rapidly in the case of a future reinfection. The antigens that the humoral immune system deals with are from freely circulating pathogens. The antibodies produced by the B-cells bind to the antigens and neutralize them through phagocytosis or lysis. **Lysis** is the dissolution or destruction of cells by an enzyme called a lysin.

Cellular immunity involves the use of T-cells to destroy infected or cancerous cells. T-cells, like B-cells, have cell membrane receptors that recognize the antigens of a pathogen, but T-cells are not directly activated by contact with the antigen. Helper T-cells release cytokines that help activated T-cells bind to the infected cells' MHC-antigen complex and differentiate the T-cell into a cytotoxic T-cell. The infected cell then undergoes lysis.

Adaptive immunity may be naturally acquired or artificially acquired. **Natural immunity** is developed when a person's own cells produce antibodies in response to a pathogen or to a vaccine. This type of immunity takes longer to develop but is long-lasting. **Artificial immunity** is developed when antibodies produced by other organisms are injected into a person to counteract an antigen. This type of immunity is developed much quicker but is not long-lasting and may have side effects. Both natural and artificial immunity may be achieved actively or passively.

Active immunity develops actively from natural exposure to pathogens and an immune response. It can also be developed artificially through **vaccinations**, where an individual is given a weakened antigen so the body can induce a response and build memory cells. **Passive immunity** elicits a temporary response when a person is given antibodies produced by another person or animal. This can be achieved actively by transfer from a mother to a fetus or infant via placenta or milk. Passive immunity can be achieved artificially through vaccines that inject preformed antibodies.

THE LYMPHATIC SYSTEM

There are some organs in the body that play a special role in the immune system. **Lymph nodes** are small glands found mainly in the thorax and abdomen. These glands help prevent disease by filtering out bacteria in the **lymph**, a watery fluid containing oxygen, proteins, and other nutrients that is formed from interstitial, or tissue, fluid. The **lymphatic system** transports lymph from the tissues of the body back to the bloodstream through lymphatic vessels. Lymph nodes are found throughout the body so that they can destroy pathogens that pass by. **Lymphocytes**, special white blood cells, are formed in response to certain antigens. If a large number of pathogens are present, the lymphocytes multiply and the lymph node grows larger, which is why swollen lymph nodes are a diagnostic sign of infection.

The lymphatic system is closely related to the circulatory system, but the lymphatic system only flows in one direction. Returning excess fluid back into the blood also helps the body maintain fluid balance. Other organs that are vital to the lymphatic system are the spleen, tonsils, and thymus. The

spleen filters bacteria in the blood. **Tonsils**, which are located at the base of the tongue, function as a filter of interstitial fluid. The **thymus gland** is pertinent for immune responses.

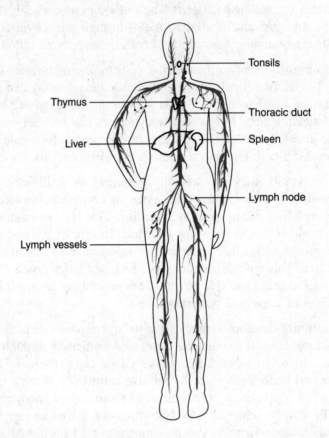

DISORDERS AND DISEASES OF THE IMMUNE SYSTEM

When the immune system is compromised, illness will occur with differing levels of severity. Sometimes the illness that manifests is the common cold, while other pathogens, such as cancer cells, evade immune responses. If the immune system mistakenly targets host cells, this leads to **autoimmune disease**. The most common immune system disorders and diseases include:

- **rheumatoid arthritis** (RA): Arthritis caused by a systemic autoimmune disorder. RA mainly affects the joints of the wrists and hands.
- **lupus** (systemic lupus erythematosus): Chronic autoimmune disorder that causes inflammation that can affect the joints, kidneys, heart, lungs, brain, and skin.
- **psoriasis**: An autoimmune disorder that affects skin cells and causes them to grow much more rapidly than usual, which results in a scaly buildup of skin cells called plaque.
- **type 1 diabetes**: Occurs when the beta cells in the pancreas stop producing insulin.

- **Hashimoto's disease** (Hashimoto's thyroiditis): An autoimmune disorder that causes the thyroid gland to become inflamed, which can damage the gland.
- **HIV/AIDS**: Human immunodeficiency virus (HIV) and autoimmune deficiency syndrome (AIDS) are viral infections that cause dysfunction of the immune system.
- **multiple sclerosis**: A systemic autoimmune disorder that damages the myelin sheath surrounding nerve cells.
- **Graves' disease**: A disorder that causes the thyroid gland to overproduce its hormones.
- **Addison's disease**: An autoimmune disorder that affects the adrenal glands, causing deficiencies of cortisol and aldosterone hormones.

REVIEW QUESTIONS

1. Which type of white blood cell protects the body by making antibodies?

A) Phagocytes
B) B-cells
C) Helper T-cells
D) Killer T-cells

2. Which of the following are functions of the lymphatic system? Select all that apply.

A) It returns excess fluid back into the blood.
B) It absorbs fats from the digestive system.
C) It reduces the level of oxygen in the blood.
D) It defends against pathogens.

3. What is a possible situation in which an autoimmune disease could develop?

A) The immune system attacks the body's own cells.
B) A person has a cold or flu.
C) Antibodies develop against a pathogen.
D) The spleen functions normally.

4. What is the function of a cytotoxic T-cell?

A) It triggers an inflammatory reaction to a pathogen.
B) It produces memory cells to remember the pathogen's antigen.
C) It finds and destroys cells that contain a pathogen's antigen signature.
D) It blocks a pathogen from entering the body.

5. Millions of different kinds of B-cells are found in the blood because they _____.

A) are needed for phagocytosis of pathogens
B) transport oxygen in addition to fighting disease
C) will no longer form after a certain age
D) each form in response to a particular pathogen

ANSWER KEY

1. B   **3.** A   **5.** D
2. A, B, and D   **4.** C

ANSWERS AND EXPLANATIONS

1. (B) Antibodies are made by B-cells.

2. (A, B, and D) The lymphatic system does not control the level of oxygen in blood; that is determined by the circulatory and respiratory systems. The lymphatic system does, however, absorb excess fluid back into the blood, absorb fats from the digestive system, and defend against pathogens.

3. (A) An autoimmune disease results when the body attacks its own cells. If a person has a cold or flu, the immune system is fighting foreign pathogens. Antibodies developing against a pathogen would be a normal immune response. The spleen filters blood and is not a vital organ.

4. (C) Cytotoxic T-cells find and destroy cells that contain a pathogen's antigen signature.

5. (D) Each pathogen triggers a particular type of B-cell. With millions of different pathogens, millions of different B-cells exist.

CHAPTER 33

The Integumentary System

The **integumentary system** is composed of the body's protective covering: the skin, hair, nails, and glands. The skin, which averages in total size about 20 square feet, performs several important functions. First and foremost, it is the body's first line of defense against pathogens. The integumentary system also regulates temperature to maintain homeostasis, communicates with the body through sensory receptors regarding outside influences, synthesizes vitamin D, and eliminates waste through perspiration.

PROTECTION

The skin is the largest organ in the body and serves as a protective barrier between the body and elements of the outside environment such as water, heat, cold, ultraviolet rays from the sun, and harmful pathogens. When the skin is intact, pathogens cannot enter the body.

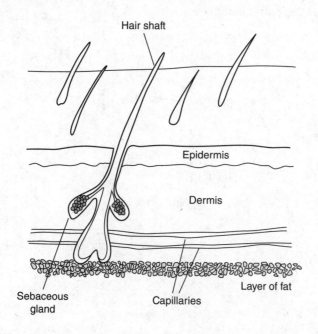

There are three layers composing the skin. The outermost layer of the skin is the **epidermis**. The epidermis prevents microbes from entering the body, which helps protect the body from disease. Epidermal cells are constantly being shed and renewed. New cells are developed in the **stratum basale** layer of the epidermis and pushed toward the top layer, the **stratum corneum**. As they move upward, the cells develop **keratin**, which provides a layer of waterproofing for the skin. The epidermis also contains melanocytes, which are specialized cells that produce the pigment **melanin**. Melanin protects the body from damage caused by the sun's ultraviolet rays.

The middle layer of the skin is the **dermis**, which is composed mainly of a protein called **collagen** that makes skin stretchy and strong. The dermis has arteries and veins for blood circulation, nerves to transmit signals about environmental conditions to the brain, sweat glands, oil glands, and hair roots and follicles. Sweat protects the surface of the skin by deterring microbes through the production of dermcidin, which has antibiotic properties. Hair growing through the skin provides protection from UV radiation and serves as a lubricant for the skin. **Lymphatic vessels**, which drain fluid from the tissues and prevent infections, are found in the dermis.

The innermost layer of the skin is the **hypodermis**, or **subcutaneous level**. Fat cells in the hypodermis form a sort of cushion to protect underlying structures and to insulate the body. The thickness of this layer varies from person to person.

The integumentary system also includes fingernails and toenails, which protect the ends of fingers and toes. The **nail plate** is a hard, flexible surface made of keratin that protects the **nail matrix**. The half-oval white area at the base of the nail is called the **lunula**, and the **cuticle** is made up of dead skin cells around the base edge of the lunula and the sides of the nail. The **nail sinus** is the base of the nail where new tissue emerges. The **nail bed** is the skin beneath the entire nail plate.

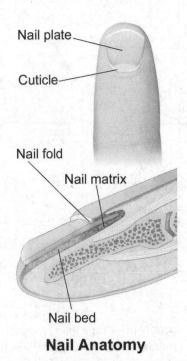

Nail Anatomy

Author: BruceBlaus. https://commons.wikimedia.org/wiki/File:Blausen_0406 _FingerNailAnatomy.png.

MAINTAINING HOMEOSTASIS

The integumentary system regulates temperature to maintain homeostasis in the body. When the body is hot, it produces sweat, which is a mixture of water, salts, and a very small amount of urea. Sweat is secreted from the sweat glands and carried up from the dermis to the epidermis, where it can evaporate, which also helps with thermoregulation. Capillaries in the dermis can also dilate to release heat from the body. When the body is cold, the capillaries in the dermis constrict to retain heat.

Layers of keratin and glycolipids in the stratum corneum of the epidermis act as a protective barrier against water loss. In addition, **sebaceous glands** in the dermis secrete an oily substance called sebum through the hair follicles that coats the hair and skin cells to prevent water loss.

COMMUNICATION

The integumentary system works with the neuromuscular system to coordinate responses to external stimuli. The skin can be classified as a sensory organ because the layers of the skin contain specialized nerve structures that detect contact with the outside world, including changes in temperature and tactile (touch) sensations. Hairs projecting from the skin can sense even small changes in the environment. Each hair follicle has sensory nerves connected to it.

The tips of the fingers have high concentrations of these receptors, so they are the most sensitive to touch. The **Pacinian corpuscle** responds to vibration. The **Meissner corpuscle** responds to light touch, and **Merkel's disks** scattered in the stratum basale are also touch receptors. **Krause end bulbs** respond to cold, and **Ruffini endings** respond to warmth. These and other receptors for pain and temperature are present throughout the skin.

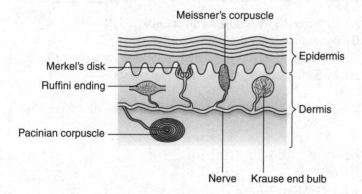

Author: CNX OpenStax. https://commons.wikimedia.org/wiki/File: Figure_36_02_02 .png.

DISORDERS AND DISEASES OF THE INTEGUMENTARY SYSTEM

The most common integumentary system disorders and diseases include:

- infections: The skin can have bacterial infections, such as cellulitis or impetigo; viral infections, such as herpes; and fungal infections, such as athlete's foot, ringworm, or candida (yeast infection).
- burns: Burn damage to the skin is caused by intense heat, radiation, electricity, or chemicals. Sunburn from UV rays is common.
- **acne**: Clogged pores can lead to inflammation and infection. Acne is common in adolescents.
- rashes: A rash is a reddened area on the skin that is often itchy. **Eczema** is an inflammatory condition that presents as a red, flaky rash. **Impetigo** is a contagious skin condition that presents as a rash. **Rosacea** is a skin disorder that also presents as a rash with breakouts. **Psoriasis** is a condition in which skin becomes thick due to an abnormal buildup of cells on the skin's surface.
- skin cancer: Overexposure to ultraviolet radiation damages DNA, which can cause cancerous lesions in the skin.

REVIEW QUESTIONS

1. Which of the following is the body's first line of defense against pathogens?

   A) Hair
   B) Tonsils
   C) Uterus
   D) Skin

2. The skin helps to maintain body temperature _____.

   A) through the action of its sweat glands
   B) by synthesizing melanin
   C) when oil glands release their secretion onto the surface
   D) by acting as a barrier against pathogens

3. Which of the following is **NOT** a component of the dermis?

   A) Arteries
   B) Veins
   C) Alveoli
   D) Sweat glands

4. What is the name of the waterproofing protein developed in the epidermis?
Write your answer in the blank: _____

5. Which of the following is **NOT** a function of the skin?

A) Assisting in the production of white blood cells
B) Protecting the body's internal environment
C) Providing protection against pathogens
D) Regulating heat loss

ANSWER KEY

1. D   **3.** C   **5.** A
2. A   **4.** keratin

ANSWERS AND EXPLANATIONS

1. (D) The skin is the body's first line of defense against pathogens. The skin also helps to maintain body temperature and communicate through sensory receptors about environmental stimuli. The tonsils and the uterus are both inside the body and would not function as the first line of defense. Hair, while protective of the body, does not protect against pathogens.

2. (A) Sweat glands in the dermis release water to the surface that evaporates in warm weather to keep the body cool.

3. (C) Alveoli are not a part of the dermis. They are tiny sacs within the lungs that perform the exchange of gases.

4. (keratin) Keratin is the waterproofing protein developed in the epidermis.

5. (A) White blood cells are produced in the bone marrow and not by the skin.

CHAPTER 34

The Reproductive System

Sexual reproduction or **procreation** in humans involves two parents: one male and one female. Two sets of DNA results in greater genetic diversity among the offspring and increases the chance of future success of the species.

The **reproductive system** has four main functions: to produce the egg and sperm cells from which an **embryo** is formed, to transport and sustain the egg and sperm cells, to produce hormones, and to nurture the developing embryo through the fetal stage until birth. Before we can discuss these functions, we need to be familiar with both the male and female reproductive organs.

MALE REPRODUCTIVE ORGANS

Gonads are the primary reproductive organs, and in males, these are the **testes**, which are small organs that produce the male sex cells called **sperm**. The testes are contained in a sac called the **scrotum**. The external reproductive organs, or **genitalia**, are the **penis** and testes. In the reproductive process, fertilization occurs when sperm and egg fuse to create a pregnancy.

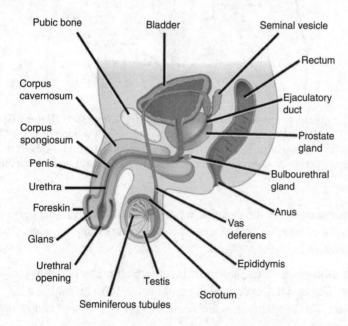

Source: Boundless. "Male Reproductive Anatomy." *Boundless Biology* Boundless, August 8, 2016. Retrieved January 12, 2017 from https://www.boundless.com/biology/textbooks/boundless-biology-textbook/animal-reproduction-and-development-43/human-reproductive-anatomy-and-gametogenesis-239/male-reproductive-anatomy-889-12140/

Sperm is produced in the testes and then stored in the **epididymis** to mature. During ejaculation, the sperm is ejected from the epididymis into the **deferent duct** and goes up through the spermatic cord into the pelvic cavity, over the ureter to the **prostate** behind the bladder. Here, the **vas deferens** joins with the **seminal vesicle** to form the **ejaculatory duct**, which passes through the prostate and empties into the **urethra**. While the sperm travels through the vas deferens, a number of glands, including the seminal and prostate glands, produce fluids to create semen. The alkaline fluid secreted by the prostate also acts to protect the sperm from the acidic environment of the female vagina. Semen exits the penis through the urethra.

FEMALE REPRODUCTIVE ORGANS

The internal organs of the female reproductive system include the ovaries, fallopian tubes, uterus, and vagina.

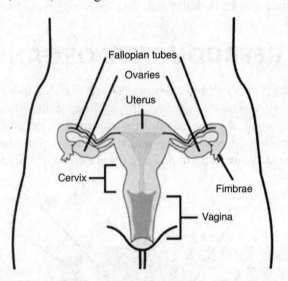

Source: Boundless. "Female Reproductive Anatomy." *Boundless Biology* Boundless, May 26, 2016. Retrieved January 12, 2017 from https://www.boundless.com/biology/textbooks/boundless-biology-textbook/animal-reproduction-and-development-43/human-reproductive-anatomy-and-gametogenesis-239/female-reproductiveanatomy-890-12141/

The female gonads are the **ovaries**, a pair of small glands in the pelvic region, where eggs, or **ova**, are developed. There is one ovary on each side of the uterus. Ovaries have three layers:

- **tunica albuginea**: The outermost layer, which protects the ovary
- **cortex**: The middle layer, which contains the follicles and ova
- **medulla**: The inner layer, which contains the nerves and blood supply for the ovary

Ovaries have two functions: to produce ova and to produce hormones.

During **ovulation**, the process by which mature eggs leave the ovaries, an egg will travel through one of the two **fallopian tubes** toward the uterus.

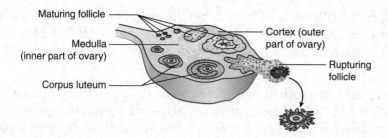

Author: CNX OpenStax. https://commons.wikimedia.org/wiki/File:Figure_43_03_04 .jpg.

Fallopian tubes are also called **uterine tubes** or **salpinges**. Each fallopian tube is made up of four segments:

- **fimbriae**: These ciliated projections at the end of the tube sweep across the ovary and capture the ova.
- **infundibulum**: The fimbriae are attached to this funnel-like opening, which is the part of the tube near the ovary.
- **ampulla**: The ampulla makes up the majority of the tube and is the widest section. Fertilization usually takes place in the ampulla.
- **isthmus**: The isthmus is the narrow part of the tube that connects it to the uterus.

The lining of each fallopian tube has small hairlike projections (cilia) that help transport an egg through the tube from the ovary to the uterus. If sperm are present, they meet with the egg in the fallopian tube and may be fertilized. The two fallopian tubes merge into the uterus.

The **uterus** is a hollow, pear-shaped muscular organ in which a fertilized egg is housed and nurtured until the offspring is ready for birth. The uterus has three layers:

- **perimetrium**: The outer serous layer
- **myometrium**: The thick middle layer mostly made of smooth muscle
- **endometrium**: The inner layer made up of glandular cells that make a mucous membrane

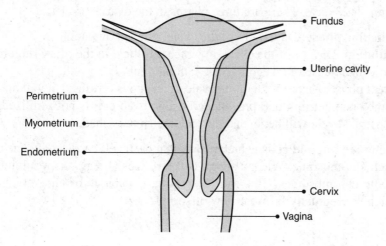

If an egg is fertilized, it will remain in the uterus, or womb, for pregnancy. If it is not, the egg will be flushed out of the body along with the endometrium. This process is called the **menstrual cycle** and typically occurs every 28 days in women.

The **vagina** is a muscular tube that connects the internal and external genitalia. It has several functions: it serves as the entry point for sperm to enter the female reproductive system, it allows menstrual fluids from the uterus to exit the body, and it serves as the birth canal during childbirth. The pH of the vagina is acidic, which discourages the growth of certain pathogens.

The **cervix** is a cylindrical neck of primarily fibromuscular tissue that connects the vagina and the uterus. Normally, the cervix is narrow. During childbirth, the cervix widens to allow the baby to pass from the uterus into the vagina, which serves as the birth canal.

The external genitalia include several accessory structures of the female reproductive system that are external to the vagina. Collectively, they are referred to as the **vulva** or **pudendum**. They include:

- **mons pubis**: A mound of fatty tissue that covers the pubic bone
- **labia majora**: The larger, outer folds of skin that extend down from the mons pubis and surround the vaginal opening
- **labia minora**: The smaller, inner folds of skin that surround the vaginal opening
- **clitoris**: A small structure above the vagina that is extremely sensitive to touch and provides sexual stimulation
- **Bartholin's glands**: Two small alveolar glands on either side of the opening of the vagina that secrete mucus to lubricate the vagina

GAMETE PRODUCTION AND TRANSPORTATION

A primary function of the reproductive system is to produce and transport **gametes**. Gametes are the egg and sperm cells and are also called **sex cells**. Eggs are produced during the ovarian cycle, which, like the menstrual cycle, lasts about 28 days. There are three phases in the ovarian cycle:

- **follicular phase**: Days 1–13 of the cycle, prior to ovulation.
- **ovulation**: Day 14 of the cycle, in which a follicle in the ovary ruptures to allow the release of an egg into the fallopian tube.
- **luteal phase**: Days 15–28 of the cycle. If an egg is fertilized, it will implant in the endometrium and pregnancy begins. If an egg is not fertilized, the menstrual cycle will begin and the endometrium is shed.

Gametes are **haploid cells**, which means that each cell carries only one copy of each chromosome. When a sperm cell fertilizes an egg, the resulting cell has both chromosomes. This cell, or **zygote**, is capable of undergoing cell division to eventually form the new offspring.

HORMONE PRODUCTION

Ovaries and testes both produce hormones. Some hormones regulate the reproductive system, some function in the maturation of the reproductive system, and some help with the development of sexual characteristics. The most important hormones include:

- follicle-stimulating hormone (FSH): In women, FSH stimulates secretion of estrogen and helps in egg production. In men, FSH is involved in sperm production.
- luteinizing hormone (LH): In women, LH stimulates estrogen and progesterone production and causes ovulation. In men, LH is involved in secreting testosterone.
- testosterone: Stimulates development of male secondary sex characteristics and sperm production.
- estrogen: Stimulates development of female secondary sex characteristics, follicle development, and pregnancy.
- progesterone: Prepares body for childbirth.

FETAL DEVELOPMENT

Another function of the (female) reproduction system is to nurture and protect offspring during **gestation**, the period of pregnancy between conception and birth.

After an egg has been fertilized, the resulting **diploid cell** is called a **zygote**. While still traveling through the fallopian tube, it begins to undergo cell division, or **cleavage**. The zygote divides into a group of smaller cells called a **blastocyst**. About five days after fertilization, the blastocyst reaches the uterus and soon implants itself in the endometrium. The blastocyst, now called an **embryo**, begins to grow and cells **differentiate** and develop into the organ and organ systems of the body. From about eight weeks until birth, the embryo is called a **fetus.**

During gestation, the embryo and then the fetus is protected inside the **amniotic sac**, a transparent pair of tough membranes that are filled with **amniotic fluid**. An organ called the **placenta** grows from the outer layer of the amniotic sac and attaches to the wall of the uterus. The **umbilical cord** grows from the placenta to what will become the navel of the baby. The umbilical cord has one vein that transports oxygen and nutrients from the placenta to the fetus and two arteries that return deoxygenated blood and waste products from the fetus back to the placenta. Before birth, the placenta also passes antibodies from the mother to the baby to protect it from infections during and for about three months after birth.

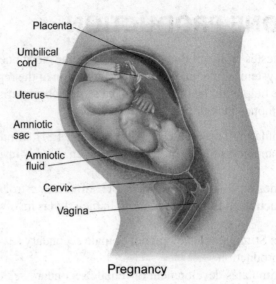

Pregnancy

Author: BruceBlaus. https://commons.wikimedia.org/wiki/File:Blausen_0747 _Pregnancy.png.

DISORDERS AND DISEASES OF THE REPRODUCTIVE SYSTEM

The most common reproductive system disorders and diseases include:

- cancers: **Breast cancer**, **cervical cancer**, **ovarian cancer**, **prostate cancer**, and **testicular cancer** are all common cancers.
- infections: **Vaginitis** is an infection of the vagina and vaginal vault. **Pelvic inflammatory disease** is an infection of the female reproductive organs including the vagina, uterus, ovaries, and fallopian tubes.
- **endometriosis**: Endometriosis is an often-painful condition in which the lining of the uterus grows outside of the uterus.
- **enlarged prostate**: Hypertrophy of the prostate gland.
- **cystocele/rectocele**: A cystocele happens when the urinary bladder pushes against weakened tissue in the vagina and the bladder drops down into the vagina. A rectocele happens when the rectum and part of the large intestine pushes against the vaginal wall.
- **erectile dysfunction**: Erectile dysfunction is a disorder in males that results in the inability to have and/or maintain an erection.

REVIEW QUESTIONS

1. Which of the following is a part of the female reproductive system?

A) Seminal vesicle
B) Fallopian tubes
C) Vas deferens
D) Scrotum

2. Which of the following hormones do **NOT** play an active role in the menstrual cycle?

A) Luteinizing hormone
B) Follicle-stimulating hormone
C) Progesterone
D) Insulin

3. If a female egg is not fertilized, what happens to the egg during the menstrual cycle?

A) It remains in the uterus.
B) It is discharged during menstruation.
C) It fuses together with sperm.
D) It travels back to the ovaries.

4. The fluid-filled sac that protects the embryo and fetus is called the _____. Write your answer in the blank.

5. The process of labor is triggered by the hormone _____.

A) Oxytocin
B) Estrogen
C) Progesterone
D) HCG

ANSWER KEY

1. B   **3.** B   **5.** A
2. D   **4.** amniotic sac

ANSWERS AND EXPLANATIONS

1. (B) Fallopian tubes are a part of the female reproductive system. Eggs are transported through the fallopian tubes from the ovaries to the uterus.

2. (D) Insulin does not play an active role in the menstrual cycle. Insulin is a hormone made in the pancreas that regulates blood glucose levels.

3. (B) If an egg, or ovum, is not fertilized, then it is discharged during menstruation. If the egg *is* fertilized, it is fused with the sperm and remains in the uterus to develop during pregnancy. The egg does not travel back to the ovaries.

4. (amniotic sac) The amniotic sac is the fluid-filled sac that provides protection and cushioning for the embryo and fetus.

5. (A) Oxytocin, produced by the posterior pituitary gland, causes the contractions of labor to begin.

Biology

CHAPTER 35

Macromolecules

Macromolecules are, as their name implies, very large molecules. Most are formed when organic molecules, or monomers, combine with covalent bonds during dehydration reactions to form biological polymers. Most of the macromolecules are groups of the same monomer or similar monomers linked together over and over.

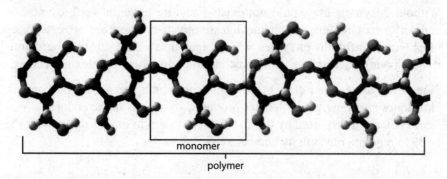

Source: Boundless. "Types of Biological Macromolecules." *Boundless Biology* Boundless, May 26, 2016. Retrieved Jan 10, 2017 from https://www.boundless. com/biology/textbooks/boundless-biology-textbook/biological-macromolecules-3/ synthesis-of-biological-macromolecules-53/types-of-biological-macromolecules-293-11426/

There are four types of macromolecules: proteins, carbohydrates, lipids, and nucleic acids. These macromolecules are the food groups needed by the body and can be broken down by hydrolysis during digestion for use by the body's cells.

PROTEINS

Proteins are long chains of amino acid monomers. The long chains are called **polypeptides**, and they sometimes fold over to form three-dimensional shapes. Different shapes have different functions.

Of the 20 primary amino acids, only 11 of these can be produced by the body itself. The remaining nine must be obtained through the diet. These nine amino acids are known as **essential amino acids**. They can be found in protein sources such as meat, eggs, fish, and some plant sources.

Nine Essential Amino Acids

- histidine
- isoleucine
- leucine
- lysine
- methionine
- phenylalanine
- threonine
- tryptophan
- valine

Enzymes are a vital class of proteins that catalyze chemical reactions. Without enzymes, life would not exist. They are essential for biosynthesis and perform many functions in the digestive system. There are two categories of enzymes: **catabolic enzymes**, which break down their substrate, and **anabolic enzymes**, which use their substrate to build more complex molecules.

Hormones are another class of proteins with which you should be familiar. Hormones are signaling molecules produced by glands in the endocrine system. They are transported by the circulatory system to organs throughout the body to regulate physiology and behavior.

Function of Proteins

Proteins have many vital functions within the body, such as:

- catalyzing chemical reactions
- synthesizing and repairing DNA
- providing structural support
- transporting materials across the cell
- responding to stimuli
- sending and receiving chemical signals

CARBOHYDRATES

Carbohydrate molecules form with a ratio of carbon to hydrogen to oxygen of 1:2:1. They can be classified into three subtypes: monosaccharides, disaccharides, and polysaccharides. A **monosaccharide** is a simple sugar, with only 3–7 carbon atoms. Glucose, fructose, and galactose are common monosaccharides. A **disaccharide** forms when two monosaccharides bond. Sucrose, lactose, and maltose are common disaccharides. A **polysaccharide** is a long chain of monosaccharides. Glycogen, cellulose, starch, and chitin are common polysaccharides.

Function of Carbohydrates

Carbohydrates are the body's source of quick fuel because they break down faster in the body than do protein and fats. Carbohydrates convert to sugar, or glucose, which is a ready source of fuel. Simple carbohydrates, such as cane sugar, break down fastest when consumed. Complex carbohydrates, such as grains and starchy vegetables, break down more slowly than simple carbohydrates and turn into sugar less quickly in the bloodstream.

Fiber is a component found in carbohydrates that cannot be digested by the body. Because it does not break down into glucose, fiber adds bulk to the diet and improves the process of transporting foods through the digestive system. Adequate fiber intake can also be helpful for controlling blood sugar levels.

While some carbohydrates perform energy storage functions, other carbohydrates perform structural functions. The polysaccharide cellulose performs an important function in plant cells. The rigid cell wall is made up mainly of cellulose. Another polysaccharide, chitin, performs an important function in arthropods: it forms an exoskeleton to protect their internal organs. Other carbohydrates, such as glycoproteins, have recognition functions.

LIPIDS

Lipids are macromolecules that contain hydrocarbons. They are highly reduced forms of carbon, and when they are metabolized, lipids are oxidized to release large amounts of energy. Lipids include:

- fats
- oils
- waxes
- sterols
- fat-soluble vitamins
- monoglycerides
- diglycerides
- triglycerides
- phospholipids

Function of Lipids

Lipids are an efficient source of fuel for the body; once digested, they break down into fatty acids and glycerol. Fats take longer to digest than either protein or carbohydrates, so they provide the body with sustained energy. **Saturated fats** are derived mainly from animal sources and tend to raise cholesterol and increase the risk of heart attack and stroke. **Unsaturated fats**—derived from certain vegetables, fish, and nuts—can lower cholesterol levels. Monounsaturated fats, such as those found in avocado and olive oil are particularly beneficial in this regard.

Lipids also have signaling functions and act as a major structural component of cell membranes.

NUCLEIC ACIDS

The nucleic acids include deoxyribonucleic acid (DNA) and ribonucleic acid (RNA).

DNA is a polymer made from a long string of repeating units called nucleotides. Nearly all DNA molecules consist of two biopolymer strands that are coiled around each other to form a double helix shape. As you probably know, DNA stores biological information and is the hereditary material in all living organisms.

RNA is also a chain of nucleotides, but it usually forms a single strand folded onto itself rather than a double-strand like DNA. RNA is mostly involved in protein synthesis. A type of RNA known as messenger RNA carries copies of the genetic information to ribosomes, where catalytic ribosomal RNA molecules and transfer RNA molecules coordinate to make a functional protein.

Function of Nucleic Acids

Nucleic acids carry out several cellular processes. They are especially involved in the regulation and expression of genes.

REVIEW QUESTIONS

1. Which of the following macromolecules breaks down most slowly in the body?

   A) Protein
   B) Lipids
   C) Simple carbohydrates
   D) Complex carbohydrates

2. Which of the following is a function of a nucleic acid?

   A) Transport
   B) Structure
   C) Storage
   D) Regulation

3. Which of the following components makes up a protein?

   A) Ribosomes
   B) Enzymes
   C) Amino acids
   D) Nucleotides

4. Which type of bond forms macromolecules? Write your answer in the blank: _____

5. Brown rice belongs primarily to which of the following categories of macromolecule?

A) Lipid
B) Nucleic acid
C) Carbohydrate
D) Protein

6. During digestion, protein breaks down into which of the following?

A) Amino acids
B) Glucose
C) Glycerol
D) Sucrose

7. Which of the following describes a function of an enzyme?

A) They store energy within a cell.
B) They catalyze chemical reactions.
C) They carry information to the ribosomes.
D) They provide structure in a cell wall.

8. Which of the following describes the process of hydrolysis?

A) Addition of H_2O to break the bond between molecules in a polymer
B) The endergonic removal of an H_2O molecule
C) Molecules joining by peptide bonds
D) Addition of a carbon atom to form an isotope

9. Cholesterol levels can be reduced by dietary intake of which of the following?

A) Simple carbohydrates
B) Saturated fats
C) Trans fats
D) Monounsaturated fats

10. Which of the following is a polysaccharide?

A) Glucose
B) Cellulose
C) Sucrose
D) Maltose

ANSWER KEY

1. B	**5.** C	**9.** D
2. D	**6.** A	**10.** B
3. C	**7.** B	
4. Covalent	**8.** A	

ANSWERS AND EXPLANATIONS

1. (B) Lipids break down more slowly in the body than either protein or carbohydrates. Complex carbohydrates break down more slowly than simple carbohydrates, but not as slowly as protein and lipids.

2. (D) The functions of nucleic acids include heredity and regulation.

3. (C) Proteins are long chains of amino acid monomers.

4. (Covalent) Macromolecules are formed by covalent bonds between monomers.

5. (C) Brown rice is a carbohydrate.

6. (A) During digestion, protein breaks down into amino acids. Carbohydrates break down into sugar or glucose, and lipids break down into fatty acids and glycerol.

7. (B) Enzymes catalyze chemical reactions.

8. (A) Hydrolysis is the process of adding water to break the bond between molecules in a polymer.

9. (D) Cholesterol levels can be reduced by dietary intake of monounsaturated fats, such as those found in avocados and olive oil. B and C are incorrect because cholesterol levels are increased by both saturated fats and trans fats. Trans fats are created through a process known as hydrogenation, in which hydrogen is added to vegetable oils to help the oils last longer.

10. (B) Cellulose is a polysaccharide. Maltose and sucrose are disaccharides, and glucose is a monosaccharide.

CHAPTER 36

The Cell

TEAS questions concerning **the cell** test your understanding of the differences between prokaryote and eukaryote cells as well as the various parts of a cell. You may also be tested on your knowledge of cell reproduction, including the processes of mitosis and meiosis.

CELLS AND LIFE

Life takes many forms, from the simplicity of bacteria to the complexity of primates. According to **cell theory**, all living things are comprised of cells. Complex life forms have more cells and more complexity to their cell structure. Cell theory goes on to state that cells are the unit of function for organisms. They are responsible for life functions like digestion, circulation, reproduction, and immunity, among others.

The life cycle depends on two different types of organisms: autotrophs and heterotrophs. The word **autotroph** comes from the Greek language and means self-feeder. Autotrophs produce glucose through photosynthesis and feed themselves and other living beings. They are mainly plants. The prefix *hetero* means different, so **heterotrophs** get their nutrition from outside sources. Animals eat plants and other animals to survive. The cell structures of autotrophs and heterotrophs differ.

PROKARYOTE AND EUKARYOTE CELLS

There are two basic types of cells that form the building blocks of all organisms: prokaryote and eukaryote cells. **Prokaryote** cells, shown in the following figure, are simpler, have no nucleus, and lack some of the complex organelles of eukaryotes. Their DNA is not tightly contained as in a eukaryote nucleus. Prokaryote cells are represented in two types of organisms: **bacteria** and **archaea**. Most organisms in these two groups are just a single cell with a **flagellum** for movement. They replicate themselves through a process called **binary fission** in which they split apart, creating two exact copies of the same cell.

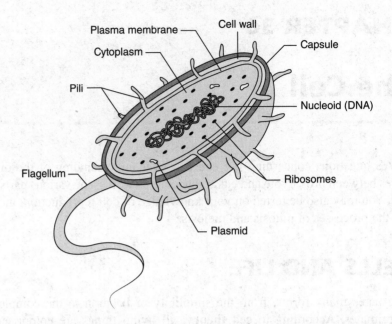

Eukaryote cells are present in almost all of the abundance of life visible to the eye, from plants and animals to fungi and even some bacteria. They have membrane-covered organelles, including a nucleus that holds the cell's DNA. They reproduce through either mitosis or meiosis.

PARTS OF THE CELL

A typical animal cell, shown below, is filled with **cytoplasm** within a **cell membrane**. The cell membrane allows select substances (proteins, enzymes, and chemicals) to pass through while keeping others out. Resting in the cytoplasm are various organelles. Organelles serve to regulate the metabolic functions of the cell.

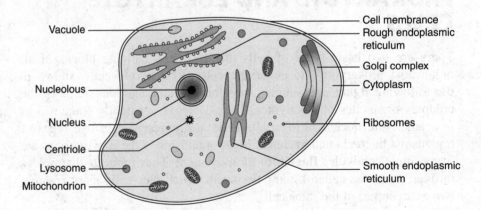

The **nucleus** is the control center of the cell and contains the **nucleolus**. The cell's DNA is contained in the nucleus, and it delivers information to control the metabolic functions of the cell. The nucleolus produces **ribosomes**. Ribosomes are found throughout the cell and synthesize proteins.

The **mitochondrion** is the energy center of the cell where glucose and oxygen are broken down into water and carbon dioxide. As a result of breaking these chemical bonds, energy in the form of adenosine triphosphate (ATP) is produced.

The **endoplasmic reticulum** of a cell is a membrane where proteins, the building blocks of cellular life, are built and stored. **Rough endoplasmic reticulum** has ribosomes attached, whereas **smooth endoplasmic reticulum** has none. Working with the **Golgi complex**, or **Golgi apparatus**, the endoplasmic reticulum assembles proteins and makes structures with those proteins.

Centrioles are organelles that assist in cell reproduction, either mitosis or meiosis.

Lysosomes capture the products of cellular function that the cell cannot use. They break down this cellular waste.

PLANT CELLS

Plant cells are similar to animal cells in most respects. They have all the same organelles, but they also have a **cell wall** and contain **chloroplasts**. Chloroplasts are organelles that aid in photosynthesis, through which plants use water, carbon dioxide, and the sun's energy to create glucose and oxygen.

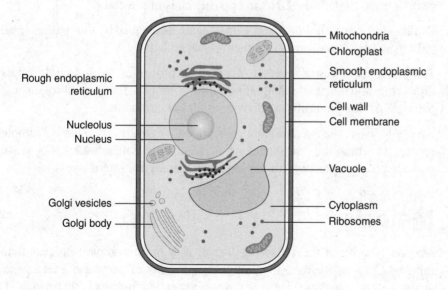

CELL REPRODUCTION

Cells proliferate in two ways, through mitosis or meiosis. **Mitosis** is the way that cells proliferate through asexual reproduction. In mitosis, cells reproduce an exact copy of themselves.

Meiosis is how cells reproduce through sexual reproduction. In this case, each daughter cell has half of the DNA of the original cell. In sexual reproduction, the daughter cells combine with such cells from another individual to form offspring, leading to genetic variation.

Cells that are thriving and conducting metabolic functions are considered to be in **interphase**. During interphase, cells' energy expenditure goes to the function of the organism.

Mitosis

Mitosis, shown in the following figure, occurs when a cell duplicates itself. This can happen in single-cell organisms, like protozoa or bacteria, and is how they reproduce. It also happens in other living organisms when they grow or heal. New cells are created with the same DNA as the original cells.

When more cells are needed or a sexual stimulus is introduced, chromosomes and centrioles are replicated.

Prophase is the first phase of mitosis. In this phase, the nuclear membrane dissolves, allowing the doubled chromosomes to float freely. Spindle fibers congregate around structures known as centrosomes to produce a spindle apparatus, which separates the floating DNA into separate poles.

Metaphase sees an orientation of the spindle apparatus, drawn by the centrosomes, to push the DNA to opposite ends of the cell.

During **anaphase**, spindle fibers retract, again influenced by the centrosomes, pulling apart chromosomes into their v-shaped halves.

Telophase ushers in a reversal of previous processes, with spindle fibers dissolving and nuclear membranes forming around the new chromosome pairings. At this point mitotic division is all but complete.

After telophase, the two daughter cells undergo **cytokinesis**. This is a simple process in which the two nuclei are divided by cell membranes. There are now identical twin cells with the same DNA ready for interphase.

Meiosis

Meiosis, shown in the following figure, is a more complex process than mitosis. Cells in meiosis go through two rounds of prophase, metaphase, anaphase, and telophase. These two stages are called **meiosis I** and **meiosis II**.

Prophase I is similar to mitotic prophase in that the nuclear membrane disappears, allowing chromosomes from each parent to mingle. In this case, chromosomes perform a crossing-over in which similar chromosomes from each parent bundle together. An allele from one parent may replace an allele from another, causing genetic variation.

Metaphase I, **anaphase I**, and **telophase I** mimic their mitotic counterparts. The new chromosomal pairings, called **tetrads**, migrate, and cytokinesis begins creating two **diploid** cells containing a full, but unique, complement of mixed DNA (46 chromosomes in humans). These two daughter cells then begin the process of meiosis II.

Prophase II, metaphase II, anaphase II, and telophase II mirror the previous process. Centrosomes and spindle fibers push apart chromosomes. When the spindle fibers retract, chromosomes are pulled apart. When telophase II begins, each daughter nucleus has only one of each pair of chromosomes (23 chromosomes rather than 46 in humans). The result is four **haploid** cells, or **gametes**.

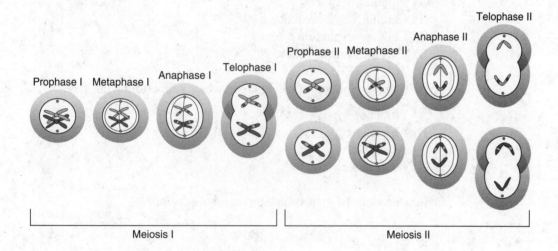

REVIEW QUESTIONS

1. A cell reproduces itself through binary fission rather than mitosis or meiosis. What kind of cell is it?

   A) Prokaryote
   B) Eukaryote
   C) Gamete
   D) Haploid

2. Which of the following is not contained within the cell membrane of a eukaryote cell?

   A) Nucleus
   B) Cytoplasm
   C) Ribosomes
   D) Flagellum

3. Which organelle works in concert with the endoplasmic reticulum to produce other organelles?

A) Centriole
B) Lysosome
C) Golgi complex
D) Cytoplasm

4. What is the function of the nucleolus?

A) Ribosome production
B) Protein storage
C) Cellular respiration
D) Reproduction

5. What is the function of lysosomes?

A) Protein transport
B) Cellular waste breakdown
C) Cellular respiration
D) Chromosome replication

6. Cells that are not reproducing are in which of the following states?

A) Prophase
B) Metaphase
C) Anaphase
D) Interphase

7. In what stage of meiosis do spindle fibers disappear?

A) Interphase
B) Prophase
C) Metaphase
D) Telophase

8. Circle the part of the diagram below that shows anaphase.

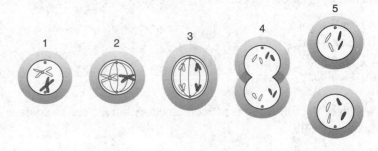

9. At the end of meiosis I, in what state is the original cell?

    A) Two haploid cells
    B) Four haploid cells
    C) Two diploid cells
    D) Four diploid cells

10. In which phase of meiosis does genetic variation take place?

    A) Prophase I
    B) Anaphase I
    C) Metaphase II
    D) Telophase II

ANSWER KEY

1. A	**5.** B	**9.** C
2. D	**6.** D	**10.** A
3. C	**7.** D	
4. A	**8.** 3	

ANSWERS AND EXPLANATIONS

1. (A) Prokaryote cells lack a nucleus. Both mitosis and meiosis begin with DNA replication in the nucleus. Binary fission is the manner in which prokaryote cells divide into two distinct but identical cells.

2. (D) The flagellum exists outside the cell membrane of single-cell organisms. These are predominately prokaryotes.

3. (C) The Golgi complex, or apparatus, uses the proteins created by the endoplasmic reticulum to build new organelles and other cellular structures.

4. (A) The nucleus contains the DNA of the cell. Within the nucleus, the nucleolus produces ribosomes, which help in protein production.

5. (B) Lysosomes capture and break down the unneeded by-products of metabolic activity, or cellular waste.

6. (D) Interphase is the name of the state that cells occupy when they are performing normal metabolic functions. DNA may be replicating in preparation for cell reproduction, but the cell is not undergoing either mitosis or meiosis.

7. (D) The last stage of meiosis I and meiosis II is telophase. The spindle apparatus has done its job of separating and orienting the chromosomes. It now dissolves to allow the cell to enter interphase and its normal metabolic functions.

8. (3) The four stages of mitosis, in order, are prophase, metaphase, anaphase, and telophase. The third part of the diagram shows anaphase, in which the sister chromatids are separated and pulled to opposite poles of the cell by the spindle fibers.

9. (C) At the end of meiosis I, the chromosomes have crossed over and then migrated to the poles. Nuclear membranes have formed around the DNA creating two diploid cells—cells with 46 chromosomes.

10. (A) In meiosis, genetic variation happens in the first phase, prophase I. The two sets of chromosomes recombine through crossing over. Homologous alleles match up, creating genetic variation.

CHAPTER 37

DNA and RNA

TEAS questions concerning **DNA and RNA** cover topics including the components of DNA and RNA, nitrogenous bases, and base pairs. You may also see questions concerning transcription and translation.

FUNCTIONS

Every living organism has instructions for growth in the form of **DNA** and **RNA**. DNA stands for **deoxyribonucleic acid**. RNA stands for **ribonucleic acid**. RNA comes in different forms, such as **mRNA** (messenger RNA), **tRNA** (transfer RNA), and **rRNA** (ribosomal RNA). DNA, the larger molecule, stores genetic information for the organism as a whole. It contains the code for creating new cells and is essential for the creation of new organisms during reproduction. RNA is smaller. In fact, it is created from the nucleic acids in DNA. Its function is to help in the creation of proteins and amino acids, and it is found in ribosomes. It also acts as a messenger carrying genetic information around a cell and beyond.

CHROMOSOMES, AMINO ACIDS, AND PROTEINS

Chromosomes are strands of DNA and related proteins that reside in the nuclei of living cells. They carry the genetic information needed to create new cells and organisms. **Amino acids** are the building blocks of organic material. They are produced by RNA as the building materials for **proteins**, which in turn are the content of cells and cellular organs. Proteins make up enzymes, which carry out the work of cellular life, like metabolic functions. Proteins also make up polymerases, which transcribe and transfer genetic material.

NUCLEIC ACIDS

Complex compounds that are present in all organic cells, **nucleic acids** are the core units of life. Both DNA and RNA are nucleic acids. A nucleic acid is composed of **nucleotides**. Nucleotides are **nucleosides** together with a phosphate group. Nucleosides are sugars (ribose or deoxyribose) combined with either a **purine** or a **pyrimidine**.

NITROGENOUS BASES

The five nitrogenous bases, **adenine (A)**, **guanine (G)**, **cytosine (C)**, **thymine (T)**, and **uracil (U)**, are needed to make nucleotides. The sequence in which they appear allows genetic information to be stored in DNA and RNA. This information comes in three nucleotide groupings called **codons**. They are written as three letters, for example CAG, to show which nitrogenous bases they are composed of. With four nitrogenous bases, this leads to a possible 64 combinations of three letters in different orders.

PURINES AND PYRIMIDINES

Purine bases, adenine and guanine, are bicyclic. Pyrimidine bases, cytosine and thymine, are monocyclic. Uracil is a form of thymine that replaces this pyrimidine in RNA. They form **hydrogen bonds** in a complementary fashion, meaning that a purine always pairs with a pyrimidine.

BASE PAIRS

Purines and pyrimidines have different structures that allow them to form hydrogen bonds, which are crucial for the formation of DNA. One purine, guanine, bonds with a pyrimidine, cytosine. This is one of the **base pairs** discovered by Watson and Crick. The other is adenine and thymine. These base pairs are held together by hydrogen bonds. Cytosine bonds with guanine using three hydrogen bonds, while adenine and thymine require only two hydrogen bonds. These bonds connect the **double helix** of DNA. These codons contain instructions for building amino acids, which are necessary for building organic structures.

DIFFERENCES BETWEEN DNA AND RNA

There are many minor differences between DNA and RNA. The major difference is their function. DNA stores and transmits genetic information for use on a cellular and organismic level. RNA transcribes and translates the genetic information into physical structures. DNA relies on four nitrogenous bases—(A) adenine, (G) guanine, (C) cytosine, and (T) thymine—whereas in RNA, (T) is replaced by (U) uracil. DNA has two strands of nucleic acid, referred to as a double helix due to its physical shape. This doubling of genetic information plays a crucial role in genetic diversity during reproduction. RNA has a single strand.

DNA comes in different forms. Mitochondrial DNA, for example, is only inherited from the mother. RNA also has different forms, such as mRNA (messenger RNA), tRNA (transfer RNA), and rRNA (ribosomal RNA).

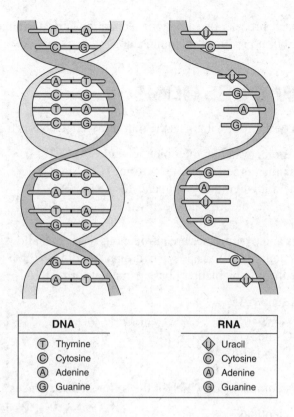

DNA		RNA	
Ⓣ	Thymine	◊	Uracil
Ⓒ	Cytosine	Ⓒ	Cytosine
Ⓐ	Adenine	Ⓐ	Adenine
Ⓖ	Guanine	Ⓖ	Guanine

TRANSCRIPTION

DNA contains all of the genetic information necessary to create living cells and organisms. **Transcription** is the process through which this genetic information is copied to make RNA (see figure above). RNA polymerase, an enzyme created from a strand of RNA, binds with a DNA sequence during the initiation phase. This binding loosens the hydrogen bonds holding the double helix together. The bound section elongates with the addition of nucleotides. Proteins called **transcription factors** provide the needed material. The process terminates with a genetic duplicate strand of mRNA being released into the cell.

TRANSLATION

At some point, genes must do their work. They contain the instructions for building amino acids and proteins and larger cellular bodies. **Translation** is the process through which that information is put into reality. Translation means making a protein. The first step in translation is transcription. After the cell's genetic code is transcribed to an mRNA molecule, the information within is unlocked in the **ribosomes**. Ribosomes are situated in the cytoplasm of a cell or in the endoplasmic reticulum and are the cell's factories for producing proteins. The mRNA carries the three base pair codons that dictate the type of amino acid needed for a particular protein. A strand of mRNA pairs with a strand of tRNA, carrying complementary codons, during translation.

The three-phase process of initiation, elongation, and termination mirrors transcription, but it produces an amino acid.

REVIEW QUESTIONS

1. Which of the following lists the four nitrogenous bases found in RNA?

   A) Alanine, cysteine, threonine, glycine (A, C, T, G)
   B) Guanine, uracil, adenine, cytosine (G, U, A, C)
   C) Adenine, thymine, guanine, cytosine (A, T, G, C)
   D) Cytosine, uracil, guanine, thymine (C, U, G, T)

2. Purines and pyrimidines are nitrogenous bases that allow DNA to form into its double helix shape via hydrogen bonding. Which of the following are the complementary base pairs that form DNA?

   A) T-C and A-G
   B) A-C and T-G
   C) G-C and A-T
   D) A-U and G-C

3. DNA is composed of which of the following substances?

   A) Nucleotides
   B) Cells
   C) Neurons
   D) Proteins

4. Which of the following is used during the transcription phase of protein synthesis?

   A) Snippets
   B) tRNA
   C) rRNA
   D) mRNA

5. During which of the following processes is tRNA active?

   A) Translation
   B) Transcription
   C) Meiosis
   D) Mitosis

6. Which of the following is inherited only from the mother?

   A) Phenotype
   B) Genotype
   C) Lysosomal DNA
   D) Mitochondrial DNA

7. Amino acids are the building blocks of which of the following?

A) Blood
B) Neurons
C) Proteins
D) Cell walls

8. DNA and RNA share almost identical nitrogenous bases. Which nitrogenous base is found only in RNA?

A) Thymine
B) Adenine
C) Uracil
D) Cytosine

9. DNA uses hydrogen bonds to hold the purines and pyrimidines together. How many hydrogen bonds are there between cytosine and guanine? Write your answer in the blank: _____

10. TAC-GGT-GTA-ACT Gene

? - ? - ? - ?   mRNA

During transcription, messenger RNA carries the code from the genes to the ribosomes. To do this, the RNA polymerase must add matching RNA nucleotides to the complementary DNA sequence. Looking at the gene sequence above, which of the following reflects the correct mRNA sequence?

A) ATG-CCA-CAT-TGA
B) CGU-AAC-ACG-GUC
C) GUC-AAG-AGU-UCG
D) AUG-CCA-CAU-UGA

ANSWER KEY

1. B	**5.** A	**9.** 3
2. C	**6.** D	**10.** D
3. A	**7.** C	
4. D	**8.** C	

ANSWERS AND EXPLANATIONS

1. (B) When RNA transcribes a codon from DNA during transcription, thymine is replaced with uracil. Thymine is less prone to mutation, which makes it a good storage vehicle for DNA. Uracil is more flexible, which makes it more suited to its temporary role in RNA. The other three nitrogenous bases, adenine, guanine, and cytosine, are used in both DNA and RNA.

2. (C) Base pairs combine in only a few ways because of the unique nature of the hydrogen bonds that hold them together. Cytosine bonds with guanine using three hydrogen bonds. Adenine and thymine require only two hydrogen bonds as do adenine and uracil in RNA. These base pairs are typically written using their letter symbols, G-C and A-T.

3. (A) Understanding the role of DNA is important in answering questions about it. DNA stores the genetic information necessary to create living matter and beings. Choices B, C, and D are all created by DNA and RNA. DNA itself is composed of nucleotides.

4. (D) Messenger RNA, called mRNA, is created during transcription. Its function is to carry the genetic code to the ribosomes for protein formation. It holds the genetic information in three base pair sequences called codons.

5. (A) Transfer RNA, called tRNA, is needed during translation. It recognizes the specific codon in mRNA needed to create a specific amino acid. There are 64 different possible codons and 20 amino acids, so only the appropriate tRNA will unlock the code and create proteins.

6. (D) Mitochondrial DNA is inherited only from the mother in almost all organisms that reproduce through sexual reproduction. Sperm cells contain mitochondrial DNA, but the egg cell's processes destroy it.

7. (C) Proteins are the engines of cellular, and thus life, function. In the form of enzymes they manage the cell's metabolic processes. DNA and RNA, through transcription and translation, build the amino acids necessary to create proteins. Without proteins, the other aspects of living material—blood, neurons, and cell walls—would not exist.

8. (C) While DNA uses thymine as a pyrimidine to bond with adenine, RNA uses uracil. Thymine is less prone to mutation, which makes it a good storage vehicle for DNA. Uracil is more flexible, which makes it more suited to its temporary role in RNA. The other three nitrogenous bases, adenine, guanine, and cytosine, are used in both DNA and RNA.

9. (3) There are only a certain number of possibilities of base pairs due to the unique nature of the hydrogen bonds that hold them together. Cytosine bonds with guanine using three hydrogen bonds. Adenine and thymine require only two hydrogen bonds, as do adenine and uracil in RNA.

10. (D) The discovery of base pairs by Watson and Crick proved that there were only certain combinations of nitrogenous bases possible. This is the meaning of the term *complementary* in the question. For example, guanine always bonds with cytosine. The three possible bonds are G-C, A-T, or A-U. In the example, the first codon is TAC, meaning that the complementary codon *must* be AUG. For the rest of the sequence, GGT-GTA-ACT, the complementary nitrogenous bases are CCA-CAU-UGA.

CHAPTER 38

Genetics

TEAS **genetics questions** cover topics including chromosomes, genes, alleles, phenotypes, and genotypes. Some questions may also test your knowledge of the use of Punnett squares.

Genetics is the discipline in biology wherein scientists focus on heredity. Whereas biology deals with individuals and groups, genetics deals with the heredity information carried in DNA.

CHROMOSOMES AND GENES

The **chromosome** is the fundamental unit of genetics. Contained in the nucleus of plant and animal cells, a chromosome is a linear strand that caries the hereditary information of the individual. It is composed of DNA and related proteins. Humans, for example, have 46 chromosomes, 23 each from their mother (through the egg cell) and from the father (carried in the sperm). All organisms that procreate through sexual reproduction are **diploid**, meaning they carry two sets of chromosomes. The two strands, connected by a single **centromere**, are referred to as **chromatids** (see figure below). The number of chromosomes differs between species, and there is no correlation between the number of chromosomes in a species and the number of genes.

The **gene** is a core unit of genetics. It contains the heredity information that, singularly or through a particular grouping of genes, leads to a characteristic. A **characteristic**, or trait, may be physical, like eye color or left-handedness. It can also be behavioral or psychological, such as a predisposition to addictive behaviors. Genes are located in a particular position on a chromosome. They are the loci of mutation, which leads to genetic variation. Mutations occur randomly or through environmental agency.

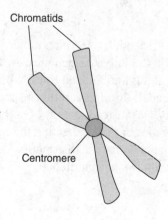

Chromatids

Centromere

ALLELES

An **allele** is a version of a gene. A gene can be composed of a pair of alleles that call for a different distinct trait. In diploid organisms there are two alleles, one from each parent. The alleles meet at a **locus**. For any pairing of alleles, we can talk about an individual's genes being **homozygous** or **heterozygous**. If the alleles are identical, the gene is homozygous. The characteristic that the gene produces will be the same as in the two parents. When the allele from each parent is different, the gene is heterozygous. Some traits are dominant, and some are recessive. The dominant trait is the one that will be expressed in the offspring.

PHENOTYPES AND GENOTYPES

Genetic variation takes place at the cellular level, but it can be seen on the surface in individuals. We can view an individual's hair color, height, and hear his or her tone of voice. These observable characteristics are known as **phenotypes**. Some traits, like blood type, are not observable to the naked eye, but they are measurable, so they fall under the phenotype rubric. This includes those traits selected through heredity and influenced by environment. An individual's height, for instance, is a product of its genes, but growing up in a poor environment with a lack of nutrition can lead to a stunting of growth. The observable height of the adult individual is part of its phenotype.

The **genotype** of an individual refers to the genetic makeup in its chromosomes. An individual may carry a recessive gene for a trait that does not appear in its phenotype but is still present and can be handed down to its genetic heirs. Although an individual's height may be inhibited by its environment, its heirs still carry the genotype for a range of height. This is not to be confused with a **genome**. A genome refers to the entire genetic material of an individual—in a human's case, all 46 chromosomes together. Genotype can refer to a specific allele. We can talk about an individual's genotype carrying DNA for both blue and brown eyes. At the phenotype level, the individual has brown eyes because the trait is dominant.

MENDEL

Many have called Gregor Mendel, a German monk who lived in the middle of the nineteenth century, the father of genetics. At the time, evolution was largely thought to work along Lamarckian lines, with traits being influenced by the environment. Mendel, through careful observation and experimentation, proved that heredity was instead at work. On the individual level, traits depended solely on the genes of the mother and the father. His work with pea plants led him to notice a mathematical distribution in traits among offspring, allowing him to codify the laws of inheritance.

He discovered that some traits are recessive, while others are dominant. He showed this by crossbreeding pea plants that varied in certain characteristics from height to color to seed shape. By tracking the appearance of phenotypic traits in the offspring, he developed a set of predictions now known as Mendel's laws of heredity.

PUNNETT SQUARES

The English geneticist Reginald Punnett created a diagram for predicting the outcomes when crossbreeding genotypes. The Punnett square is used to show how the genes of parents (the genes of which are already known) might combine in their offspring. It is a simple box of four squares. The alleles of one parent are placed across the top, and the alleles of the other are placed along the side. The four boxes show all the possible distributions of alleles in offspring (first filial generation, or Fl) of the two homozygous parents (parental generation, or P).

	H	**H**
h	*Hh*	*Hh*
h	*Hh*	*Hh*

H = tall (dominant); h = short (recessive)

In the Punnett square above, there is a 100% chance that the offspring will exhibit the dominant gene, becoming a tall pea plant.

In the following Punnett square, between two heterozygous parents with one dominant and one recessive allele, the offspring are shown to have a 25% chance of exhibiting the recessive gene.

	H	**h**
H	*HH*	*Hh*
h	*Hh*	*hh*

H = tall (dominant); h = short (recessive)

When a homozygous parent with two recessive alleles and a parent with heterozygous alleles are crossed, the results are as shown below:

	H	**h**
h	*Hh*	*hh*
h	*Hh*	*hh*

H = tall (dominant); h = short (recessive)

Even though the recessive alleles represent 75% of the genetic material, the dominant gene will be represented in the phenotype 50% of the time. This demonstrates the difference between an organism's genotype and phenotype.

MONOHYBRID INHERITANCE

Mendel's first law relates to monohybrid inheritance and is also known as the **law of segregation**. This law predicts the inheritance of a single trait. Punnett squares are useful tools for calculating the outcomes of crossbreeding.

In a typical monohybrid cross, we only record one trait. Let's look at eye color. Both parents are **homozygous**, which means that they have both genes the same. One parent has the dominant trait and one has the recessive trait. In this case, brown eyes (B) are dominant and blue eyes (b) are recessive, so one parent is BB and one is bb. Since each parent donates only one gene to the offspring, there is only one possible combination result for the first generation of offspring—one dominant and one recessive gene: Bb. This means that the F_1 generation is **heterozygous**, but the phenotype is the dominant brown eyes gene.

The first generation is then self-crossed to produce the second generation, F_2. For this generation, a Punnett square becomes useful for tracking the combinations. The parents are both Bb and the offspring are BB, Bb, Bb, and bb. The monohybrid ratio of the phenotypes here is 3:1.

	B	b
B	*BB*	*Bb*
b	*Bb*	*bb*

DIHYBRID INHERITANCE

Mendel's second law relates to dihybrid inheritance and is also known as the **law of independent assortment**. This law predicts the simultaneous inheritance of two separate and independent traits. Let's look at eye color (brown or blue) and thumb shape (straight or curved). The parent generation begins with one parent homozygous and dominant for both traits and one parent homozygous and recessive for both traits. We will use BBTT for brown eyes and straight thumbs and bbtt for blue eyes and curved thumbs. The F_1 generation will inherit BT from one parent and bt from the other to get BbTt, which will result in brown eyes and straight thumbs. Gametes from the F_1 generation can have BT, Bt, bT, or bt genotypes. When the F_1 generation is self-crossed, we get the Punnett square shown below.

	BT	Bt	bT	bt
BT	*BBTT*	*BBTt*	*BbTT*	*BbTt*
Bt	*BBTt*	*BBtt*	*BbTt*	*Bbtt*
bT	*BbTT*	*BbTt*	*bbTT*	*bbTt*
bt	*BbTt*	*Bbtt*	*bbTt*	*bbtt*

Looking at the Punnett square, we can count nine outcomes in which both B and T are dominant. There are three outcomes with B dominant and one recessive.

There are three outcomes with b recessive and T dominant. There is only one outcome with both b and t recessive. This means a dihybrid cross has a 9:3:3:1 phenotype ratio.

There are also non-Mendelian inheritances that do not follow the 3:1 and 9:3:3:1 ratios due to codominance, incomplete dominant-recessive relationships, multiple alleles, or epistasis.

REVIEW QUESTIONS

1. Which of the following reflects the genetic makeup of an organism?

A) Mitochondrion
B) Protein
C) Phenotype
D) Genotype

2. Which of the following reflects the outward observable expression of an organism's genetic makeup?

A) Phenotype
B) Allele
C) Genotype
D) Codon

3. Diploid organisms contain alleles that code for a specific gene. Which of the following terms describes two identical alleles at the same locus?

A) Heterozygous
B) Recessive
C) Homozygous
D) Dominant

4. Which of the following terms describes two different alleles at the same locus?

A) Heterozygous
B) Homozygous
C) Recessive
D) Dominant

5. A homozygous individual (RR) procreates with an individual who is heterozygous for a recessive trait (Rr). Which of the following is the correct percentage of offspring who will be carriers of the recessive trait?

A) 0%
B) 25%
C) 50%
D) 100%

6. A homozygous individual (NN) procreates with an individual who is heterozygous for a recessive trait (Nn). Which of the following is the correct percentage of offspring who will express the recessive trait?

A) 0%
B) 25%
C) 50%
D) 100%

7. A specific disease is carried on allele (s), which is recessive to the general condition of (S). If a heterozygous male (Ss) procreates with a female who is also heterozygous for the recessive trait (Ss), what percentage of offspring will have the disease?

8. A specific disease is carried on allele (X), which is dominant to the normal condition of (x). If a heterozygous male (Xx) procreates with a female who is normal homozygous (xx), which of the following is the correct percentage of offspring who will have the disease?

A) 0%
B) 25%
C) 50%
D) 100%

9. When two F_1 generation flowers with the genotype AaBb are crossed, the F_2 offspring are found to have which of the following phenotype ratios?

A) 3:1
B) 6:1:3:1
C) 6:3:3:1
D) 9:3:3:1

10. An individual's genome is composed of which of the following?

A) Only sex chromosomes
B) Only mitochondrial DNA
C) All of the DNA
D) All of the RNA polymerase

ANSWER KEY

1. D	**5.** C	**9.** D
2. A	**6.** A	**10.** C
3. C	**7.** B	
4. A	**8.** C	

ANSWERS AND EXPLANATIONS

1. (D) The question forms a general definition of the term *genotype*. It is the genetic material of the organism whether or not those genes have been expressed in the phenotype, choice C. These genes are available to be passed on to offspring. The mitochondrion, choice A, is the organelle in the cell that converts sugar into usable energy. Protein, choice B, is the building block of cellular life.

2. (A) The phenotype comprises the observable traits of an organism. A person may have brown hair. This is a phenotypic description. The person's genotype might have alleles for blond hair and brown hair. The dominant gene shows up in the phenotype, but the person's offspring may get the allele for blond hair. A codon is a grouping of DNA that correlates with an amino acid.

3. (C) When two alleles at the same locus are identical, we call this gene homozygous. Heterozygous means that the alleles are different. One allele will be dominant, which means that it will override the other, recessive, allele in the phenotype of the individual. In a homozygous gene, both alleles are the same, so the trait will exhibit itself phenotypically in the individual.

4. (A) A diploid organism has two sets of chromosomes, one from each parent. The genes from each match up at a place called the locus. The allele from one parent will meet its paired allele from the other parent at the locus. If the two alleles are identical, the gene is homozygous. When they are different, they are heterozygous. One allele is dominant, meaning it will exhibit its characteristics over the recessive trait.

5. (C) For this answer we can use a Punnett square to show the probability being sought.

	R	**R**
R	*RR*	*RR*
r	*Rr*	*Rr*

R = dominant; r = recessive

Half of the possible offspring of the two parents are Rr, meaning they carry the recessive allele r. Phenotypically, they will show the dominant trait, no disease, but their offspring might exhibit it. According to the Punnett square, 50% will be carriers of the trait.

6. (A) This answer basically uses the same Punnett square as the answer before. The only change is that the letters referring to the traits are different, and the question is asking about the phenotype, not the genotype.

	N	N
N	NN	NN
n	Nn	Nn

N = dominant; n = recessive

Just as in the last question, half of the possible offspring of the two parents are heterozygous, meaning they carry the recessive allele n. None of them show the recessive trait phenotypically, though. According to the Punnett square, 0% will exhibit the disease phenotypically.

7. (B) This answer also can be achieved through the use of a Punnett square.

	S	s
S	SS	Ss
s	Ss	ss

S = disease (dominant); s = no disease (recessive)

The Punnett square shows that only the ss, which is one in four offspring, or 25%, will exhibit the disease phenotypically. Three in four offspring, or 75%, Ss and ss, will be carriers, while SS, 25%, won't have any trace of the disease. The question asks what percentage will have the disease, rather than what percentage will be carriers of the disease. According to the Punnett square, 25% will have the disease.

8. (C) This answer, as well, can be solved by turning to a Punnett square.

	X	x
x	Xx	xx
x	Xx	xx

X = disease (dominant); x = no disease (recessive)

Half of the offspring of these two individuals have the dominant, disease-carrying allele. These offspring will exhibit the disease phenotypically. According to the Punnett square, 50% will have the disease.

9. (D) The ratio for a dihybrid cross is 9:3:3:1. If you cannot remember the ratio, you can always draw a Punnett square to find the ratio.

	AB	Ab	aB	ab
AB	*AABB*	*AABb*	*AaBB*	*AaBb*
Ab	*AABb*	*AAbb*	*AaBb*	*Aabb*
aB	*AaBB*	*AaBb*	*aaBB*	*aaBb*
ab	*AaBb*	*Aabb*	*aaBb*	*aabb*

10. (C) The term *genome* refers to the complete set of genetic material available to an individual or a group. The important unit of genetic material as it pertains to both genotype and phenotype is DNA. An individual's genome is all of its DNA.

Chemistry

CHAPTER 39

The Atom

Atoms questions on the TEAS test your understanding of the components of an atom. You may also be asked to identify parts of atoms based on their atomic number and mass number, and you may be asked to calculate an atom's overall mass. You may see questions regarding isotopes and the overall charge of an atom as well.

ATOMIC COMPONENTS

An atom is the smallest unit of an element that still possesses all of the properties of that element. Atoms contain three component parts: protons, neutrons, and electrons. **Protons** are positively charged particles located in the **nucleus**, or center, of the atom. **Neutrons** are also located in the nucleus of the atom along with the protons, but neutrons have a neutral electrical charge.

Electrons are negatively charged particles that orbit around the nucleus of the atom. Valence electrons are those in the outermost shell of an atom that can participate in the formation of a chemical bond with another atom. The figure below shows the four main components of an atom:

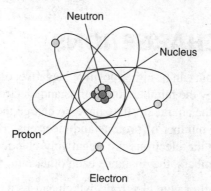

In terms of size, protons and neutrons are roughly the same size, and they are much larger than electrons.

ATOMIC NUMBER AND MASS NUMBER

The **atomic number** of an element is an identifying number that indicates the number of protons found in atoms of that element. An atom of an element with an atomic number of 8 would have 8 protons in its nucleus; an atom with an atomic number of 14 has 14 protons. The atomic number is equivalent to the number of protons.

The **mass number** of an element is an identifying number that indicates the number of protons plus the number of neutrons found in atoms of that element. An atom with an atomic number of 8 and a mass number of 17 would have 8 protons and 9 neutrons. To calculate the number of neutrons that an atom possesses, subtract the number of protons from the mass number:

Mass number − number of protons = number of neutrons

An atom with 12 protons and a mass number of 24 would have 24 − 12, or 12, neutrons.

Protons and neutrons each have a mass of 1 **atomic mass unit** (AMU). To determine the approximate overall mass of an atom in AMUs, we add the number of protons and neutrons. Electrons are left out of this equation because the mass of electrons is so small relative to that of protons and neutrons.

ISOTOPES

Atoms of a given element always have the same number of protons, but the number of neutrons may vary. One atom of nitrogen may have 7 protons and 7 neutrons, while another atom may have 7 protons and 8 neutrons. These different versions of atoms are called **isotopes**. In the nitrogen example given, the first isotope would be referred to as nitrogen-14 or N-14. The second isotope, with a mass number of 15, would be referred to as nitrogen-15 or N-15.

ATOMIC CHARGE/IONS

The charge of an atom can be either positive, negative, or neutral. The **atomic charge** is affected by the numbers of protons and electrons in the atom; neutrons do not affect the charge, as they have no charge themselves. A **neutral atom** has the same number of protons and electrons. The protons are positively charged, and the electrons are negatively charged, so when they are present in equal numbers, they balance each other out.

An atom can give off or gain electrons, which causes its charge to shift from neutral to positive or negative. An atom that has an electrical charge is known as an **ion**. If an atom gives off electrons, it will have fewer electrons than protons, and its charge will be positive (**cation**). If an atom gains electrons, it will have more electrons than protons, so its charge will be negative (**anion**).

A neutral isotope of nitrogen-14 would have 7 protons, 7 neutrons, and 7 electrons. The atomic number of nitrogen is 7, so we know that it has 7 protons, and the mass number of the nitrogen-14 isotope is 14. This means the number of neutrons is 14 − 7, or 7. The isotope is neutral, so it must have the same number of electrons as protons.

A negatively charged isotope of nitrogen-14 would have more electrons than protons. If the charge was −1, the isotope would have 7 protons, 7 neutrons, and 8 electrons. The −1 charge tells us that this isotope contains 1 more electron than the number of protons. In shorthand, this −1 charge would be written as N^-. An ion with a positive charge of +1 would be written as N^+.

Atoms are stable when they have full valence shells (like the noble gases do). They gain or lose electrons, forming ions, in pursuit of that stability. Bonds that form between oppositely charged atoms via the transferring of electrons are **ionic bonds**. Compounds that have ionic bonds can conduct electricity and are water soluble. Bonds that form between atoms via the sharing of electrons are **covalent bonds**. Bonds with partially covalent and partially ionic characteristics are **polar covalent bonds**.

REVIEW QUESTIONS

1. Which of the following indicates the number of protons and neutrons in an atom with an atomic number of 6 and a mass number of 14?

A) 6 protons and 6 neutrons
B) 6 protons and 8 neutrons
C) 8 protons and 6 neutrons
D) 12 protons and 14 neutrons

2. The mass and electrical charge of a neutron can best be described by which of the following statements?

A) A neutron has the same mass as a proton and a negative charge.
B) A neutron has the same mass as a proton and a neutral charge.
C) A neutron has the same mass as an electron and a neutral charge.
D) A neutron has the same mass as an electron and a positive charge.

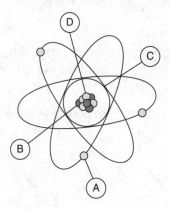

3. In the model of the atom shown above, circle the lettered label that identifies a negatively charged particle.

4. Which of the following reflects the overall charge of an atom with 10 protons, 12 neutrons, and 11 electrons?

   A) −2
   B) −1
   C) +1
   D) +2

5. What is the approximate overall mass of an atom with 19 protons and 23 neutrons?

   A) 19 AMU
   B) 23 AMU
   C) 38 AMU
   D) 42 AMU

6. Which of the following indicates the number of protons in an atom with an atomic number of 21 and a mass number of 55?

   A) 21
   B) 23
   C) 24
   D) 27

7. Which of the following describes isotopes?

   A) Two atoms have the same number of neutrons and the same number of protons.
   B) Two atoms have different numbers of neutrons but the same number of protons.
   C) Two atoms have the same number of neutrons but different numbers of protons.
   D) Two atoms have the same number of neutrons but different numbers of electrons.

8. An atom has 47 protons, 48 neutrons, and 49 electrons. This atom has an overall charge of _____ and an overall mass of approximately _____ AMU.

   Which of the following correctly completes the sentence above?

   A) +2; 96
   B) +2; 95
   C) −2; 96
   D) −2; 95

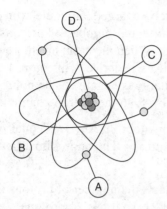

9. In the model of an atom shown above, circle the lettered label that shows the nucleus of the atom.

10. A neutral atom isotope has an atomic number of 16 and a mass number of 34. How many protons, neutrons, and electrons does the atom have?

A) 16 protons, 16 neutrons, and 16 electrons
B) 16 protons, 16 neutrons, and 18 electrons
C) 16 protons, 18 neutrons, and 16 electrons
D) 18 protons, 16 neutrons, and 18 electrons

ANSWER KEY

1. B   **5.** D   **9.** C
2. B   **6.** A   **10.** C
3. A   **7.** B
4. B   **8.** D

ANSWERS AND EXPLANATIONS

1. (B) The atomic number reflects the number of protons in the atom. So an atom with an atomic number of 6 would have 6 protons. The mass number reflects the number of protons and neutrons added together. So an atom with 6 protons and a mass number of 14 would have $14 - 6$, or 8, neutrons.

2. (B) Protons and neutrons have approximately the same mass, and neutrons have a neutral charge. Electrons are much smaller in mass than protons and neutrons.

3. (A) In the model of the atom, label A indicates an electron. Electrons orbit around the nucleus of the atom and have a negative charge.

4. (B) In an atom, protons are positively charged, and electrons are negatively charged. When an atom has an equal number of protons and electrons, its overall charge will be neutral. When the atom has more electrons than protons, its overall charge will be negative. This atom has 11 electrons and 10 protons, so its overall charge is negative. The number of electrons exceeds the number of protons by 1, so the overall charge is −1.

5. (D) The approximate overall mass of an atom, in AMU, is equal to the number of protons plus the number of neutrons. The approximate overall mass of this atom is 19 + 23, or 42, AMU.

6. (A) The atomic number of an atom reflects the number of protons in the atom. This atom has an atomic number of 21, so it has 21 protons.

7. (B) Two atoms are said to be isotopes when they have different numbers of neutrons but the same number of protons.

8. (D) This atom has more electrons than protons. It therefore has a negative charge, which eliminates choices A and B. The mass in AMU is determined by adding the number of protons and neutrons: 47 + 48 = 95.

9. (C) In the model shown, label C indicates the nucleus, which contains protons and neutrons.

10. (C) The atom has an atomic number of 16, so it has 16 protons. The atom has a mass number of 34, so it has 34 − 16, or 18, neutrons. The isotope is neutrally charged, so it has the same number of electrons as protons, or 16 electrons.

CHAPTER 40

The Periodic Table

Periodic table questions test your understanding of how to read the periodic table of elements. You may also be tested on various properties shared by different groups of elements. Other questions may address atomic radii, ionization potential, and electronegativity, based on an element's location on the periodic table.

READING THE PERIODIC TABLE

The **periodic table** is a table of chemical elements arranged by atomic number. Here is an example:

Periodic Table of the Elements

1 IA	2 IIA	3 IIIB	4 IVB	5 VB	6 VIB	7 VIIB	8	9 VIIIB	10	11 IB	12 IIB	13 IIIA	14 IVA	15 VA	16 VIA	17 VIIA	18 0
H 1 1.0079																	He 2 4.0026
Li 3 6.941	Be 4 9.0122											B 5 10.811	C 6 12.011	N 7 14.007	O 8 15.999	F 9 18.998	Ne 10 20.180
Na 11 22.990	Mg 12 24.305											Al 13 26.982	Si 14 28.086	P 15 30.974	S 16 32.065	Cl 17 35.453	Ar 18 39.948
K 19 39.098	Ca 20 40.078	Sc 21 44.956	Ti 22 47.867	V 23 50.942	Cr 24 51.996	Mn 25 54.938	Fe 26 55.845	Co 27 58.933	Ni 28 58.693	Cu 29 63.546	Zn 30 65.39	Ga 31 69.723	Ge 32 72.61	As 33 74.922	Se 34 78.96	Br 35 79.904	Kr 36 83.80
Rb 37 85.468	Sr 38 87.62	Y 39 88.906	Zr 40 91.224	Nb 41 92.906	Mo 42 95.94	Tc 43 (98)	Ru 44 101.07	Rh 45 102.91	Pd 46 106.42	Ag 47 107.87	Cd 48 112.41	In 49 114.82	Sn 50 118.71	Sb 51 121.76	Te 52 127.60	I 53 126.90	Xe 54 131.29
Cs 55 132.91	Ba 56 137.33	57-70 *	Lu 71 174.97	Hf 72 178.49	Ta 73 180.95	W 74 183.84	Re 75 186.21	Os 76 190.23	Ir 77 192.22	Pt 78 195.08	Au 79 196.97	Hg 80 200.59	Tl 81 204.38	Pb 82 207.2	Bi 83 208.98	Po 84 (209)	At 85 (210)	Rn 86 (222)
Fr 87 (223)	Ra 88 (226)	89-102 **	Lr 103 (262)	Rf 104 (261)	Db 105 (262)	Sg 106 (266)	Bh 107 (264)	Hs 108 (269)	Mt 109 (268)	Uun 110 (271)	Uuu 111 (272)	Uub 112 (277)	Uuq 114 (289)				

*Lanthanide series	La 57 138.91	Ce 58 140.12	Pr 59 140.91	Nd 60 144.24	Pm 61 (145)	Sm 62 150.36	Eu 63 151.96	Gd 64 157.25	Tb 65 158.93	Dy 66 162.50	Ho 67 164.93	Er 68 167.26	Tm 69 168.93	Yb 70 173.04
**Actinide series	Ac 89 (227)	Th 90 232.04	Pa 91 231.04	U 92 238.03	Np 93 (237)	Pu 94 (244)	Am 95 (243)	Cm 96 (247)	Bk 97 (247)	Cf 98 (251)	Es 99 (252)	Fm 100 (257)	Md 101 (258)	No 102 (259)

The elements on the periodic table are listed in order of their atomic number. Some periodic tables provide the atomic mass of the element as well:

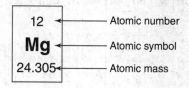

12 ← Atomic number
Mg ← Atomic symbol
24.305 ← Atomic mass

From the periodic table, by reading the atomic number, you can determine the number of protons and electrons in a neutral atom of an element. The number of neutrons can also be determined if the mass number of the atom is known.

PERIODS AND GROUPS

Elements of the periodic table are arranged in periods and in groups. **Periods** of the periodic table are organized horizontally across the table in rows. In the table shown, the shaded row represents a period:

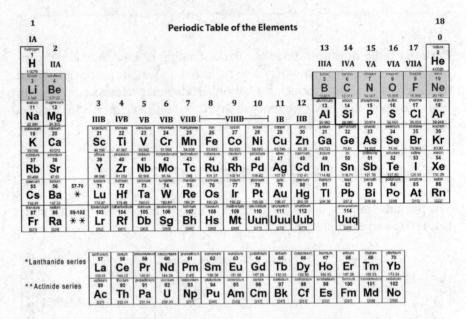

Groups in the periodic table are organized vertically down the table in columns. (Groups may also be referred to as families.) In the table shown, the shaded column represents a group:

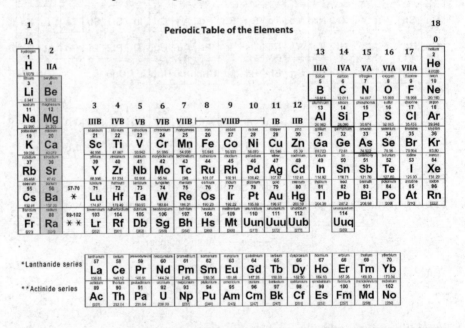

Elements in different groups share certain properties. The **alkali metals** in group 1 are shiny, soft, and highly reactive. The **alkaline earth metals** in group 2 are fairly soft and fairly reactive. The **transition metals** in groups

3 to 12 are hard and have low to negligible reactivity. The **halogens** in group 17 are extremely reactive, whereas the **noble gases** in group 18 are extremely stable. Metals overall tend to be malleable and highly conductive of heat and electricity, whereas nonmetals break easily and are generally poor conductors. **Metalloids,** such as boron, silicon, and germanium, have properties between those of metals and nonmetals.

ATOMIC RADII

The **atomic radius** of an atom is the measure of the distance from the center of the atom to its outermost orbital shell. Atoms with greater numbers of orbital shells have larger atomic radii because the outermost electrons are farther away from the nucleus. The length of the atomic radii decreases as you move from left to right across a period (row) of the table. The length of the atomic radii increases as you move down a group (column) of the table.

IONIZATION POTENTIAL AND ELECTRONEGATIVITY

The term **ionization energy** is used to refer to the amount of energy required for the removal of one electron from an atom. The ionization energy of an atom increases as the atomic radius of the atom decreases. This means that ionization energy increases as you move from left to right across a period (row) of the table. It also decreases as you move down a group (column) of the table.

The term **electronegativity** is used to refer to the tendency of an atom to want to bond with other atoms by taking electrons from those atoms. Like ionization energy, the electronegativity of an atom increases as the atomic radius of the atom decreases. This means that electronegativity increases as you move from left to right across a period (row) as atomic radius decreases, and it decreases as you move down a group (column) of the table as the atomic radius increases.

ORBITALS

The periodic table can also show the orbitals for the elements. An orbital is an area around the nucleus of a cell where electrons can be located. There are four types for orbitals.

An *s* **orbital** has the lowest level of energy and forms a symmetrical sphere around the nucleus. It can have a maximum of two electrons.

A *p* **orbital** has like an hourglass shape with the nucleus at the center. The *p* orbital has a maximum of six electrons.

D **orbitals** are more complex, but most look like four pear shapes connected by the nucleus at the center. The *d* orbital has a maximum of 18 electrons.

F orbitals are even more complex and are very difficult to visualize. The *f* orbital has a maximum of 32 electrons.

As the period numbers on the periodic table increase, the number of orbitals available also increases. Period 1 has only one orbital, *s*, with a maximum of two electrons. Period 2 elements have both an *s* orbital and a *p* orbital. Period 3 can have *s*, *p*, and *d* orbitals. Period 4 can have *s*, *p*, *d*, and *f* orbitals. Below is a version of the periodic table that shows which elements have which type of orbitals.

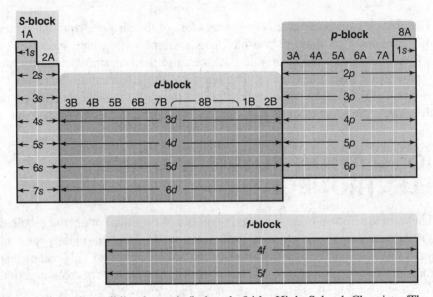

Source: https://en.wikibooks.org/w/index.php?title=High_School_Chemistry/The_Periodic_Table_and_Electron_Configurations&oldid=2991517

REVIEW QUESTIONS

1. Which of the following elements is most highly reactive?

   A) Argon (Ar)
   B) Neon (Ne)
   C) Radon (Rn)
   D) Fluorine (F)

2. Which of the following indicates the number of electrons in a neutral atom of zinc (Zn)?

   A) 16
   B) 20
   C) 30
   D) 40

3. Which of the following elements is the best heat conductor?

A) Iron (Fe)
B) Phosphorus (P)
C) Sulfur (S)
D) Selenium (Se)

4. Which of the following atoms is the most stable?

A) Nitrogen, because the elements in Group 15 can form anions
B) Argon, because the noble gases have full valence shells
C) Sodium, because alkali metals can form cations
D) Magnesium, because alkaline earth metals have a high melting point

5. Tungsten (W) has greater electronegativity than which of the following?

A) Tin (Sn)
B) Chromium (Cr)
C) Hafnium (Hf)
D) Molybdenum (Mo)

6. The greatest number of protons is found in an atom of which of the following elements?

A) Chromium (Cr)
B) Cobalt (Co)
C) Lithium (Li)
D) Carbon (C)

7. Atoms of which of the following elements have the highest ionization energy?

A) Potassium (K)
B) Nickel (Ni)
C) Calcium (Ca)
D) Manganese (Mn)

8. Which of the following statements is true about the relationship between mercury (Hg) and lead (Pb)?

A) Mercury atoms have fewer protons and a larger atomic radius than lead atoms.
B) Mercury atoms have more protons and a smaller atomic radius than lead atoms.
C) Mercury atoms have fewer protons and a higher ionization energy than lead atoms.
D) Mercury atoms have a smaller atomic radius and a higher ionization energy than lead atoms.

9. Which of the following atoms has the smallest atomic radius?

A) Rubidium (Rb)
B) Radium (Ra)
C) Strontium (Sr)
D) Barium (Ba)

10. Order the following elements from lowest (1) to highest (3) electronegativity.

_____ Vanadium (V)
_____ Manganese (Mn)
_____ Titanium (Ti)

ANSWER KEY

1. D	**5.** C	**9.** C
2. C	**6.** B	**10.** 2, 3, 1
3. A	**7.** B	
4. B	**8.** A	

ANSWERS AND EXPLANATIONS

1. (D) Fluorine is a member of the halogen group, whose elements are highly reactive. Argon, neon, and radon are members of the noble gases group, whose elements are extremely stable.

2. (C) Zinc is found in the fourth row of the periodic table with an atomic number of 30. Its atoms therefore have 30 protons. A neutral atom of zinc would have the same number of electrons as protons, or 30 electrons.

3. (A) Metals are better conductors of heat and electricity than are nonmetals. Iron is the only metal among the answer choices. Phosphorus, sulfur, and selenium are all nonmetals.

4. (B) Argon and the other noble gases have the most chemically inert atoms because they have full valence shells with no electrons that need to seek bonding.

5. (C) Tungsten is located on the sixth row of the periodic table, and it has an atomic number of 74. Electronegativity increases as you move from left to right across a period (row) of the table, and it decreases as you move down a group (column) of the table. Hafnium is located to the left of tungsten on the sixth row, so it has a lower electronegativity value.

6. (B) Cobalt has an atomic number of 27, so it contains 27 protons. Chromium has 24 protons, lithium has 3 protons, and carbon has 6 protons.

7. (B) Ionization energy increases as you move from left to right across a period (row) of the table. Nickel is the element located the farthest to the right of the four elements mentioned, which all lie on the fourth row of the periodic table. Nickel therefore has the highest ionization energy.

8. (A) Mercury has an atomic number of 80, while lead has an atomic number of 82, so mercury has fewer protons than lead. Mercury is located to the left of lead on the sixth row of the table, so its atoms have a larger atomic radius than lead atoms.

9. (C) The length of the atomic radius decreases as you move from left to right across a period (row) of the table, and it increases as you move down a group (column) of the table. Strontium is located to the right of rubidium on the fifth row and above barium and radium in the second column, so its atoms have the smallest atomic radii.

10. (2, 3, 1) Electronegativity increases as you move from left to right across a period (row) of the table, and it decreases as you move down a group (column) of the table. Titanium, vanadium, and manganese are listed in order of their positions from left to right on the fourth row of the table, so they are listed in order of least to greatest electronegativity.

CHAPTER 41

Properties and States of Matter

Matter questions on the TEAS test your knowledge of chemical properties and processes. You may be asked questions about states of matter, properties of matter, phase changes, chemical solution concentrations and diffusion, and the special properties of water, and acids and bases.

STATES OF MATTER

Matter is made up of microscopic particles that move at different speeds depending on the energy they are exposed to. We measure this energy as temperature. The molecules can move either quickly and randomly or hardly at all.

When the energy is high, matter takes the form of a **gas**, in which molecules are moving about quickly and are far apart. Gases have no fixed form. Molecules are free to move at random past each other, and they tend to fill any container that holds them. If a gas is not contained, its molecules will disperse.

Lower temperatures result in a **liquid**, in which molecules cohere but are fluid. **Coherence** means that the molecules remain close together, but they can change position by sliding over one another. In liquids, molecules move less freely than in a gaseous state, and they slide past one another. They have a fixed volume but will flow freely unless they fill a portion of a container.

When the temperature is low, matter takes the form of a **solid**, in which molecules are packed closely together and retain their positions. Solid matter is rigid, and molecules retain a uniform spacing. A solid has a defined form, which is brittle. It can be broken into pieces but tends to stay together.

A somewhat unusual state of matter is **plasma**, which is like a gas in many of its properties but carries an electric charge. The TEAS focuses on solids, liquids, and gases.

PHASE CHANGES

The state of matter depends on temperature and pressure. Higher temperatures cause molecules to energize and move farther apart. Increasing pressure forces molecules closer together. Changes in temperature or pressure can cause matter to change from one state to another, which is called a **phase change**. **Melting** is the phase change from solid to liquid, and **boiling** is the phase change from liquid to gas. There is also a direct change from solid to gas known as **sublimation**. The phase change from gas to liquid is **condensation**, and the change from liquid to solid is **freezing**. A direct change from gas to solid is **deposition**.

PROPERTIES OF MATTER

All types of matter can be described in terms of the physical and chemical properties each substance has. **Physical properties** are observable, and there is an extensive list of physical properties that one could observe about a substance. A few examples are density, the temperatures at which the substance undergoes phase changes, malleability, conductivity, specific heat capacity, mass, volume, color, and many other properties. Physical properties are further divided into intensive and extensive properties. An **intensive property** does not depend on the size or amount of matter in the object, while an **extensive property** does depend on the amount of matter in the object. For example, mass is extensive because the measurement would change with the size of the sample. Boiling point is intensive because the temperature at which the object boils is not dependent on its volume.

Chemical properties describe how a substance behaves during and following a chemical reaction. For example, we can categorize wood as flammable because it becomes heat, ash, and carbon dioxide when heated in the presence of oxygen. Chemical properties include oxidation, flammability, radioactivity, toxicity, reactivity with other chemicals, chemical stability, and others.

The properties of an unknown substance can be used to identify it. You may be asked to do this using a chart showing various characteristics.

CHEMICAL SOLUTIONS

A chemical solution is a group of chemical compounds evenly distributed in a state of matter. The solution is a **homogenous mixture** where one chemical compound is completely dissolved in the others. This is most easily achieved in a liquid state.

The **solute** is the compound dissolved in the **solvent**. Liquids make excellent solvents. The **solubility** of a solvent depends on the nature of the liquid as well as external factors like temperature. The **concentration** of the solution is the amount of solute in the solution. The **mole** is the unit of measurement for chemical reactions and refers to a compound's molecular mass.

Diffusion is the movement of molecules from an area of higher concentration to an area of lower concentration. When two liquids are mixed to make a solution, diffusion takes place until they are homogenous, meaning the concentration of each substance is the same throughout the mixture. The process of diffusion allows the molecules of the two liquids to mix and become evenly distributed, resulting in a homogenous solution. The rate of diffusion depends on factors such as the temperature, concentration gradient, and the properties of the molecules involved.

Diffusion is slightly different from **osmosis**, which is the movement of water molecules across a selectively permeable membrane from an area of lower solute concentration to an area of higher solute concentration.

There are mixtures that are not solutions. A **heterogeneous mixture** maintains separation between two substances, like oil and water.

ACIDS AND BASES

Many acids and bases can be understood from the perspective of the theory developed by Arrhenius, a Swedish scientist. In this view, an **acid** is a substance that gives off hydrogen (H^+) ions when it is dissolved in water. A **base**, or alkaline substance, is a substance that gives off hydroxide (OH^-) ions when it is dissolved in water. Acidic solutions have higher concentrations of hydrogen ions, whereas alkaline solutions have lower concentrations of hydrogen ions.

The presence of acids and bases can be tested using tools known as **indicators**. One indicator in common use is litmus paper. **Litmus paper** turns red in the presence of an acid and blue in the presence of a base.

Here are some examples of acids and their chemical formulas:

Acid	Chemical Formula
Acetic acid	$HC_2H_3O_2$
Phosphoric acid	H_3PO_4
Citric acid	$H_3C_6H_5O_7$
Hydrochloric acid	HCL
Sulfuric acid	H_2SO_4

Here are some examples of bases and their chemical formulas:

Base	Chemical Formula
Ammonium hydroxide	NH_4OH
Lithium hydroxide	LiOH
Magnesium hydroxide	$Mg(OH)_2$
Potassium hydroxide	KOH
Sodium hydroxide	NaOH

The acidity or alkalinity of a solution is measured using a scale known as the **pH scale**. The following figure shows examples of substances and lists where they fall on the pH scale:

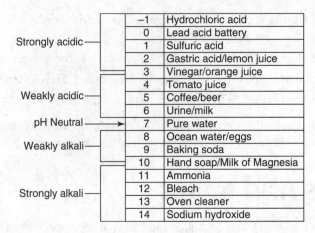

Strongly acidic	−1	Hydrochloric acid
	0	Lead acid battery
	1	Sulfuric acid
	2	Gastric acid/lemon juice
	3	Vinegar/orange juice
Weakly acidic	4	Tomato juice
	5	Coffee/beer
	6	Urine/milk
pH Neutral →	7	Pure water
Weakly alkali	8	Ocean water/eggs
	9	Baking soda
	10	Hand soap/Milk of Magnesia
Strongly alkali	11	Ammonia
	12	Bleach
	13	Oven cleaner
	14	Sodium hydroxide

Each step of the pH scale has 10 times the difference in concentration of hydrogen (H^+) ions as the step before or after it. So a solution with a pH of 7 will have 10 times more hydrogen ions than a solution with a pH of 8 and 10 times fewer hydrogen ions than a solution with a pH of 6.

SPECIAL PROPERTIES OF WATER

Water is a very important and unique substance with many physical and chemical properties that make it essential for life on Earth.

Physical properties:

- Water is a liquid at room temperature, which means it can flow and take on the shape of its container.
- It is transparent, meaning that light can pass through it.
- It has a high boiling point and melting point compared to other substances of similar size and weight, which means it can exist in all three states of matter (solid, liquid, and gas) under normal conditions.
- It has a high **surface tension**, which allows small insects and other objects to float on its surface.
- **Cohesiveness** allows water to travel through tiny capillaries, and cohesiveness creates surface tension on the surface of a body of water.
- **Adhesiveness** allows water to stick to other molecules and dissolve them, making it known as the "universal solvent."
- **Capillary action** is the ability of water (or any liquid) to flow upward against the force of gravity in narrow spaces, such as in thin tubes or narrow gaps in porous materials. This occurs due to the combined effects of adhesion and cohesion. As water molecules are attracted to the walls of the narrow tube, they form a concave shape at the edges of the water surface. This shape creates a surface tension that pulls the water up the tube or through the narrow gaps in the material, against the force of gravity. Capillary action is important for many natural processes, such as the movement of water from the roots to the leaves of plants and the movement of water through soil and other porous materials.

Chemical properties:

- Water is a very good solvent; it can dissolve many substances such as salts, sugars, and acids.
- It is a neutral substance with a pH of 7.
- It is a polar molecule, meaning it has a slightly positive and slightly negative end. This polarity allows it to form hydrogen bonds with other water molecules and with other polar molecules, making it an important part of many chemical reactions.
- The **polarity** of water allows it to exhibit both cohesive and adhesive properties.
- H_2O is a covalent compound because oxygen and hydrogen are nonmetals. It has eight total valence electrons (six from oxygen and one from each hydrogen). Breaking the bonds requires a lot of energy, so water has a very high specific heat and heat of vaporization. The molar mass of water is 18.02 g/mol.
- The high specific heat of water allows it to absorb a lot of heat energy without changing temperature very much. This property helps to regulate the temperature of the Earth's surface and protect living organisms from sudden changes in temperature.
- Water also has a unique property called **osmosis**, which is a specific type of diffusion in which water moves passively through a semipermeable membrane to equalize water concentration on both sides of the membrane. This is how water moves through cell walls in the body.

REVIEW QUESTIONS

1. A solution with a pH of 13 is considered to be which of the following?

   A) Weak acid
   B) Strong acid
   C) Weak base
   D) Strong base

2. Which of the following describes the phase change of sublimation?

   A) Solid to liquid
   B) Liquid to gas
   C) Solid to gas
   D) Liquid to solid

3. A solid item (X) with the density of 0.917 g/cm³ is placed in a beaker containing an aqueous substance (Y) with the density of 1.0000 g/cm³. Which of the following things do you expect to happen?

   A) X will float on the surface.
   B) X will sink halfway down the beaker.
   C) X will sink to the bottom of the beaker.
   D) X and Y have such close density that X will move around freely within Y.

4. Liquids have the capability of flowing. Which of the following statements below explains this phenomenon?

A) The spacing of the particles is close together.
B) The spacing of the particles is far apart.
C) The particles can glide over one another.
D) The particles are attracted to one another.

5. In which of the following states of matter are molecules located closest together?

A) Gas
B) Liquid
C) Plasma
D) Solid

6. A _____ is the standard scientific unit for measuring large quantities of tiny substances such as atoms and molecules. Write your answer in the blank.

7. Which of the following properties are responsible for water's capillary action? Select all that apply.

A) Adhesion
B) Density
C) Cohesion
D) Surface tension

8. Which of the following is an alkaline substance? Select all that apply.

A) H_2CO_3
B) LiOH
C) H_3PO_4
D) CaOH

9. Circle the part of the phase change graph that shows an increase in kinetic energy.

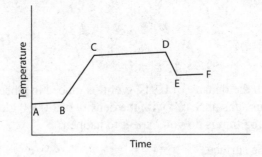

10. Why are droplets of water spherical?

A) Because of the high surface tension of water.
B) Because water is an inorganic molecule.
C) Because water is an excellent solvent.
D) Because of water's high heat of vaporization.

ANSWER KEY

1. D   **5.** D   **9.** B to C
2. C   **6.** mole   **10.** A
3. A   **7.** A, C, and D
4. C   **8.** B and D

ANSWERS AND EXPLANATIONS

1. (D) A solution with a pH of 13 is a strong base. Household bleach and oven cleaner are two examples of strong bases.

2. (C) Sublimation is the process in which a solid skips the liquid state and becomes a gas immediately. This somewhat rare phase change is seen in special compounds like dry ice, which goes from a solid to steam at room temperature. Choice A, solid to liquid, is known as melting. Choice B, liquid to gas, can be characterized as vaporization, evaporation, or even boiling, depending on the energy input. Choice D, liquid to solid, is typically known as freezing.

3. (A) The relative densities of solids and liquids are important for determining how they will react. A solid that is denser than a liquid will sink when placed in it. A solid that is less dense will float.

4. (C) Choice A could apply to both liquids and solids. Choice B could apply relatively to both gases and liquids. Choice D could apply to solids as well as liquids. The ability of particles to move fluidly is what describes the viscosity of liquids.

5. (D) The differences between the three main states of matter is the distance between molecules and their motion. These are caused by the energy put into the system. Lower energy means less movement and smaller distances between molecules, which describes solids. Plasma is closer to a gas than any other state.

6. (mole) Large quantities of very small substances are measured in moles.

7. (A, C, and D) The capillary action of water is caused by a combination of adhesion, cohesion, and surface tension.

8. (B and D) Alkaline substances (bases) usually have OH or H attached to a metal, as with LiOH (lithium hydroxide) and CaOH (calcium hydroxide). Acids usually start with a hydrogen and are attached to a nonmetal as with H_2CO_3 (carbonic acid) and H_3PO_4 (phosphoric acid).

9. (B to C) The temperature of a substance is directly proportional to the average kinetic energy of its particles, so as temperature increases, so does kinetic energy. This increase is shown between points B and C on the chart.

10. (A) Drops of water are spherical in shape because of the property of surface tension. The surface tension pulls the water molecules at the surface of the droplet equally in all directions, creating a symmetrical, rounded shape. A sphere is the shape that minimizes the surface area of the droplet while still containing the same volume of water.

CHAPTER 42

Chemical Reactions

CHEMICAL BONDING

A **chemical compound** is created when two or more atoms join to form a **chemical bond** that leaves the atoms in a less excited state than they were in before the bond. Such bonds form in two ways: covalent and ionic bonds.

A **covalent** bond occurs when nonmetallic atoms share electrons between them. This type of bond is common between two atoms of the same element, as in hydrogen (H_2) or in similar elements. When a molecule shares a pair of electrons in a stable state, it has formed a covalent bond. Alkanes, for example, share a single bond. In some compounds, one atom takes the shared electron for more time, due to its structure, forming a **polar covalent bond**. This molecule is partly negatively charged and partly positively charged. Some molecules form a **double bond**, sharing four electrons as opposed to two. These bonds are commonly represented in the alkenes, hydrocarbons with twice as many hydrogen molecules as carbon molecules. It is possible to form triple bonds, as seen in a group of hydrocarbons called alkynes.

An **ionic bond** is created between atoms when one atom gives an electron to the other. These bonds typically take place between metals and nonmetals due to the unique electron configuration of metals, with the metal giving an electron to the nonmetal. This transfer creates a positive charge and a negative charge at the ends of the compound. The positive charge, or **cation**, is created by the giver of an electron. The negative charge, or **anion**, is located at the receiving end of the electron. The **net charge** of the compound remains balanced at zero.

REACTION TYPES

To create a new chemical compound from other elements and compounds, a **chemical reaction** is needed. Two or more reactants are added together, often with an input of energy, creating one or more products and by-products. Photosynthesis occurs, for instance, when a plant cell combines carbon dioxide and water. The sun's rays provide the energy. The chemical reaction produces sugar and oxygen.

Chemical reactions are shown with equations and have a basic pattern: reactants go on the left and products go on the right, with the reaction sign (an arrow) showing the direction of the reaction in the middle. Here is an example showing the formation of water molecules:

$$2H_2 + O_2 \rightarrow 2H_2O$$

Equations for chemical reactions must be balanced; there must be the same number of atoms of each element on both sides of the reaction. Notice in the equation above that there are four hydrogen atoms and two oxygen atoms on each side. Only their arrangement is changed.

There are five basic types of chemical reactions:

- Synthesis
- Decomposition
- Combustion
- Single replacement
- Double replacement

Reaction rates depend on the likelihood of collision between particles. The reaction rate can be altered by changing the following factors:

- Concentration—The more particles there are, the higher the chance of collisions.
- Temperature—Particles excite at higher temperatures, so more collisions are likely and will have more energy.
- Pressure—Increased pressure forces particles together, so collisions are more likely.
- Surface area—In a solid, only particles at the surface can collide. The bigger the surface, the faster is the reaction. Breaking up a sample into smaller particles provides more surface area for collisions.
- Catalysts—A catalyst is a substance that changes the rate of a chemical reaction but is chemically unchanged at the end of the reaction.

CATALYSTS AND ENZYMES

Chemical reactions occur in nature and in the laboratory. Catalysts and enzymes are substances that speed up chemical reactions by lowering the activation energy required for the reaction to occur.

A **catalyst** is a substance that increases the rate of a chemical reaction by providing an alternative pathway for the reaction to occur. The catalyst itself is not consumed in the reaction, but it enables the reaction to occur more quickly and efficiently by reducing the amount of energy needed to initiate the reaction. Catalysts can be used in a variety of applications, from industrial processes to everyday products like catalytic converters in cars.

Enzymes are specialized biological catalysts that are produced by living organisms to speed up biochemical reactions in the body. Enzymes play a crucial role in many biological processes, including digestion, metabolism, and DNA replication. They work by binding to specific molecules, called **substrates**, and converting them into products. Enzymes are highly specific, meaning that each enzyme is designed to catalyze only one type of reaction. This specificity allows enzymes to carry out complex biochemical reactions with high efficiency and accuracy.

An example of an enzyme in action is the enzyme lactase, which is produced in the small intestine and helps to break down lactose, a sugar found in milk and other dairy products. Lactase catalyzes the hydrolysis of lactose into glucose and galactose, which can be easily absorbed into the bloodstream and used for energy. Without lactase, lactose would not be efficiently broken down and absorbed, leading to lactose intolerance and digestive discomfort.

BALANCING EQUATIONS

The TEAS Science section may contain questions that ask you to balance chemical equations. We will outline the steps in this process later in this chapter.

One of the most important chemical equations for humans is the one that represents photosynthesis. Without the following equation, there would be no life on Earth:

$$CO_2 + H_2O \rightarrow C_6H_{12}O_6 + O_2$$

This equation shows how green plant cells, with the help of the sun's energy, convert carbon dioxide (CO_2) and water (H_2O) into glucose and oxygen (O_2). The two **reactants**, carbon dioxide and water, are on the left side of the arrow. The arrow shows the direction of production. The two **products**, sugar and oxygen, are on the right side of the arrow.

According to the **law of the conservation of mass**, in a chemical reaction, no energy is lost, but neither is mass destroyed. The amount of reactant must match the amount of products that are made, even if those products escape as a gas or a liquid.

In the photosynthesis equation, there is a difference in the number of atoms on the right and left sides:

Element	Reactants	Products
C	1	6
H	2	12
O	3	8

To produce sugar and oxygen requires more reactants than we have on the left side. The solution is to balance the two sides.

We can multiply any molecule with a number called a **coefficient**. We cannot change the subscript, however, without changing the nature of the molecule. By adding coefficients to the reactants and products, we can balance the equation in a few simple steps.

The best way to do this is by balancing each element in turn. Start with the carbon. The right side has 6 carbon atoms, so the left side needs 6:

$$\underline{6}CO_2 + H_2O \rightarrow C_6H_{12}O_6 + O_2$$

Here we have multiplied the CO_2 by 6 to result in 6 carbon atoms on the left side. When we multiply CO_2 by 6, this also changes the number of oxygen atoms on the left side from 3 to 13. There are now 12 oxygen atoms in the CO_2 molecule, plus 1 in the H_2O molecule, for a total of 13. The two changed numbers are shown underlined in the following table.

Element	Reactants	Products
C	**6**	6
H	2	12
O	**13**	8

Now the carbon is equal, but the hydrogen remains unequal, and the oxygen has changed in number. Next, fix the hydrogen:

$$\underline{6}CO_2 + \underline{6}H_2O \rightarrow C_6H_{12}O_6 + O_2$$

Here we multiplied the H_2O molecule by 6 to result in 12 hydrogen 2 atoms on the left side. When we multiply H_2O by 6, this further changes the 2 number of oxygen atoms on the left side from 13 to 18. There are now 12 oxygen atoms in the CO_2 molecule, plus 6 in the H_2O molecule, for a total of 18.

Element	Reactants	Products
C	**6**	6
H	**12**	12
O	**18**	8

The last remaining imbalance rests with the oxygen. At this point, there is plenty of oxygen in the reactants. We can balance the equation by producing more O_2.

$$\underline{6}CO_2 + \underline{6}H_2O \rightarrow C_6H_{12}O_6 + \underline{6}O_2$$

In this step, the O_2 molecule on the right side was multiplied by 6. This resulted in 18 oxygen atoms on the right side. The equation is now balanced. Each element has the same number of atoms on the left and right sides.

Element	Reactants	Products
C	**6**	6
H	**12**	12
O	**18**	**18**

REVIEW QUESTIONS

1. A molecule that is acted upon by an enzyme is called a _____.
   Write your answer in the blank.

2. A hydrocarbon with one triple bond is called an _____.

   Which of the following correctly completes the sentence above?

   A) Alkyne
   B) Alkane
   C) Alkene
   D) Anion

3. ___Mg + ___HNO_3 → ___H_2 + ___$Mg(NO_3)_2$

Which of the following correctly balances the equation above?

A) $2Mg + HNO_3 → H_2 + Mg(NO_3)_2$
B) $Mg + 2HNO_3 → H_2 + Mg(NO_3)_2$
C) $Mg + 2HNO_3 → 2H_2 + Mg(NO_3)_2$
D) $2Mg + HNO_3 → H_2 + 2Mg(NO_3)_2$

4. Which of the following is the chemical formula for pentane?

A) C_6H_{12}
B) C_8H_{12}
C) C_5H_{12}
D) C_7H_{12}

5. Which of the following represents an example of ionic bonding?

A) The bonding of nonmetal atoms
B) The sharing of electrons
C) The transfer of electrons
D) The bonding of metal atoms

6. Which of the following hydrocarbons contains double bonds?

A) C_2H_8
B) C_6H_8
C) C_8H_6
D) $C_{12}H_{24}$

7. Which of the following is a function of enzymes?

A) Stop a reaction
B) Speed up the reaction rate
C) Slow down the reaction rate
D) Reduce the number of reactions

8. ___H_3PO_4 + ___$LiOH$ → ___H_2O + ___Li_3PO_4

Which of the following correctly balances the acid-base reaction above?

A) $H_3PO_4 + LiOH → 3H_2O + 2Li_3PO_4$
B) $H_3PO_4 + 3LiOH → 2H_2O + Li_3PO_4$
C) $2H_3PO_4 + LiOH → 3H_2O + Li_3PO_4$
D) $H_3PO_4 + 3LiOH → 3H_2O + Li_3PO_4$

9. ___C_2H_6 + ___O_2 → ___CO_2 + ___H_2O

Which of the following correctly balances the combustion reaction above?

A) $2C_2H_6 + 8O_2 \rightarrow 4CO_2 + 4H_2O$
B) $2C_2H_6 + 7O_2 \rightarrow 4CO_2 + 6H_2O$
C) $6C_2H_6 + 5O_2 \rightarrow 3CO_2 + 2H_2O$
D) $6C_2H_6 + 7O_2 \rightarrow 4CO_2 + 2H_2O$

10. Acids provide H^+ ions in water, while bases provide OH^- ions. Which of the following is a pair of bases?

A) HCl, HNO_3
B) H_2SO_4, HNO_3
C) $NaOH$, KOH
D) $Ba(OH)_2$, H_3PO_4

ANSWER KEY

1. Substrate	**5.** C	**9.** B
2. A	**6.** D	**10.** C
3. B	**7.** B	
4. C	**8.** D	

ANSWERS AND EXPLANATIONS

1. (substrate) Enzymes are proteins that act as catalysts to speed up chemical processes. Enzymes act upon a molecule known as a substrate.

2. (A) An alkane has a single bond. An alkene has a double bond. Alkynes are characterized by a triple bond. An anion refers to the negatively charged end of an ionic bond.

3. (B) To balance the equation, we must make the left side have the same number of elements as the right:

___Mg + ___HNO_3 → ___H_2 + ___$Mg(NO_3)_2$

The elements in this example number as follows:

Element	Reactants	Products
Mg	1	1
H	1	2
N	1	2
O	3	6

The Mg (magnesium) is already balanced. We move on to the next element, H (hydrogen). We double it in the reactants and look at the result:

$$\underline{\quad}Mg + \underline{2}HNO_3 \rightarrow \underline{\quad}H_2 + \underline{\quad}Mg(NO_3)_2$$

Element	Reactants	Products
Mg	1	1
H	**2**	2
N	**2**	2
O	**6**	6

The two sides are balanced by adding the coefficient 2 to the second reactant.

4. (C) The chemical formula for pentane is C_5H_{12}. A member of the alkane family, it has five carbon atoms, giving it its name.

5. (C) Ionic bonds differ from covalent bonds in that they transfer an electron from one compound to another rather than sharing electrons. They occur between metals and nonmetals in conjunction.

6. (D) Hydrogen bonds come in different forms. Double bonds form among hydrocarbons in different ways, as well, but the ratio is always one carbon atom for every two hydrogen atoms. The basic form is C_1H_2. $C_{12}H_{24}$ is the only example given that fits this 2:1 ratio.

7. (B) Enzymes serve as catalysts in chemical reactions. They speed up reaction times by lowering the energy required to activate a reaction. They change the environment in which a reaction takes place without being altered by the reaction themselves.

8. (D) To balance the equation, we must make the left side have the same number of elements as the right:

$$\underline{\quad}H_3PO_4 + \underline{\quad}LiOH \rightarrow \underline{\quad}H_2O + \underline{\quad}Li_3PO_4$$

The elements in this example number as follows:

Element	Reactants	Products
H	4	2
P	1	1
O	5	5
Li	1	3

The Li (lithium) stands out as being unbalanced. Adding a coefficient of 3 to the reactant gets us this distribution:

$$\underline{\quad}H_3PO_4 + \underline{3}LiOH \rightarrow \underline{\quad}H_2O + \underline{\quad}Li_3PO_4$$

Element	Reactants	Products
H	**6**	2
P	1	1
O	**7**	5
Li	**3**	3

Since the Li is balanced, we want to change the other molecule in the product, like this:

$$\underline{}H_3PO_4 + 3LiOH \rightarrow \underline{3}H_2O + \underline{}Li_3PO_4$$

The elements in this example now number:

Element	Reactants	Products
H	6	**6**
P	1	1
O	7	**7**
Li	3	3

The two sides are balanced by adding the coefficient 3 to the product.

9. (B) To balance the equation, we must make the left side have the same number of elements as the right:

$$\underline{}C_2H_6 + \underline{}O_2 \rightarrow \underline{}CO_2 + \underline{}H_2O$$

The elements in this example number as follows:

Element	Reactants	Products
C	2	1
H	6	2
O	2	3

Let's start by balancing H (hydrogen):

$$\underline{}C_2H_6 + \underline{}O_2 \rightarrow \underline{}CO_2 + \underline{3}H_2O$$

That gives us the following distribution:

Element	Reactants	Products
C	2	1
H	6	**6**
O	2	**5**

Now, C (carbon):

$$\underline{}C_2H_6 + \underline{}O_2 \rightarrow \underline{2}CO_2 + \underline{}3H_2O$$

That gives us the following distribution:

Element	Reactants	Products
C	2	**2**
H	6	6
O	2	**7**

To balance O (oxygen), we would need to multiply the reactant by 3.5. Coefficients must be whole numbers. We can double everything to fix the problem:

$$\underline{2}C_2H_6 + \underline{7}O_2 \rightarrow \underline{4}CO_2 + \underline{6}H_2O$$

That gives us the following distribution:

Element	Reactants	Products
C	<u>4</u>	<u>4</u>
H	<u>12</u>	<u>12</u>
O	<u>14</u>	<u>14</u>

The answer is:

$$2C_2H_6 + 7O_2 \rightarrow 4CO_2 + 6H_2O$$

10. (C) Sodium hydroxide (NaOH) and potassium hydroxide (KOH) are both bases. Barium hydroxide ($Ba(OH)_2$) is also a base, but it is paired with phosphoric acid (H_3PO_4), so choice D is incorrect. Choice A contains hydrochloric acid (HCl) and nitric acid (HNO_3), while choice B contains sulphuric acid (H_2SO_4) and nitric acid (HNO_3).

PART IV

ENGLISH AND LANGUAGE USAGE

The **TEAS English and Language Usage section** tests your understanding of English in three main areas: the conventions of standard written English, your knowledge of language and the writing process, and vocabulary. The review that follows covers the grammatical components you'll need to know, as well as important considerations concerning clarity and style. The final chapter helps you increase your ability to determine the meaning of vocabulary words in context.

CHAPTER 43

Parts of Speech

Parts of speech questions address the differences between subjects, verbs, nouns, pronouns, adjectives, adverbs, conjunctions, articles, and prepositions. You must identify these parts of speech in a sentence. These questions also test the difference between singular and plural nouns.

In the English language, we use different parts of speech to convey different types of information in sentence form. The parts of speech identify the role that a particular word or words play in a sentence. Essentially, parts of speech are sentence components.

SUBJECTS AND VERBS

The most important sentence components are subjects and verbs. **Subjects** convey who or what is performing the action in a sentence. **Verbs** describe the action that is taking place:

> Matt couldn't keep a secret.

In this sentence, the subject of the sentence is *Matt*. The verb is *couldn't*, a contraction for *could not*. Consider this example:

> Sarah's brother couldn't keep a secret.

In this sentence, the subject of the sentence is *Sarah's brother*. The verb is *couldn't*.

Here's a subject that's slightly more complex:

> Sarah's sincere but talkative little brother couldn't keep a secret.

In this form of the sentence, the subject is *Sarah's sincere but talkative little brother*. The verb is still *couldn't*, as in the previous two examples.

NOUNS AND PRONOUNS

A **noun** is a person, place, or thing, and a **pronoun** is a word that refers to a noun:

> Jamie entered the room before she saw Charles.

This sentence contains three nouns: *Jamie*, *the room*, and *Charles*. The word *she* is a pronoun that refers to *Jamie*.

Nouns and pronouns often make up the subjects of sentences, but they aren't always the subjects. Sometimes a form of a verb may be the subject of the sentence:

Laughing is contagious in our household.

In this example, the word *laughing* is a form of the verb *to laugh*. *Laughing* is the subject of the sentence, followed by the verb *is*.

Nouns can be singular or plural. A **singular** noun represents only one person, place, or thing. A **plural** noun represents more than one person, place, or thing being described.

Pronouns can also be singular or plural, depending on the noun they refer to:

Laughing is contagious in our household, especially when we are watching television.

In this example, *household* is a singular noun: it describes only one household. *Television* is also a singular noun, indicating one TV. The pronoun *we* is plural. It indicates more than one person watching TV.

ADJECTIVES AND ADVERBS

Adjectives and adverbs are descriptive words. In grammatical parlance, we say that **adjectives** modify nouns, and **adverbs** modify verbs. That just means that adjectives describe nouns, and adverbs describe how the action of a verb is taking place.

Adverbs can also modify adjectives and other adverbs.

The beach had massive waves.

In this sentence, the word *massive* is an adjective. It modifies the noun *waves*. Consider this example:

The beach's massive waves immediately caused a scare.

In this sentence, the word *massive* is still an adjective modifying *waves*. The word *immediately* is an adverb, modifying the verb *caused*. *Immediately* is used to describe how the action of causing a scare took place.

CONJUNCTIONS, ARTICLES, AND PREPOSITIONS

Other important parts of speech to know are conjunctions, articles, and prepositions. These components are less central to the meaning of a sentence than are subjects and verbs, but they must be included in order to make the meaning understood. **Conjunctions** are connecting words. They join together the ideas in a sentence. **Articles** are identifiers; they let us know if a noun is specific or general. Finally, **prepositions** indicate relationships between components of a sentence, often showing the location or direction of action. Prepositions are commonly included as parts of prepositional phrases.

The weather was cool and inviting.

In this sentence, the word *and* is a conjunction. It joins the words *cool* and *inviting.* In the following sentence, the word *a* is an article. It identifies the noun *golf cart.*

Leonard decided to go shopping for a golf cart.

Let's consider the following example, which contains the preposition *to.*

Hayley went to the library.

This preposition is part of the prepositional phrase *to the library.* The phrase indicates where Hayley went, showing the direction of her action.

INTERJECTIONS

An **interjection** is a word added to a sentence to show sudden or strong emotion. For example, the interjection might express surprise, joy, excitement, enthusiasm, pain, or disgust. It usually comes at the beginning of the sentence, although there is no set rule.

Hey, give me back my cookie!

In this sentence, the word *hey* is an interjection.

Introductory words, such as *yes*, *no*, or *well*, are also considered interjections.

No, I will not give back your cookie.

REVIEW QUESTIONS

1. The <u>severe</u> thunderstorm developed <u>later</u> than predicted, so we had time to finish our picnic.

Which of the following correctly identifies the parts of speech in the underlined portions of the sentence above?

A) Noun; adverb
B) Adjective; adverb
C) Adverb; adjective
D) Adjective; noun

2. Antibacterial soap should be used to help prevent the spread of germs.

Circle the adjective in the sentence above.

3. Although the plumber repeatedly attempted to fix the drainpipe, it still remains clogged.

   The word *repeatedly* serves as which of the following parts of speech in the sentence above?

   A) Verb
   B) Noun
   C) Adverb
   D) Preposition

4. Which of the following plural nouns is written in the correct form?

   A) Alumni
   B) Mouses
   C) Phenomeni
   D) Syllabuses

5. After the team played <u>its</u> championship game, the coach <u>treated</u> the children to ice cream.

   Which of the following correctly identifies the parts of speech in the underlined portions of the sentence above?

   A) Pronoun; verb
   B) Adjective; adverb
   C) Adverb; noun
   D) Adjective; verb

6. Surveillance videos reveal suspicious activity <u>behind</u> the store around midnight.

   The underlined word in the sentence above is an example of which of the following parts of speech?

   A) Article
   B) Pronoun
   C) Preposition
   D) Verb

7. Dolphins are social creatures and tend to live in pods ranging in size from ten to over one hundred animals.

   The word *social* serves as which of the following parts of speech in the sentence above?

   A) Adjective
   B) Preposition
   C) Verb
   D) Noun

8. Which of the following plural nouns is written in the correct form?

A) Patioes
B) Melodies
C) Geeses
D) Cactuses

9. When the cruise ship pulled into port, the seaside town was flooded with tourists.

Which of the following are nouns in the sentence above? Select all that apply.

A) Seaside
B) Cruise
C) Port
D) Ship

10. Samuel left <u>his</u> riding boots at the stable last week.

The underlined word in the sentence above is an example of which of the following parts of speech?

A) Preposition
B) Noun
C) Adverb
D) Pronoun

11. This year's concert series features rock, folk, and country music.

The word *features* serves as which of the following parts of speech in the sentence above?

A) Noun
B) Verb
C) Adverb
D) Adjective

12. Which of the following plural nouns is written in the correct form?

A) Nucleuses
B) Childs
C) Criteria
D) Potatos

13. Each <u>exquisite</u> necklace is <u>meticulously</u> crafted by hand.

Which of the following correctly identifies the parts of speech in the underlined portions of the sentence above?

A) Noun; adverb
B) Adjective; adverb
C) Adverb; adjective
D) Adverb; adverb

14. Constructed with sustainable materials, the new music building on campus is powered by <u>an</u> array of solar panels.

The underlined word in the sentence above is an example of which of the following parts of speech?

A) Article
B) Noun
C) Preposition
D) Pronoun

15. Mechanics generally advise motorists to have their cars serviced every 3,000 miles.

The word *motorists* serves as which of the following types of speech in the sentence above?

A) Pronoun
B) Article
C) Preposition
D) Noun

ANSWER KEY

1. B	**6.** C	**11.** B
2. Antibacterial	**7.** A	**12.** C
3. C	**8.** B	**13.** B
4. A	**9.** C and D	**14.** A
5. A	**10.** D	**15.** D

ANSWERS AND EXPLANATIONS

1. (B) Since the word *severe* modifies the noun *thunderstorm*, it functions as an adjective in this sentence. The word *later* functions as an adverb in this sentence, modifying the verb *developed*.

2. (Antibacterial) The word *antibacterial* is an adjective that modifies the word *soap*.

3. (C) Because the word *repeatedly* modifies the verb *attempted*, it is used as an adverb in this sentence. Therefore, choice C is the correct answer.

4. (A) The word *alumni* is the plural form of the nouns *alumnus* and *alumna*. The other answer choices are incorrect because *mice* is the plural of *mouse; phenomena* is the plural of *phenomenon;* and *syllabi* is the plural of *syllabus*.

5. (A) The word *its* refers back to the noun previously introduced in the sentence, *team,* so it is a pronoun. The main action of the sentence is described by the verb *treated*.

6. (C) The word *behind* links the prepositional phrase *behind the store* to the rest of the sentence and therefore acts as a preposition in this sentence.

7. (A) Since the word *social* modifies the noun *dolphins,* it serves as an adjective in this sentence. Therefore, choice A is the correct answer.

8. (B) The word *melodies* is the plural form of the noun *melody.* The other answer choices are incorrect because *patios* is the plural of *patio; geese* is the plural of *goose;* and *cacti* is the plural of *cactus.*

9. (C and D) The words *ship, port, town,* and *tourists* are the nouns in the sentence. *Seaside* and *cruise* are adjectives.

10. (D) Because the word *his* refers to the noun antecedent *Samuel,* the word *his* functions as a pronoun in this sentence.

11. (B) The word *features* presents the main action in this sentence and therefore serves as a verb, making choice B the correct answer.

12. (C) The word *criteria* is the plural form of the noun *criterion.* The other answer choices are incorrect because *nuclei* is the plural of *nucleus; children* is the plural of *child;* and *potatoes* is the plural of *potato.*

13. (B) Since the word *exquisite* modifies the noun *necklace,* it functions as an adjective in this sentence. The word *meticulously* functions as an adverb in this sentence, modifying the verb *crafted.*

14. (A) Choice A is correct because the word *an* is an article that modifies the word *array.*

15. (D) The word *motorists* serves as the direct object of the noun *Mechanics* in this sentence and functions as a noun. Therefore, choice D is the correct answer.

CHAPTER 44

Subject-Verb Agreement

The subject of a sentence must always agree with its verb. This means that the subject and verb must both be either singular or plural. **Subject-verb agreement questions** address whether there is a match between single and plural subjects and verbs.

Consider the following sentence:

> Her niece was never in the mood to play hopscotch. ✓ CORRECT

The subject of this sentence, *her niece*, is singular. The verb, *was*, is also singular. This sentence has subject-verb agreement because the subject and verb are both singular. Now look at this sentence:

> Her nieces was never in the mood to play
> hopscotch. ✗ INCORRECT

In this case, the subject is plural: *her nieces* refers to more than one niece. This sentence therefore requires the plural verb *were*:

> Her nieces were never in the mood to play
> hopscotch. ✓ CORRECT

The singular verb *was* in the incorrect sentence has been replaced by the plural verb *were*. Now the subject and the verb are both plural, so the subject and verb agree. Here's another example:

> Why doesn't your grandfather like to fish? ✓ CORRECT

The subject here, *grandfather*, is singular. The verb, *doesn't like*, is also singular. This sentence has subject-verb agreement.

This sentence, on the other hand, is incorrect:

> Why doesn't your grandfather and grandmother like
> to fish? ✗ INCORRECT

Whenever a subject contains two nouns joined by the word *and*, this makes the subject plural. Since the subject of the sentence is now plural, the sentence needs a plural verb:

> Why don't your grandfather and grandmother
> like to fish? ✓ CORRECT

The singular verb *doesn't like* from the sentence above has been replaced with the plural verb *don't like*. The subject and the verb are both in plural form, so they now agree.

REVIEW QUESTIONS

1. Which of the following sentences has correct subject-verb agreement?

   A) After a heavy rainfall, the dry creek beds often overflows.
   B) The barns surrounding the farmhouse were painted shades of red and brown.
   C) Many trees in this orchard produces a variety of delicious apples.
   D) Freezing temperatures last winter is blamed for the lackluster harvest.

2. Which of the following sentences contains subject-verb agreement?

   A) Both Jenna and Patrick is interested in playing soccer this year.
   B) Brian and Eileen expects to hear their favorite song at the dance tonight.
   C) The dog and the cat is both due for their annual veterinary visits.
   D) My aunt and my uncle plan to visit our family over the holidays.

3. Which of the following sentences provides an example of correct subject-verb agreement?

   A) The herd of elephants are being driven from their natural habitat.
   B) The flock of baby ducks search for bread crumbs near the edge of the pond.
   C) The pride of lions is traveling across the plains in search of fresh water.
   D) The pack of hungry wolves follow their prey until the early morning hours.

4. Which of the following sentences contains a correct example of subject-verb agreement?

   A) Neither Howard nor Phillip likes to play board games.
   B) Either the host or hostess greet guests when they arrive at the restaurant.
   C) Sally or Brenda volunteer at the hospital nearly every weekend.
   D) Hiking or jogging provide excellent cardiovascular exercise.

5. Which of the following sentences contains an example of correct subject-verb agreement?

   A) Both of the children prefer pink lemonade to iced tea.
   B) Everyone attend orientation meetings before the start of the semester.
   C) Somebody mow the grass regularly even though the house is vacant.
   D) All of the students enjoys the school trip at the end of the year.

6. Which of the following sentences has correct subject-verb agreement?

A) Topics included in the manual ranges from welding to pipefitting.
B) Captains of the ship rotates their time on and off duty.
C) Dates for each club meeting is posted by the door.
D) Numbers for current program enrollment indicate a high degree of interest.

7. Which of the following sentences contains subject-verb agreement?

A) After practice this Saturday, the team play its season opener.
B) Before the pool opens for the season, the waterpark staff provides lifeguard training.
C) As classical music enthusiasts, the audience tend to favor works by Baroque composers.
D) In addition to geometry and algebra, the class study calculus this year.

8. Which of the following sentences provides an example of correct subject-verb agreement?

A) The list of standing committees is in the folder.
B) One reason for college visits are to help students narrow down the many choices available.
C) Peter's collection of model airplanes were started by gifts from his grandfather.
D) A rare volume of classic folktales were donated to the library.

9. Which of the following sentences provides an example of correct subject-verb agreement?

A) Street signs depicting small children at play is visible all over the neighborhood.
B) Students pursuing degrees in healthcare take anatomy and physiology courses.
C) Vendors selling food at the state fair undergoes regular safety inspections.
D) Politicians running for office in this town frequently visits with local residents.

10. Which of the following sentences contains an example of correct subject-verb agreement?

A) Julia and David performs solo pieces in this evening's choral concert.
B) Brian or Alice plan to assist at the school science fair next week.
C) Mary and her sisters browse antique stores for unique gift items.
D) Donald or his brother stop at the grocery store on Fridays to pick up milk and bread.

11. Which of the following sentences has correct subject-verb agreement?

   A) Visitors who toured the botanical garden was impressed with its lush beauty.
   B) Members of the honor society are chosen based on academic achievement.
   C) Archaeologists working at the excavation site has discovered evidence of ancient civilizations.
   D) Lawyers at the firm serves as mentors to law student interns.

12. Which of the following sentences contains subject-verb agreement?

   A) Charles and Katherine, veteran news reporters, interview the mayoral candidate.
   B) Charles and Katherine, veteran news reporters, interviews the mayoral candidate.
   C) Several veteran news reporters interviews the mayoral candidate.
   D) Veteran news reporters, Charles and Katherine, interviews the mayoral candidate.

13. Which of the following sentences provides an example of correct subject-verb agreement?

   A) The damaged wiper blades on the truck is being replaced.
   B) The two mailboxes in front of the house overflows with newspapers.
   C) The bright rays of the sun are strongest between 10 A.M. and 2 P.M.
   D) The many pickets of the backyard fence is painted white.

14. Which of the following sentences contains a correct example of subject-verb agreement?

   A) Everyone who hears that song comment on its catchy rhythm.
   B) Anyone who cares about the environment recycles plastic water bottles.
   C) Somebody who listens to that radio station call in every morning.
   D) Both professors who are on sabbatical intends to write a book this year.

15. Which of the following sentences contains an example of correct subject-verb agreement?

   A) Because of the excellent school district, houses for sale in this area sells quickly.
   B) Since there are many clouds this evening, stars in the night sky is not visible.
   C) With the excellent park system, visitors to the area enjoys many recreational activities.
   D) Despite the disappointing stock report, investors in the company remain optimistic.

ANSWER KEY

1. B	**6.** D	**11.** B
2. D	**7.** B	**12.** A
3. C	**8.** A	**13.** C
4. A	**9.** B	**14.** B
5. A	**10.** C	**15.** D

ANSWERS AND EXPLANATIONS

1. (B) Since the subjects of these sentences are plural, the accompanying verbs must also be plural. Choices A, C, and D present plural subjects with singular nouns, making these answer choices incorrect.

2. (D) Choice D provides an example of a sentence containing subject-verb agreement since the compound subject, *aunt and uncle,* is considered a plural subject. Therefore, the verb must also be plural, as is the case with the verb *plan.*

3. (C) These sentences' subjects are collective nouns that indicate group unity and are singular in number. Only choice C pairs its singular subject with a singular verb.

4. (A) Compound subjects with multiple nouns are still considered singular if they are joined with words like *or* or *nor.* Therefore, choice A is correct because it links a singular subject, *Howard nor Phillip,* with the singular verb *likes.*

5. (A) Indefinite pronouns that are singular, such as *everyone* and *somebody,* require a singular verb; indefinite pronouns that are plural, including *both* and *all,* need a plural verb. Choice A's plural subject, *Both,* agrees with its plural verb, *prefer.*

6. (D) Choice D contains correct subject-verb agreement since the subject *Numbers* is plural, and the verb *indicate* is also plural. The other answer choices present plural subjects with singular verbs and are therefore incorrect.

7. (B) Each of these sentences contains a collective noun that indicates group unity. Since this type of noun is considered a singular noun, the proceeding verb must also be singular.

8. (A) Choice A correctly conjugates the singular subject *list* with the singular verb *is*; the other answer choices incorrectly link plural verbs to plural nouns in the preceding prepositional phrases rather than to the singular subjects of these sentences.

9. (B) Each of these sentences contains a plural subject that requires a plural verb. Only choice B correctly pairs the plural subject *Students* with the plural verb *take*; the other sentences all use plural subjects with singular verbs.

MCGRAW HILL TEAS REVIEW

10. (C) Compound subjects joined by the word *and* are considered plural and require plural verbs; compound subjects linked with the word *or* are considered singular and must be followed by singular verbs. Therefore, only choice C is correct.

11. (B) Choice B contains correct subject-verb agreement since the subject *Members* is plural, and the verb *are chosen* is also plural. The other answer choices present plural subjects with singular verbs and are therefore incorrect.

12. (A) Choice A is the only sentence that correctly uses a plural subject, *Charles and Katherine,* with a plural verb, *interview.* The other answer choices connect plural subjects with singular verbs.

13. (C) Choice C's plural subject *rays* is correctly paired with the plural verb *are.* Since choices A, B, and D use plural subjects along with singular verbs, they are incorrect.

14. (B) Choice B is correct because the singular verb *cares* is paired with its singular subject, *Anyone.* Most indefinite pronouns are singular and require singular verbs, except for certain pronouns, such as *both* and *all.*

15. (D) Choices A, B, and C are examples of incorrect subject-verb agreement in which plural subjects, separated from verbs with prepositional phrases, are incorrectly paired with singular verbs. Choice D correctly links a plural subject with a plural verb.

CHAPTER 45

Verb Tenses

Verb tenses are used to show when the action is taking place in the sentence.

SIMPLE TENSES

The most common verb tenses are past, present, and future. If the action of the sentence is taking place in the past, the verbs showing that action should be in the past tense. If the action of the sentence is taking place in the present, the verbs showing that action should be in the present tense, and so on.

Verb tenses questions address the correct use of verb tenses and whether a verb phrase matches the tense used in the rest of the sentence.

The following example is written in the past tense. It contains the past tense phrase *yesterday*:

Andrew received his class award yesterday.   ✓ CORRECT

The verb *received* correctly indicates that the action of the sentence took place in the past.

The following example is incorrect because the past tense verb *received* does not make sense in the context of the sentence. Here we have a future tense phrase, *tomorrow*:

Andrew received his class award tomorrow.   ✗ INCORRECT

The correct verb for this sentence is *will receive*, to place this sentence in the future tense:

Andrew will receive his class award tomorrow.   ✓ CORRECT

The following sentence also contains a reference to show that the action took place in the past. The phrase *before the movie* shows that some action took place prior to the movie. That action therefore needs a past tense verb.

Before the movie, the group went out to dinner.   ✓ CORRECT

This sentence is correct as written. The past tense verb *went* shows that the group had dinner before seeing the film.

Here's a sentence that correctly shows its action taking place in the present. It contains the present tense phrase *today*, and it uses the present tense verb *is choosing*:

She is choosing between her top two colleges today.   ✓ CORRECT

The following example also contains the present tense verb phrase *is choosing*. However, the phrase *last week* indicates that the action of the sentence took place in the past. This sentence, as written, is therefore incorrect:

She is choosing between her top two colleges last week. ✗ INCORRECT

The sentence should read that she *chose* between her top two colleges last week, to show clearly that the action took place in the past:

She chose between her top two colleges last week. ✓ CORRECT

PROGRESSIVE TENSES

Progressive tenses are the present progressive, past progressive, and future progressive. They show that an action is in progress. These tenses are also sometimes called **continuous** tenses.

Present progressive is formed: Subject + *am / is / are* + -*ing* verb + object. My teacher is assigning us a mountain of homework.

Past progressive is formed: Subject + *was / were* + -*ing* verb + object. The rabbit was running for hours.

Future progressive is formed: Subject + *will be* + -*ing* verb + object. I will be sleeping when you get back.

PERFECT TENSES

Perfect tenses are the present perfect, past perfect, and future perfect.

Present perfect tense shows action that was recently completed or was completed at an indefinite time in the past.
The tense is formed: Subject + *has / have* + past participle verb + object. My teacher has assigned a mountain of homework.

Past perfect tense shows an action that was completed directly before another action was completed.
The tense is formed: Subject + *had* + past participle verb + object. The rabbit had run for hours until it found shelter.

Future perfect tense shows an action that will happen before another action happens.
The tense is formed: Subject + *will have* + past participle verb + object. I will have fallen asleep by the time you get back.

PERFECT PROGRESSIVE TENSES

Perfect progressive tenses are the present perfect progressive, past perfect progressive, and future perfect progressive. They show that an action in the perfect tense is in progress. These tenses are also sometimes called **perfect continuous** tenses.

Present perfect progressive is formed: Subject + *has / had been* + *-ing* verb + object.
My teacher has been assigning us a mountain of homework all year.

Past perfect progressive is formed: Subject + *had been* + *-ing* verb + object.
The rabbit had been running for hours.

Future perfect progressive is formed: Subject + *will have been* + *-ing* verb + object.
I will have been sleeping for hours by the time you get home.

REVIEW QUESTIONS

1. Because of the frost warning issued yesterday, Henry _____ to take his houseplants off the back porch and bring them indoors last night.

   Which of the following verbs correctly completes the sentence above?

   A) has decided
   B) decide
   C) decided
   D) will decide

2. For the family reunion next weekend, Elizabeth and her sisters _____ apple, cherry, and blueberry pies the morning of the event.

   Which of the following verbs correctly completes the sentence above?

   A) will bake
   B) bake
   C) baked
   D) have baked

3. Students who register for classes today may _____ their class schedules online.

   Which of the following verbs correctly completes the sentence above?

   A) will view
   B) view
   C) viewed
   D) have viewed

4. When Judy arrives at the station later this evening, she _____ the late train to Washington, D.C.

   Which of the following verbs correctly completes the sentence above?

   A) boarding
   B) board
   C) boarded
   D) will board

5. Despite the large crowds at the zoo last Friday, Matthew and his mother _____ to see the new snow leopard cubs.

Which of the following verbs correctly completes the sentence above?

A) manage
B) managed
C) will manage
D) have managed

6. Until I broke my leg, I _____ running a mile a day.

A) had been
B) has been
C) was
D) used to be

7. Katie's parents _____ her school supplies after updated supply lists are posted next week.

Which of the following verbs correctly completes the sentence above?

A) had purchased
B) purchase
C) purchased
D) will purchase

8. Typically, student council meetings are held the first Wednesday of the month, and the foreign language club _____ twice a month on Fridays.

Which of the following verbs correctly completes the sentence above?

A) had met
B) meets
C) met
D) will have met

9. It is estimated that within the next decade, temperatures _____ to escalate, and coastal areas will be more vulnerable to rising waters.

Which of the following verbs correctly completes the sentence above?

A) continued
B) continue
C) will continue
D) had continued

10. With the addition of a third highway lane a few months ago, traffic congestion between the two cities was significantly _____.

    Which of the following verbs correctly completes the sentence above?

    A) reduced
    B) reduce
    C) will reduce
    D) reducing

11. Even though Janice has a gym membership, she _____ to take long walks outside when the weather is so pleasant.

    Which of the following verbs correctly completes the sentence above?

    A) preferred
    B) will prefer
    C) prefers
    D) had preferred

12. The upcoming school trip to the natural history museum _____ an excellent opportunity for students to learn more about many dinosaur species.

    Which of the following verbs correctly completes the sentence above?

    A) had provided
    B) will provide
    C) provided
    D) provide

13. Jacob _____ piano very well; in fact, he is currently mastering one of Bach's two-part inventions.

    Which of the following verbs correctly completes the sentence above?

    A) playing
    B) will play
    C) played
    D) plays

14. He _____ eaten all the candy by the end of the night.

    A) will have
    B) has
    C) would
    D) is

15. In anticipation of increased demand, the local food bank _____ its stock of nonperishable goods at its annual canned food drive next month.

Which of the following verbs correctly completes the sentence above?

A) had replenished
B) replenished
C) will replenish
D) replenish

ANSWER KEY

1. C	**6.** A	**11.** C
2. A	**7.** D	**12.** B
3. B	**8.** B	**13.** D
4. D	**9.** C	**14.** A
5. B	**10.** A	**15.** C

ANSWERS AND EXPLANATIONS

1. (C) This sentence is written in the past tense, as indicated by the word *yesterday* and the phrase *last night*. Therefore, the correct answer must also be in the past tense.

2. (A) Because this sentence describes an action that will take place in the future, as indicated by the phrases *next weekend* and *morning of the event*, a verb in the future tense is required.

3. (B) The content of this sentence, which includes the word *today*, pertains to the present tense, so choice B is correct. Choice D is not correct since the verb is in the present perfect tense, indicating an action that happened at some unspecified time before the present.

4. (D) Because the time frame indicated by this sentence is revealed by the phrase *later this evening*, the correct answer must be a verb in the future tense. Therefore, choice D is the correct answer.

5. (B) The phrase *last Friday* places the action in this sentence in the past tense. Therefore, choice B is the best answer since a verb in the past tense is needed.

6. (A) Since the sentence indicates an action process (*running*) that occurred before another action (*I broke my leg*), the past perfect progressive tense should be used.

7. (D) The time frame suggested in this sentence is in the future, as shown by the word *after* and the phrase *next week*. Choice D contains a verb in the future tense and is the correct answer.

8. (B) This sentence describes an action that is continuing, so verbs must be written in the present tense. The correct answer, choice B, is a present tense verb.

9. (C) Phases such as *within the next decade* and *will be more vulnerable* place this sentence's time frame in the future. Therefore, a verb written in the future tense is required.

10. (A) This sentence pertains to an action completed in the past, as indicated by the phrase *a few months ago*. Choice A, a verb in the past tense, is the best answer.

11. (C) This sentence is written in the present tense, as indicated by the present tense verbs in the sentence, *has* and *is*. Therefore, the correct answer must also be in the present tense.

12. (B) Because the museum trip mentioned in this sentence is described as *upcoming*, the event must take place in the future. Choice B presents a verb written in the future tense.

13. (D) This sentence is written in the present tense, as revealed by the phrase *is currently mastering*. Therefore, the correct answer must also be in the present tense.

14. (A) The phrase *by the end of the night* indicates an action that will happen in the future, so you know you need one of the future tenses. Since the action (eating candy) will happen before another action (the night ends), you need a future perfect verb to go with the past participle *eaten*.

15. (C) Since the action of this sentence will take place in the future, as suggested by the phrases *In anticipation* and *next month*, the correct answer must be a verb written in the future tense.

CHAPTER 46

Pronouns

Pronouns are words used to refer to nouns. Usually a pronoun will be used after a noun has already been given in the sentence or paragraph. The noun that the pronoun refers to is called the **antecedent**.

> <u>Sasha</u> is a vegetarian, so <u>she</u> will order a nonmeat entrée.

In this example, the pronoun *she* is used to refer to Sasha. *Sasha* is the antecedent of the pronoun.

Similarly, in the following sentence, the pronoun *him* is used to refer to Jorge. *Jorge* is the antecedent of the pronoun:

> <u>Jorge</u> loves all the gifts that the bowling team gave <u>him</u>.

In the following example, the pronoun *their* is used to refer to the Rudolphs. *The Rudolphs* is the antecedent in this sentence.

> <u>The Rudolphs</u> have an apple tree in <u>their</u> backyard.

PRONOUN FORMS

When a pronoun is used, it must be in the correct form. Pronouns can act as **subjects** doing the action. They can also act as **objects** receiving the action, and they can show **possession**.

In the following sentence, the pronoun *she* is used as a subject. *She* is completing the action of ordering, so the subjective form of the pronoun is used correctly.

> <u>Sasha</u> is a vegetarian, so <u>she</u> will order a nonmeat
> entrée.   ✓ CORRECT

It wouldn't sound right to use an object form of the pronoun in this sentence:

> <u>Sasha</u> is a vegetarian, so <u>her</u> will order a nonmeat
> entrée.   ✗ INCORRECT

Instead, the object form should be used when the pronoun is receiving the action of the verb, as in this example:

> <u>Sasha</u> is a vegetarian, so the waiter brought <u>her</u> a
> nonmeat entrée.   ✓ CORRECT

Here is a list of subjective, objective, and possessive forms of pronouns.

	Subjective	Objective	Possessive
First Person	I	me	my, mine
	we	us	our, ours
Second Person	you	you	your, yours
Third Person	he	him	his
	she	her	her
	it	it	its
	they	them	their, theirs

These forms of pronouns are also called **cases**.

GENDER AND NUMBER

Pronouns can show both gender and number. In other words, they can be masculine or feminine, and they can be singular or plural. Pronouns should match their antecedent in both respects. If a noun is singular feminine, the pronoun should be singular feminine as well. If a noun is plural neutral, the pronoun should be plural neutral as well, and so on.

Jorge loves all the gifts that the bowling team gave him.

In this sentence, the antecedent *Jorge* is masculine and singular. The pronoun *him* is also masculine and singular.

In the following example, the antecedent *The Rudolphs* is plural. The pronoun *their* is also plural.

The Rudolphs have an apple tree in their backyard.

Finally, the following sentence shows an example of a gender-neutral antecedent, *the table*. The table has no gender, so it is referenced using the gender-neutral possessive pronoun *its*:

The table was polished to show off the beautiful grain of its wood.

In cases where a single person is being discussed but that person's gender has not been made clear, the singular pronoun phrase *he or she* should be used.

Each camper must make sure that he or she packs enough warm clothes for the week. ✓ CORRECT

In this example, *each camper* is the antecedent. This antecedent is singular, but the gender is not clear. The phrase *he or she* is used correctly to refer back to *each camper*.

It may be tempting to use the pronoun *they* when the gender of a singular antecedent is not specified; however, this is incorrect.

The word *they* is a plural pronoun, so it should not be used with singular antecedents.

<u>Each camper</u> must make sure that <u>they</u> pack enough warm clothes for the week.   ✗ INCORRECT

It would be correct to use *they* if the antecedent was also plural, as in the sentence below:

<u>All campers</u> must make sure that <u>they</u> pack enough warm clothes for the week.   ✓ CORRECT

RELATIVE PRONOUNS

Pronoun questions on the TEAS also test relative pronouns (*who, which,* and *that*) and the correct usage of *who* versus *whom*. Regarding these pronouns, there are two points to keep in mind.

> The relative pronoun *who* is always used to refer to people, whereas *which* and *that* are used to refer to things.

<u>Principal Smith</u> is the one <u>who</u> ordered the extra copies.   ✓ CORRECT

<u>Principal Smith</u> is the one <u>that</u> ordered the extra copies.   ✗ INCORRECT

In these sentences, *Principal Smith* is the antecedent. Since *Principal Smith* is a person, the pronoun *who* should be used.

Here's an example of a relative pronoun that refers back to a thing:

To Kill a Mocking Bird is the book <u>that</u> I told you about.   ✓ CORRECT

To Kill a Mockingbird is the book <u>whom</u> I told you about.   ✗ INCORRECT

> The word *who* is used when the pronoun is the subject completing the action, and the word *whom* is used when the pronoun is a direct object receiving action.

<u>The teacher</u> is a knowledgeable instructor <u>who</u> truly cares about her students.   ✓ CORRECT

<u>The teacher</u> is a knowledgeable instructor <u>whom</u> truly cares about her students.   ✗ INCORRECT

These sentences use relative pronouns to refer back to the noun *the teacher*. In this case, the teacher is performing an action: she truly cares about her students. Because she is performing the action shown by the verb *cares,* the pronoun *who* should be used.

The following examples show a relative pronoun used as the direct object of an action. In this case, the pronoun *whom* should be used. Here, Carol performed the action of speaking. The person to *whom* she spoke was the recipient of her action.

Carol was not sure to <u>whom</u> she was speaking.   ✓ CORRECT

Carol was not sure to <u>who</u> she was speaking.   ✗ INCORRECT

REVIEW QUESTIONS

1. When <u>Joseph</u> arrives at the bookstore, _____ will look for a birthday gift for his niece.

   Which of the following options is the correct pronoun for the sentence above? The antecedent of the pronoun to be added is underlined.

   A) we
   B) he
   C) him
   D) they

2. The high school band will perform _____ new set at the first football game.

   Which of the following is the correct pronoun to complete the sentence above?

   A) their
   B) our
   C) one's
   D) its

3. Steven is a dedicated student _____ always completes his class assignments on time.

   Which of the following correctly completes the sentence above?

   A) whom
   B) which
   C) who
   D) that

4. Since that medical office is so busy, <u>patients</u> often schedule _____ appointments months in advance.

   Which of the following is the correct pronoun for the sentence above? The antecedent of the pronoun to be added is underlined.

   A) their
   B) they're
   C) it's
   D) its

5. Which of the following is an example of a grammatically correct sentence?

   A) Summer courses are offered to students that want to learn more about filmmaking.
   B) Summer courses are offered to students who want to learn more about filmmaking.
   C) Summer courses are offered to students which want to learn more about filmmaking.
   D) Summer courses are offered to students whom want to learn more about filmmaking.

6. After <u>Wendy and Daniel</u> gather their fishing gear, _____ will walk to the pond.

   What is the correct pronoun for the sentence above? The antecedent of the pronoun to be added is underlined. Write your answer in the blank.

7. Many doctors advise _____ patients to get plenty of daily exercise and rest.

   Which of the following is the correct pronoun to complete the sentence above?

   A) their
   B) they're
   C) one's
   D) his

8. After the professor agreed to write a letter of recommendation, she asked to _____ it should be sent.

   Which of the following correctly completes the sentence above?

   A) which
   B) whom
   C) who
   D) that

9. If the <u>team</u> loses tonight's game, _____ chances for playing in the state finals decrease.

   Which of the following is the correct pronoun for the sentence above? The antecedent of the pronoun to be added is underlined.

   A) they're
   B) their
   C) its
   D) it's

10. Which of the following is an example of a grammatically correct sentence?

A) The store manager forgot whom she issued a refund.
B) The store manager forgot who she issued a refund to.
C) The store manager forgot to who she issued a refund.
D) The store manager forgot to whom she issued a refund.

11. If <u>Maria</u> locks her keys in the car, _____ will have to call a locksmith to open the doors.

Which of the following options is the correct pronoun for the sentence above? The antecedent of the pronoun to be added is underlined.

A) she
B) we
C) her
D) they

12. <u>Jason and his friends</u> arrived at _____ destination about an hour later than expected.

Which of the following is the correct pronoun to complete the sentence above? The antecedent of the pronoun to be added is underlined.

A) its
B) their
C) they're
D) his

13. Extra boxed lunches will be given to _____ might want them.

Which of the following correctly completes the sentence above?

A) whoever
B) whichever
C) whatever
D) whomever

14. <u>Terence and Sonia</u> refused to ride the roller coaster because _____ afraid of heights.

Which of the following is the correct pronoun and verb for the sentence above? The antecedent of the pronoun to be added is underlined.

A) it's
B) they're
C) their
D) its

15. Which of the following is an example of a grammatically correct sentence?

 A) The pharmacist which filled my prescription gave me information about the medication.

 B) The pharmacist that filled my prescription gave me information about the medication.

 C) The pharmacist who filled my prescription gave me information about the medication.

 D) The pharmacist whom filled my prescription gave me information about the medication.

ANSWER KEY

1. B	**6.** they	**11.** A
2. D	**7.** A	**12.** B
3. C	**8.** B	**13.** D
4. A	**9.** C	**14.** B
5. B	**10.** D	**15.** C

ANSWERS AND EXPLANATIONS

1. (B) Since the antecedent, *Joseph,* is singular and masculine, the correct answer must also be singular and masculine. Therefore, choice B, the pronoun *he,* is the correct answer.

2. (D) This sentence has a singular antecedent since the noun *band* refers to one unified body. Therefore, the singular pronoun *its* is needed.

3. (C) In this sentence, the subjective case form *who* is needed since *who* is the subject of the clause *always completes his assignments on time.* The pronouns *that* and *which* refer to things, not people, and *whom* is an objective case pronoun for direct and indirect objects.

4. (A) In this sentence, the antecedent *patients* is a plural noun that requires a plural possessive pronoun before the noun *appointments* to show ownership. Choice B is incorrect because *they're* is a contraction for *they are* and not a plural possessive pronoun.

5. (B) Choice B is grammatically correct since the subjective case pronoun *who* is needed as the subject of the clause modifying the noun *students.* Choices A and C incorrectly use pronouns that refer to objects, and choice D incorrectly uses the objective case pronoun *whom.*

6. (they) Since the antecedent, *Wendy and Daniel,* is plural, the correct answer must also be plural. Therefore, the pronoun *they* is the correct answer.

7. (A) This sentence has a plural antecedent, *doctors,* so it requires a plural pronoun. Therefore, choice A is the best answer.

8. (B) In this sentence, the objective case form *whom* is needed since *whom* serves as the direct object of the sentence. The pronouns *that* and *which* refer to things, not people, and *who* is the subjective case form used for subjects of sentences and clauses.

9. (C) In this sentence, the antecedent *team* is a collective and therefore singular noun that requires a singular possessive pronoun. Choice B is incorrect because it is a plural possessive pronoun. Choices A and D are incorrect since they are contractions for *they are* and *it is* and not relevant to this sentence.

10. (D) Choice D is grammatically correct since the objective case pronoun *whom* is needed as the direct object of the clause modifying the noun *manager*. Choice C uses a subjective case pronoun and is incorrect.

11. (A) Since the antecedent, *Maria*, is singular and feminine, the correct answer must also be singular and feminine. Therefore, choice A, the pronoun *she*, is the correct answer.

12. (B) The antecedent *Jason and his friends* is plural, so the possessive pronoun *their* is needed to complete this sentence. The other options are either singular or do not show possession.

13. (D) An objective case pronoun is needed in this sentence to serve as the direct object, so choice D, *whomever*, is correct. Choice A presents a subjective case pronoun, and choices B and C are pronouns used to refer to things, not people.

14. (B) In this sentence, the antecedent *Terence and Sonia* is a plural noun that requires a plural pronoun and verb, so *they're*, a contraction for *they are*, is correct. Choice C is incorrect because *their* is a plural possessive pronoun used to show ownership and not relevant to this sentence.

15. (C) Choice C is grammatically correct since the subjective case pronoun *who* is needed as the subject of the clause modifying the noun *pharmacist*. Choices A and B incorrectly use pronouns that refer to objects, and choice D incorrectly uses the objective case pronoun *whom*.

CHAPTER 47

Sentence Structure

Sentence structure questions address clarity of expression, subordinating conjunctions, and how to combine sentences into a single sentence. You must also be able to distinguish between simple sentences, complex sentences, compound sentences, and sentence fragments.

SIMPLE SENTENCES

A **simple sentence** has one independent clause and expresses a complete thought:

Ezra went to the store.

This sentence is considered simple because it expresses a complete thought and contains only one independent clause and no dependent clauses. The following sentence is longer, but it is also a simple sentence:

Ezra went to the store and bought some chocolate milk for his sister.

SUBORDINATING CONJUNCTIONS

In the chapter on punctuation, we will review the use of coordinating conjunctions. These are connecting words, such as *and*, *but*, *so*, and *for*, which may be used to join two independent clauses:

Ezra went to the store, and he bought some milk.

When a coordinating conjunction is used to join two independent clauses, as we saw earlier, the conjunction must always be preceded by a comma:

Ezra went to the store and he bought some milk.   ✗ INCORRECT

Ezra went to the store, and he bought some milk.   ✓ CORRECT

Independent clauses are considered independent because they can stand as complete sentences on their own. When we join two independent clauses with a coordinating conjunction, we are joining two clauses of equal weight. Neither is dependent on the other.

Dependent clauses, on the other hand, do not form complete sentences on their own. They start with connecting words known as subordinating conjunctions:

Dependent Clauses

Because she left early

Although the package was heavy

While Mr. Galloway waited

When the game was over

After the crowd dispersed

Subordinating conjunctions are connecting words used to start dependent clauses. They include the words *because*, *although*, *while*, *when*, *after*, *before*, *until*, *since*, *as*, *if*, and *once*, among others. Subordinating conjunctions can be used to join two clauses in a way that places emphasis on one of the clauses over the other:

> Because its batteries had run low, the alarm clock suddenly stopped working.

In the example above, the underlined clause is an independent clause. It is placed at the end of the sentence, after the dependent clause *Because its batteries had run low*. This combination and ordering of clauses emphasizes the information at the end of the sentence. Here are a few more examples:

> Although pizza is high in calories, it's my favorite food.

> While the teacher was away, the students talked loudly.

> Until it started to snow, the weather had been gorgeous.

COMPLEX SENTENCES

Complex sentences contain an independent clause and one or more dependent clauses.

> When Ezra went to the store, he bought some milk.

In this example, the underlined clause is an independent clause. The dependent clause is at the beginning of the sentence: *When Ezra went to the store*.

The following examples are all complex sentences too:

> Although pizza is high in calories, it's my favorite food.

> While the teacher was away, the students talked loudly.

> Until it started to snow, the weather had been gorgeous.

Each of these examples contains an independent clause (underlined) plus a dependent clause with a subordinating conjunction.

COMPOUND SENTENCES

Compound sentences contain two or more independent clauses. They can be joined by a semicolon or by a comma and a coordinating conjunction.

> The professor gave a great lecture today; we thoroughly enjoyed it.

> The professor gave a great lecture today, and we thoroughly enjoyed it.

SENTENCE FRAGMENTS

A **sentence fragment** is a group of words that cannot stand on its own as a complete sentence. Sentence fragments often consist of solitary dependent clauses:

> After Martin thought it over.   Fragment

This example is a fragment, because the clause *After Martin thought it over* doesn't provide enough information to stand on its own. We can change this fragment into a simple or complex sentence:

> Martin thought it over.   Simple sentence

> After Martin thought it over, he decided to attend.   Complex sentence

Sentence fragments can also be created if a sentence is missing its subject or its verb:

> Thinking it over in the middle of the afternoon.   Fragment

> Martin, who spent a lot of time thinking it over.   Fragment

As with the earlier sentence fragment, these examples do not stand as complete sentences on their own. One way to correct these examples would be to add a subject to the first sentence and a main verb to the second:

> Martin was thinking it over in the
> middle of the afternoon.   Simple sentence

> Martin, who spent a lot of time thinking it
> over, eventually decided to attend.   Simple sentence

RUN-ON SENTENCES

A **run-on sentence** is a sentence in which two or more independent clauses are joined without an appropriate conjunction or punctuation. There are two types of run-on sentences: **fused sentences** and **comma splices**. A fused sentence has two independent clauses joined together with no conjunction or punctuation.

> The cat likes milk she drinks it as often as she can.   ✗ INCORRECT

A comma splice incorrectly joins two independent clauses with a comma.

The cat likes milk, she drinks it as often as she can.   ✗ INCORRECT

To correct a run-on sentence, you have four options:

1. Separate the two independent clauses into two sentences.

The cat likes milk. She drinks it as often as she can. ✓ CORRECT

2. Correctly join the two independent clauses with a semicolon or with a comma and coordinating conjunction.

The cat likes milk; she drinks it as often as
she can.   ✓ CORRECT

The cat likes milk, so she drinks it as often
as she can.   ✓ CORRECT

3. Subordinate one of the two independent clauses so that you have a complex sentence.

Because the cat likes milk, she drinks it as often
as she can.   ✓ CORRECT

4. Change the sentence into a simple sentence with only one independent clause.

The cat likes to drink milk as often as she can.   ✓ CORRECT

DICTION

Diction refers to the choice and use of words. In the Reading section of this book, you learned about how writers choose words to achieve a certain tone in their writing. Writers also vary their diction according to their purpose and audience. **Formal diction** is used in formal situations such as business writing and scholarly works. **Informal diction** is used in informal situations such as writing to our friends. **Colloquial diction** uses words common in the everyday speech of a time and region. **Slang** is the use of words that are newly coined, very informal, or impolite.

You will need to be able to distinguish between formal and informal modes of writing and identify slang.

REVIEW QUESTIONS

1. The puppy barked. The puppy rolled over on his back. I realized the puppy wanted attention. I petted the puppy's head.

   To improve sentence fluency, which of the following best states the information above in a single sentence?

   A) When the puppy barked and I petted the puppy's head and realized he wanted attention, he rolled over on his back.
   B) I petted the puppy's head as I realized he wanted attention and rolled over on his back, and the puppy barked.
   C) When the puppy barked and rolled over on his back, I realized the puppy wanted attention, so I petted his head.
   D) I realized the puppy wanted attention, so the puppy rolled over on his back, and I petted the puppy's head, and the puppy barked.

2. Which of the following is a simple sentence? Select all that apply.

   A) Jane's vegetable garden receives plentiful sunshine.
   B) Receives plentiful sunshine and produces ample tomatoes, cucumbers, and green beans.
   C) Because it receives plentiful sunshine, Jane's vegetable garden produces ample tomatoes, cucumbers, and green beans.
   D) Jane's vegetable garden receives plentiful sunshine and produces ample tomatoes, cucumbers, and green beans.

3. College tuition costs have continued to escalate rapidly. Many more students are applying for financial aid.

   Which of the following uses a conjunction to combine the sentences above so that the focus is more on students applying for financial aid and less on escalating tuition costs?

   A) Since college tuition costs have continued to escalate rapidly, many more students are applying for financial aid.
   B) College tuition costs have continued to escalate rapidly, and many more students are applying for financial aid.
   C) College tuition costs have continued to escalate rapidly; many more students are applying for financial aid.
   D) College tuition costs have continued to escalate rapidly, many more students are applying for financial aid.

4. Which of the following sentences uses slang that identifies the setting as the United States in the late 1960s or early 1970s?

   A) He's a hottie, but don't mess with that—he's a scrub.
   B) That party was far out, man. We had a gas!
   C) That moll has quite a kisser on her. She thinks she's the cat's pajamas.
   D) The vicar is droning on up there in his cackle-tub.

5. The barber shop on Main Street _____.

Which of the following completions for the above sentence results in a simple sentence structure?

A) decided to relocate since its lease expired at the shopping plaza.

B) welcomed many new customers after its grand opening last weekend.

C) is hiring several more employees, and applicants should inquire within.

D) is a local landmark located in the city's historic district downtown.

6. Which of the following is a simple sentence?

A) Mary was interested in archaeology before she studied paleontology.

B) Since Dan and his friends enjoy skiing, they've decided to try snowboarding.

C) Shingles on Jenna's garage roof are starting to come loose and must be replaced.

D) Red apple varieties tend to be sweet, and green apples are crisp and tart.

7. Which of the following is an example of a simple sentence?

A) The girl with the long, blond ponytail and pink jeans played on the elementary school playground after she completed her homework.

B) The girl with the long, blond ponytail and pink jeans played on the elementary school playground.

C) The girl with the long, blond ponytail and pink jeans playing on the elementary school playground.

D) The girl with the long, blond ponytail and pink jeans.

8. Phil prepared for the final exam. He reviewed his lecture notes. He read chapters in his textbook. He attended a study session.

Which of the following choices best uses grammar for style and clarity to combine the sentences above?

A) Phil prepared for the final exam though he reviewed his lecture notes and read chapters in his textbook; he attended a study session.

B) After Phil prepared for the final exam, he reviewed his lecture notes and read chapters in his textbook when he attended a study session.

C) To prepare for the final exam, Phil reviewed his lecture notes, read chapters in his textbook, and attended a study session.

D) Once Phil prepared for the final exam and he reviewed his lecture notes, then he read chapters in his textbook or attended a study session.

9. Which of the following is an example of a complex sentence?

A) Before Ken may ride the bicycle he purchased from the yard sale, he must put air in the tires and fix the broken kickstand.
B) Ken may ride the bicycle he purchased from the yard sale.
C) Ken must put air in the bicycle's tires and fix the broken kickstand.
D) Ken may ride the bicycle he purchased from the yard sale, but he must put air in the tires and fix the broken kickstand.

10. The man who walks his Labrador retriever by our house _____.

Which of the following allows the above sentence to be completed as a simple sentence?

A) sometimes stops to talk about mutual friends in the neighborhood.
B) sometimes stops to talk, and he likes to discuss mutual friends.
C) sometimes stops to talk although he only discusses mutual friends.
D) sometimes stops to talk when he wants to discuss mutual friends.

11. Which of the following sentences is most clear and correct?

A) The twins were adopted when they were two years old by Larry.
B) Larry adopted his twin sons when they were two years old.
C) Larry adopted his twin sons at the age of two years.
D) Two years old, Larry adopted his twin sons.

12. Samantha forgot to set her alarm clock. Her mother had to drive her to school.

Which of the following uses a conjunction to combine the sentences above so that the focus is more on Samantha's mother driving her to school and less on Samantha forgetting to set her alarm clock?

A) Because Samantha forgot to set her alarm clock, her mother had to drive her to school.
B) Samantha forgot to set her alarm clock, and her mother had to drive her to school.
C) Samantha forgot to set her alarm clock; her mother had to drive her to school.
D) Samantha forgot to set her alarm clock since her mother had to drive her to school.

13. Which of the following is a compound sentence?

A) My neighbor's porch light shines brightly at night and often keeps me awake.
B) Because my neighbor's porch light shines brightly at night, it often keeps me awake.
C) My neighbor's porch light shines brightly at night, and it often keeps me awake.
D) When my neighbor's porch light shines brightly at night, it often keeps me awake.

14. In the Northern Hemisphere, the winter solstice occurs _____ .

Which of the following allows the above sentence to be completed as a simple sentence?

A) in late December, and it is the shortest day of the year.
B) in late December; it is the shortest day of the year.
C) in late December; furthermore, it is the shortest day of the year.
D) in late December and is the shortest day of the year.

15. Which of the following is an example of a complex sentence?

A) Jamie enjoys socializing with friends, but he also appreciates quiet time alone.
B) Although Jamie enjoys socializing with friends, he also appreciates quiet time alone.
C) Jamie enjoys socializing with friends; conversely, he also appreciates quiet time alone.
D) Jamie enjoys socializing with friends and also appreciates quiet time alone.

ANSWER KEY

1. C	**6.** C	**11.** B
2. A and D	**7.** B	**12.** A
3. A	**8.** C	**13.** C
4. B	**9.** A	**14.** D
5. D	**10.** A	**15.** B

ANSWERS AND EXPLANATIONS

1. (C) Choice C retains the intent of the original group of sentences by using dependent clauses and transitional words to subordinate the puppy's actions to the subject's response. The other choices muddle the meaning of the original sentences and place them in nonlinear sequences.

2. (A and D) Choices A and D are examples of simple sentences. Since it contains a dependent clause, choice C is a complex sentence. Choice B does not contain both a subject and a verb and is not a complete sentence.

3. (A) Through the use of the subordinating conjunction *Since,* choice A positions the dependent clause pertaining to college tuition as secondary to the independent clause addressing students applying for financial aid.

4. (B) *Far out, man*, and *gas* are all slang terms that indicate the setting is the late 1960s or early 1970s in America. Choice A would imply a setting of 1990s America, while choice C indicates the 1920s. Choice D may be unfamiliar, but the use of *vicar* indicates that this is a British saying rather than an American one. *Cackle-tub* is a Victorian slang word for *pulpit*.

5. (D) Choice D provides an example of a simple sentence completion since it connects one verb, *is,* to one subject, *shop.* Choices A and B are complex sentences containing subordinating conjunctions, and choice C is a compound sentence.

6. (C) Even though this sentence contains a compound verb, it is composed of one independent clause and is therefore a simple sentence. Choices A and B are complex sentences with dependent clauses, and choice D is a compound sentence.

7. (B) Choice B presents a simple sentence containing one subject, *girl,* and one verb, *played.* Choice A contains a dependent clause and is therefore a complex sentence, and choices C and D are sentence fragments lacking a verb.

8. (C) Choice C retains the intent of the original group of sentences by using a dependent clause to introduce the purposeful sequence of actions performed by the subject, Phil. The other choices distort the meaning of the original sentences through inappropriate subordinate conjunctions.

9. (A) Choice A consists of a dependent clause followed by an independent clause, making it a complex sentence. Choices B and C are examples of a simple sentences, and choice D is a compound sentence.

10. (A) Choice A provides an example of a simple sentence completion since it connects one verb, *stops,* to one subject, *man.* Choice B is a compound sentence, and choices C and D are complex sentences containing dependent clauses.

11. (B) Choice B clearly and correctly relates the writer's intent, connecting the plural pronoun *they* to the plural antecedent, *twins.* Choice A is less succinct, and choices C and D distort the writer's meaning through confusing word order.

12. (A) Through the use of the subordinating conjunction *Because,* choice A positions the dependent clause pertaining to Samantha's forgetting to set her alarm clock as secondary to the independent clause about her mother driving her to school. The use of the subordinating conjunction *since* in choice D changes the sentences' original intent.

13. (C) Choice C is a compound sentence. It contains two independent clauses joined by a comma and the coordinating conjunction *and.* The first independent clause is *My neighbor's porch light shines brightly at night.* The second independent clause is *it often keeps me awake.* Both of these clauses can stand as complete sentences on their own.

14. (D) Choice D provides an example of a simple sentence completion since it contains one subject, *solstice,* and one compound verb, *occurs* and *is.* The other choices are compound sentences connecting two independent clauses.

15. (B) Choice B consists of a dependent clause followed by an independent clause, making it a complex sentence. Choices A and C are examples of compound sentences, and choice D is a simple sentence.

CHAPTER 48

Spelling

Spelling is important in written communication, so you should be familiar with the conventions of standard English spelling. There are several common rules that you may already be familiar with, and there are some common mistakes that you can learn to avoid. First, let's look at the most common rules of English spelling.

VOWEL SOUNDS

Rules about vowel sounds include the famous "*i before e except after c or when sounding like a as in neighbor or weigh.*" Unfortunately, that rule has many exceptions!

i **before** *e* **rule:** *achieve, relief, grief, belief*

Exceptions:

- except after *c*: *deceive, perceive, conceive*
- sounding like *a*: *neighbor, weigh, their, reign*
- other exceptions: *weird, neither*

Short vowel rule: Only one letter is needed to spell a short vowel sound: *red, hot, bad, sit, shut.*

Oi **or** *oy* **rule:** Use *oi* in the middle of a word (*boil, soil*) and use *oy* at the end of a word (*joy, toy*).

Ou **or** *ow* **rule:** Use *ou* in the middle of a word (*house, found*) and use *ow* at the end of words other than those that end in *n* or *d* (*borrow, chow, throw*).

CONSONANTS

Double consonant rule: When *b, d, g, m, n,* or *p* appear after a short vowel in a word with two syllables, double the consonant: *rabbit, ladder, haggle, tummy, banner, dipper.*

Ch **sound rule:** At the beginning of a word, use *ch* (*chide, chair*). At the end of a word, use *tch* (*batch, ditch*). When the *ch* sound is followed by *ure* or *ion,* use *t* (*picture, caption*).

ADDING SUFFIXES

A **suffix** is a word ending, such as *ing* or *ed*. There are several important rules about adding suffixes.

Drop final *e* rule: When you add a suffix to a word that ends in a silent *e*, drop the *e* if the suffix begins with a vowel: *come = coming, drive = driving*.

Exceptions: *duly, truly, peaceable*

Change final *y* to *i* rule: When you add a suffix to a word that ends in a *y* preceded by a consonant, change the *y* to an *i* (unless the suffix begins with an *i*): *deny = denial, party = partier,* but *deny = denying* and *party = partying*. Words that end in a *y* preceded by a vowel can add the suffixes *ed* and *ing* without any changes: *stray = straying, strayed*.

Doubling the final consonant rule: When you add a suffix that begins with a vowel to a word that ends in *y* preceded by a single consonant AND is a one-syllable word or a multisyllable word with the final syllable accented, then double the final consonant before adding the suffix: *cap = capping, occur = occurring*.

CREATING PLURALS

Here are some basic rules for making a word plural:

For most regular plurals, just add *s*: *medicine = medicines, doctor = doctors*

For words ending in *s*, *sh*, *ch*, *x*, or *z*, add *es*: *gas = gases, wash = washes, church = churches, tax = taxes, waltz = waltzes*

For some words that end in *f* or *fe*, use *ves*: *self = selves, life = lives, wife = wives, knife = knives*

Some words have the same singular and plural forms: *series, species, aircraft,* many animals such as *deer, moose, sheep,* and *shrimp*

COMMONLY CONFUSED WORDS

Homophones are words that sound the same but are spelled differently and have different meanings. Common homophones include the words *it's/its* and *their/there/they're*. Homophones can be easily confused, as can other words that sound similar.

The table below shows commonly confused words in English and their definitions.

Words	Definitions
anecdote/antidote	An **anecdote** is a story; an **antidote** is a remedy for an illness or problem.
blue/blew	**Blue** is a color; **blew** is the past tense of the verb *to blow*.
capital/capitol	A **capital** letter is a letter written in upper case or the primary political city in a state; a **capitol** is a building or group of buildings used for state governance.
confident/confidant	**Confident** is an adjective meaning self-assured. A **confidant** is a trusted friend or advisor.
creek/creak	A **creek** is a small body of water. A **creak** is a sound: the wooden floor *creaked* when she stepped on it.
edition/addition	An **edition** is a version of text; **addition** is an operation in math.
effect/affect	The word *effect* is commonly used as a noun. An **effect** is the result produced by some causal factor. The word *affect* is commonly used as a verb. To **affect** something means to have an impact on it.
for/four	**For** is a preposition showing purpose; **four** is a number.
here/hear	The word **here** indicates location; the word **hear** means to perceive sound.
insure/ensure	**Insure** is generally used to refer to insurance; when you insure something, you protect it against harm. To **ensure** means to make certain.
its/it's	The word **its** is a possessive pronoun. The word **it's** is the contraction for *it is*.
meet/meat	The verb **meet** means to come together; the noun **meat** refers to animal protein.
pair/pare/pear	The noun **pair** means two of something: he bought a *pair* of socks. The verb **pare** means to cut away or reduce: he *pared* down his possessions to just the essentials. The noun **pear** is a fruit.
pale/pail	The word **pale** means light in color; the word **pail** means a bucket.
peace/piece	The word **peace** indicates harmony or lack of conflict; the word **piece** means a portion.
peek/peak	**Peek** means to take a look or to spy; **peak** means the top or highest point.
principal/principle	A **principal** is a person who is the head or leader. A **principle** is a rule or guideline.
site/cite	The word **site** is a noun meaning location. The word **cite** is a verb meaning to give credit to a source.

Homophones	Definitions
sole/soul	**Sole** is an adjective meaning only. **Soul** is a noun that refers to a person's spiritual nature.
stationary/stationery	**Stationary** means motionless or fixed in place. **Stationery** is fine paper used for writing.
their/there/they're	The word **their** is a possessive pronoun: they gave us the address of *their* new home. The word **there** indicates location: we will see you *there*. **They're** is a contraction for *they are*.
then/than	The word **then** indicates order in a sequence: first this happened, *then* that happened. The word **than** indicates comparison: she is taller *than* him.
too/two/to	**Too** means also. **Two** refers to the number 2. **To** is a preposition.
week/weak	The noun **week** is a time interval of seven days. The adjective **weak** means not strong.
whale/wail	A **whale** is a large sea mammal. To **wail** means to scream or cry.
which/witch	The word **which** is a relative pronoun: *which* side of the family are you related to? The word **witch** is a noun: she dressed as a *witch* for Halloween.
whole/hole	**Whole** is an adjective meaning entire. **Hole** is a noun meaning a gap or an opening.
whose/who's	The word **whose** is a relative pronoun: *whose* side are you on, anyway? The word **who's** is a contraction for *who is*: Sherrie is the one *who's* calling.
your/you're	**Your** is a possessive pronoun: is that *your* dog? **You're** is a contraction for *you are*.

HOMOGRAPHS

Homographs are words that are spelled the same but have different meanings. Here are just a few common ones:

bear	(v) to carry or endure	(n) the animal
fair	(adj.) just; pleasing	(n) exhibition or event
tear	(v) to pull or rip apart	(n) salty liquid from the eye
hide	(v) keep out of sight	(n) animal skin
wind	(v) to twist or wrap	(n) moving air
content	(adj.) happy, peaceful	(n) things held or included in something

REVIEW QUESTIONS

1. Which of the following underlined words is an example of correct spelling?

   A) Flooding along the <u>creak</u> has caused the embankment to erode.
   B) At the <u>peek</u> of his career, the artist was exhibiting many watercolors.
   C) Seafood will be offered as an alternative to <u>meet</u> dishes at the dinner.
   D) Prior to our trip to England, we will spend a <u>week</u> in Ireland.

2. _____ planning a fall road trip when the leaves start to exhibit _____ fall color.

   Which of the following options correctly completes the sentence above?

   A) They're; their
   B) Their; they're
   C) They're; there
   D) There; they're

3. The class rehearsed for several weeks before _____ annual holiday performance.

   Which of the following correctly completes the sentence above?

   A) they're
   B) their
   C) its
   D) it's

4. Following recent personnel changes, the company decided that _____ time to update _____ website.

   Which of the following sets of words should be used to fill in the blanks in the sentence above?

   A) its; its
   B) it's; its
   C) it's; it's
   D) its; it's

5. At the antiquarian book sale, a signed first _____ of that novel sold for nearly one thousand dollars.

   Which of the following is the correctly spelled word to complete the sentence?

   A) edition
   B) eddition
   C) addition
   D) adition

6. Which of the following underlined words is an example of correct spelling?

   A) Drivers must proceed cautiously in this area because of the large <u>dear</u> population.
   B) Veronica's collection of greeting cards from family members is very <u>deer</u> to her.
   C) At the petting zoo, children may visit with <u>deers</u>, goats, and many other animals.
   D) Although it remains controversial, <u>deer</u> hunting is now legal in this county.

7. If we are going to watch _____ hockey game this evening, we'll need to get _____ before 7 P.M.

   Which of the following options correctly completes the sentence above?

   A) there; they're
   B) they're; their
   C) their; there
   D) they're; there

8. Aerobic exercise is necessary for optimal physical health, but _____ also important to perform weight-bearing exercises.

   Which of the following correctly completes the sentence above?

   A) its
   B) there
   C) their
   D) it's

9. My coffee mug has lost _____ handle, and now _____ starting to chip along the rim.

   Which of the following sets of words should be used to fill in the blanks in the sentence above?

   A) its; it's
   B) it's; its
   C) it's; it's
   D) its; its

10. Although they have only been friends for a few months, Jarrod is Emily's trusted confident.

   Circle the word in the sentence that is spelled incorrectly.

11. Which of the following underlined words is an example of correct spelling?

    A) Children should drink plenty of milk to <u>insure</u> healthy bone development.
    B) Jack decided to <u>ensure</u> his valuable painting for the full replacement cost.
    C) Getting enough rest has a positive <u>affect</u> on one's ability to concentrate.
    D) Headaches are a reported side <u>effect</u> of this particular medication.

12. Molly and Landon mentioned that _____ is a problem with _____ microwave that _____ trying to fix.

    Put the following words in the order that they should appear in the sentence above.

    _____ their
    _____ there
    _____ they're

13. Students participating in the science fair should submit project entries by Friday to _____ a grade.

    Which of the following correctly completes the sentence above?

    A) recieve
    B) receive
    C) receve
    D) receev

14. Since the levy will be placed on the November ballot, _____ time to recruit volunteers to support _____ passage.

    Which of the following sets of words should be used to fill in the blanks in the sentence above?

    A) it's; its
    B) its; it's
    C) it's; it's
    D) its; its

15. Even though I would like to include that country in my travel itinerary, the current political unrest makes it much _____ dangerous to visit.

    Which of the following is the correctly spelled word to complete the sentence?

    A) to
    B) two
    C) too
    D) tow

ANSWER KEY

1. D	6. D	11. D
2. A	7. C	12. 2, 1, 3
3. C	8. D	13. B
4. B	9. A	14. A
5. A	10. confident	15. C

ANSWERS AND EXPLANATIONS

1. (D) Choice D is the only sentence with correct usage of the underlined word. Choices A, B, and C provide examples of words that sound like the intended word choices but are incorrect.

2. (A) Choice A is the correct combination of words to complete this sentence. The first part of the sentence requires the contraction *They're* for *They are*, and the second part of the sentence needs the possessive plural pronoun *their* to refer back to the plural antecedent, *leaves*.

3. (C) Because the antecedent *class* is a singular, collective noun, the singular pronoun *its* is the correct answer. Choice B is a plural possessive pronoun, and choice D is the contraction for *it is*, so these choices are incorrect.

4. (B) In the first part of the sentence, the contraction *it's* is needed in place of the words *it is*. The second part of the sentence should be completed with the possessive pronoun *its*, which is not written with an apostrophe.

5. (A) In this sentence, the word *edition* is needed, which is spelled correctly in choice A.

6. (D) Choice D is the only sentence with correct usage of the underlined word. Choices A and B are homophones that sound like the intended word choice but are spelled differently. Choice C has an incorrect plural.

7. (C) Choice C is the correct combination of words to complete this sentence. The first part of the sentence requires the possessive pronoun *their*; the second part of the sentence needs the adverb *there*, which typically indicates placement (in this case, the ice rink or site of the hockey game).

8. (D) In this sentence, the contraction for *it is*, or *it's*, is needed. Choice A presents the singular possessive pronoun *its* and is therefore incorrect in this sentence.

9. (A) The first part of the sentence should be completed with the possessive pronoun *its*, which is not written with an apostrophe. In the second part of the sentence, the contraction *it's* is needed in place of the words *it is*.

10. (confident) In this sentence, the word *confidant* is needed instead.

11. (D) Choice D is the only sentence with correct usage of the underlined word. Choices A, B, and C provide examples of words that sound like the intended word choice but are incorrect.

12. (2, 1, 3) *There, their, they're* is the correct combination of words to complete this sentence. The first part of the sentence requires the adverb *there,* the second part requires the possessive plural pronoun *their,* and the third part of the sentence needs the contraction *they're* for *they are.*

13. (B) The correct spelling is *receive.* This word follows the rule "*i* before *e* except after *c* or when sounding like *a* as in *neighbor* and *weigh.*"

14. (A) In the first part of the sentence, the contraction *it's* is needed in place of the words *it is.* The second part of the sentence should be completed with the possessive pronoun *its,* which is not written with an apostrophe.

15. (C) In this sentence, the adverb *too* is needed, which is spelled correctly in choice C.

CHAPTER 49

Capitalization

Capitalization questions address capitalization rules involving proper nouns. You must know how to apply capitalization rules to publication titles, individual names, professional titles, names of events, organizations, and geographic locations. Months, days, and holidays may also be tested.

A **proper noun** is the name of a specific person, place, or thing, such as an organization or a landmark. In the English language, proper nouns are always capitalized. Several specific examples of proper noun capitalization are shown in this chapter.

PUBLICATION TITLES

When referring to a publication, such as a book or magazine, the first word in the title should be capitalized, as should all major words in the title. Minor words, such as *of* and *the*, are not capitalized.

✓ CORRECT	✗ INCORRECT
The Wall Street Journal	*the Wall Street Journal*
A Wrinkle in Time	*A Wrinkle In Time*
The Cat in the Hat	*The Cat In The Hat*

INDIVIDUAL NAMES

The names of specific people should be capitalized. Words that indicate family titles are capitalized if they are used to refer to a specific person.

✓ CORRECT	✗ INCORRECT
Jim Pearson	Jim pearson
Aunt Sally	aunt Sally
his only living uncle	his only living Uncle

PROFESSIONAL TITLES

Professional titles, such as doctor or professor, are capitalized when they are used to refer to the name of a specific individual:

Regina was looking for a good doctor, so I sent
her to Dr. Cole.   ✓ CORRECT

The professor asked the students to call him
Professor Thomas.   ✓ CORRECT

GEOGRAPHIC LOCATIONS AND EVENT NAMES

The names of geographic locations are capitalized if they refer to a specific place. This includes national landmarks and historical monuments, such as Lincoln's Memorial. The names of directions—east, west, north, and south—are capitalized if they refer to a specific geographical region or are used as part of a place name. If they are used as adjectives, they should be lowercase.

Capitalize	Don't Capitalize
Germany	southern fried chicken
Main Street	east of the city
Hoover Dam	western style
the old West	head north on the highway
South Dakota	

Formal titles of events should be capitalized. Examples include Macy's Thanksgiving Day Parade, Boston Marathon, and Super Bowl Sunday.

ORGANIZATIONS

The names of organizations should be capitalized. Be sure to capitalize all major words in the title.

The pilot went to work for American Airlines.   ✓ CORRECT

The pilot went to work for American airlines.   ✗ INCORRECT

Professor Carter graduated from Princeton university.   ✗ INCORRECT

Professor Carter graduated from Princeton University.   ✓ CORRECT

MONTHS, DAYS, AND HOLIDAYS

The full names of months, days, and holidays are all capitalized.

✓ CORRECT	✗ INCORRECT
January	January
Tuesday	tuesday
St. Patrick's Day	St. Patrick's day
New Year's Eve	New Year's eve

The names of seasons—winter, spring, summer, and fall—are not normally capitalized, unless the season is included as part of a proper noun.

Don't Capitalize

spring flowers

winter snow

a summer day

changing fall colors

Capitalize

Spring Fling

Winter Solstice Festival

Summer Concert Series

Autumn Harvest Celebration

REVIEW QUESTIONS

1. Which of the following phrases follows the rules of capitalization?

   A) Eastern Michigan
   B) aunt Becky
   C) Sergeant Smith
   D) Labor day

2. Which of the following book titles is correctly capitalized?

   A) *the Little Prince*
   B) *The Catcher In The Rye*
   C) *Anne of green gables*
   D) *Gone with the Wind*

3. Which of the following sentences uses capitalization rules correctly?

   A) I traveled with Aunt Lucy, Uncle Frank, and my Sister to Key West in southern Florida.
   B) I traveled with Aunt Lucy, Uncle Frank, and my sister to Key West in southern Florida.
   C) I traveled with aunt Lucy, uncle Frank, and my sister to Key West in southern Florida.
   D) I traveled with Aunt Lucy, Uncle Frank, and my sister to Key West in Southern Florida.

4. When our train arrived in New York City, Andrew's mother asked the station manager for directions to the Empire State building.

   Circle the word or words in the sentence above that should be capitalized.

5. Which of the following phrases follows the rules of capitalization?

   A) Italian bistro
   B) Art class
   C) professor Thomas
   D) Fourth of july

6. To garner support from democrats, each candidate made a campaign stop in the western part of the state.

   Which of the following words in the sentence above should be capitalized?

   A) democrats
   B) candidate
   C) western
   D) state

7. Which of the following phrases follows the rules of capitalization?

   A) their Cousin
   B) your Uncle
   C) my brother John
   D) aunt Barbara

8. Which of the following phrases follows the rules of capitalization?

   A) aunt Jane
   B) Chancellor Jones
   C) Eastern Connecticut
   D) New Year's day

9. Which of the following book titles is correctly capitalized?

   A) *War And Peace*
   B) *The Witch of blackbird pond*
   C) *Mansfield park*
   D) *Tuesdays with Morrie*

10. Which of the following sentences uses capitalization rules correctly?

A) Last summer, my Family visited Redwood National Park in northern California.

B) Last summer, my family visited Redwood National Park in Northern California.

C) Last summer, my family visited Redwood National Park in northern California.

D) Last summer, my family visited Redwood national park in northern California.

11. As part of their annual Class trip to Washington, DC, students from Jefferson High School visited the Smithsonian National Air and Space Museum.

Which of the following words in the sentence above should *not* be capitalized?

A) Class

B) Jefferson

C) Smithsonian

D) Museum

12. Which of the following phrases follows the rules of capitalization?

A) irish heritage

B) president Cooper

C) music lessons

D) Columbus day

13. To provide greater access to a college education, president Benson of Springside University has announced plans to add a satellite campus to the southeastern part of the state.

Circle the word or words in the sentence above that should be capitalized.

14. Which of the following book titles is correctly capitalized?

A) *the Millionaire Next Door*

B) *Last-Minute retirement planning*

C) *Investing On a Shoestring*

D) *Personal Finance for Dummies*

15. Which of the following sentences uses capitalization rules correctly?

A) Made up of three large waterfalls, Niagara Falls is located between western new york in the United States and southern Ontario in Canada.

B) Made up of three large waterfalls, Niagara Falls is located between western New York in the United States and southern ontario in Canada.

C) Made up of three large waterfalls, Niagara Falls is located between western New York in the United States and southern Ontario in Canada.

D) Made up of three large waterfalls, niagara falls is located between western New York in the United States and southern Ontario in Canada.

ANSWER KEY

1. C	**6.** A	**11.** A
2. D	**7.** C	**12.** C
3. B	**8.** B	**13.** president
4. building	**9.** D	**14.** D
5. A	**10.** C	**15.** C

ANSWERS AND EXPLANATIONS

1. (C) Since a specific title is used with a named person in choice C, it is considered a proper noun and should be capitalized. For choice A, the word *eastern* should not be capitalized since this word is used an as adjective instead of a place name. Choices B and D require capitalization of both words since each is a proper noun.

2. (D) Choice D is the only example of a correctly capitalized book title. Choice A fails to capitalize the first word in the title; choice B capitalizes a preposition and an article in the title, which is unnecessary; and choice C does not capitalize two major words in the title.

3. (B) Choice B correctly capitalizes *Aunt Lucy*, *Uncle Frank*, *Key West*, and *Florida* since these words are used as proper nouns in this sentence. Choice A incorrectly capitalizes the word *sister*, which is used as a common noun, and choice D incorrectly capitalizes the word *southern*, which is used as an adjective and not a place name in this sentence.

4. (building) Because the word *building* is part of a proper noun describing a specific place, it should be capitalized in this sentence.

5. (A) Since nationalities and their languages are capitalized, choice A is correct. Choice B does not require capitalization since it is not a specific course name. Choices C and D are incorrect because professional titles of named individuals and full names of holidays should be capitalized.

6. (A) Since the word *democrats* refers to a specific political party, it should be capitalized. Choices B, C, and D are used as common nouns in this context and therefore do not require capitalization.

7. (C) Words showing family relationships should only be capitalized when they are used as proper nouns. If the name is preceded by a possessive pronoun, the name is capitalized but not the word showing the family relationship: *Callie spoke with her aunt Barbara.*

8. (B) Since a specific title is used in front of a person's name in choice B, it is considered a proper noun and should be capitalized. Choices A and D require capitalization of both words since each is a proper noun. For choice C, the word *eastern* should not be capitalized since this word is used an as adjective instead of a place name.

9. (D) Choice D is the only example of a correctly capitalized book title in which the first word and all other important words are capitalized. Choice A is incorrect since the article *and* is capitalized, and choices B and C fail to capitalize major words in the title.

10. (C) Choice C correctly capitalizes *Redwood National Park* since these words describe a specific place. Choice A incorrectly capitalizes the word *family,* which is not used as a proper noun, and choice B incorrectly capitalizes the word *northern,* which is used as an adjective and not a place name in this sentence.

11. (A) The word *class* does not require capitalization since it is used as a common noun. Choices B, C, and D are all words describing a particular place name, so these proper nouns must all be capitalized.

12. (C) Because choice C is not the name of a specific class, there is no need to capitalize these words. Choices A, B, and D are incorrect because names of languages, professional titles of people, and full names of holidays are always capitalized.

13. (president) The word *president* should be capitalized since it is used as a proper noun referring to a specific person.

14. (D) Choice D is the only example of a correctly capitalized book title in which the first word and all other important words are capitalized. Choices A and C are incorrect since the article *the* and the preposition *on* are capitalized, and choice B fails to capitalize major words in the title.

15. (C) Choice C correctly capitalizes *Niagara Falls* since these words describe a specific place. Choices A and B are incorrect because the specific geographic place names, *New York* and *Ontario,* should be capitalized.

CHAPTER 50

Punctuation

Punctuation questions address the correct use of punctuation in regular text and quotations. You must know the appropriate use of periods, question marks, exclamation points, commas, semicolons, colons, apostrophes, hyphens, double quotation marks, and single quotation marks.

PERIODS, QUESTION MARKS, AND EXCLAMATION POINTS

Periods are used at the end of a complete sentence. **Question marks** are used at the end of a question, and **exclamation points** are used to mark the end of a forceful command or a statement that expresses strong emotions.

Amira went skating Sunday.	Period
Did you know Amira went skating Sunday?	Question mark
I'm shocked that Amira went skating Sunday!	Exclamation point

DEPENDENT AND INDEPENDENT CLAUSES

In order to understand the correct use of commas and semicolons, you must first understand the difference between a dependent and an independent clause. **Clauses** are groups of words that make up sentences. A **dependent clause** can't stand as a complete sentence on its own, whereas an **independent clause** forms a complete sentence and can stand on its own.

　　She forgot her sunglasses at the library

The clause in this example is an independent clause because it forms a complete or **simple sentence**. It can stand entirely on its own.

The clause in the following example, by contrast, is a dependent clause. It does not form a complete sentence; we need more information to understand the full meaning being conveyed.

　　Because she was rushing to get to school

Here are a few more examples of dependent and independent clauses:

After the football game ended	Dependent
The committee voted against the bill	Independent

You really should learn to tie your shoelaces	Independent
Although Laura drove all over town	Dependent

COMMAS, SEMICOLONS, AND COLONS

Dependent and independent clauses are important in understanding how and when to use commas and semicolons. A **comma** is a punctuation mark that shows a pause between ideas. Among other uses, commas can be used to separate items in a list and to join parts of sentences.

The following example of a **simple sentence** uses commas correctly to separate three items in a list:

Rashid bought school supplies, water, and a backpack at the store.

Now consider this sentence, which uses commas correctly to join parts of a sentence:

Even though it was cold outside, we went camping anyway.

Notice that here we have a **complex sentence** and the comma is being used to join a dependent clause—*Even though it was cold outside*—with an independent clause, *we went camping anyway*.

Commas can also be used to join two independent clauses in a **compound sentence**, but the comma must be followed by a connecting word such as *and*, *but*, *for*, or *so*. These connecting words are called **coordinating conjunctions**. There are seven coordinating conjunctions that can be used to join independent clauses:

Coordinating Conjunctions

for

and

nor

but

or

yet

so

Coordinating conjunctions can be remembered by using a memory phrase. The first letter of each conjunction spells out the word *FANBOYS*.

If you use a coordinating conjunction to join two independent clauses in a compound sentence, a comma must come directly before the conjunction:

A crowd gathered outside the building, and the protesters began to seem restless.	✓ CORRECT
A crowd gathered outside the building, the protestors began to seem restless.	✗ INCORRECT
A crowd gathered outside the building and the protesters began to seem restless.	✗ INCORRECT

The first example uses the coordinating conjunction *and,* which is correctly preceded by a comma. The second sentence is incorrect because it omits the coordinating conjunction. The last example is incorrect because it omits the comma before the coordinating conjunction.

Semicolons can be used to join two independent clauses without a coordinating conjunction. The second example above could be could be corrected by replacing the comma with a semicolon as follows:

A crowd gathered outside the building; the protesters began to seem restless.	✓ CORRECT

Semicolons are not used to join independent clauses with coordinating conjunctions, but they can be used with transitional words, such as *however, nevertheless,* and *therefore.* Whenever a semicolon joins two independent clauses with the help of a transitional word, a comma must follow the transitional word:

The evidence against the defendant was strong; nevertheless, the defendant was acquitted.	✓ CORRECT

In the preceding example, the transitional word *nevertheless* is preceded by a semicolon and followed by a comma. Without both of these punctuation marks, the sentence would be punctuated incorrectly:

The evidence against the defendant was strong; nevertheless the defendant was acquitted.	✗ INCORRECT
The evidence against the defendant was strong nevertheless, the defendant was acquitted.	✗ INCORRECT

Similar to semicolons, **colons** can also be used to join independent clauses. For a colon to be used, the second independent clause must expand upon the ideas in the first independent clause, as in the following sentence:

The evidence against the defendant was strong: the prosecution had gathered testimony from multiple eye witnesses.	✓ CORRECT

Colons can also be used to introduce elements in a list:

Three items should accompany you on every rafting trip: a rain poncho, a waterproof lunch kit, and a sturdy life jacket.	✓ CORRECT

APOSTROPHES AND HYPHENS

Apostrophes are used to show possession and to form contractions. To show possession, we normally add an apostrophe followed by an *s*:

Noun Form	Possessive Form	Example
the sun	the sun's	the sun's rays
a dog	a dog's	a dog's toy
our car	our car's	our car's horn

If the noun that is showing possession is a plural that ends in the letter *s*, normally only an apostrophe is used:

Noun Form	Possessive Form	Example
the families	the families'	the families' picnic baskets
the windows	the windows'	the windows' panes
your sneakers	your sneakers'	your sneakers' laces

Hyphens are used to separate some prefixes from the main part of the word, or root word. Hyphens should always be used following the prefixes *all*, *ex*, and *self*. They should also be used after prefixes that precede a proper noun or a proper adjective:

Prefixes	Proper Nouns and Adjectives
all-seeing	trans-Siberian
ex-employer	mid-Atlantic
self-supporting	un-American

Hyphens are also used with compound adjectives that come before the word they modify.

Emma was a strong-willed person.	✓ CORRECT
Treats are an often-used incentive at the vet's office.	✓ CORRECT
Sunday's game was full of record-breaking plays.	✓ CORRECT

Hyphens are not used, however, in compound adjectives that start with adverbs ending in -*ly*:

✗ INCORRECT	✓ CORRECT
a frequently-made error	a frequently made error
a flimsily-built house	a flimsily built house
an awfully-loud noise	an awfully loud noise

In the left column in the table above, the words *frequently*, *flimsily*, and *awfully* are all adverbs ending in -*ly*. Hyphens should not be used following these words, as shown in the column on the right.

QUOTATION MARKS

Quotation marks can come in double or single form, each with its own specific uses. **Double quotation marks** are used to signal direct quotations.

> Sarah said, "It's a lovely day to go hiking."

A comma should also follow the direct quotation if the phrase is a statement:

> "It's a lovely day to go hiking," Sarah said.

If the quoted phrase is a question, it should end with a question mark:

> "Would you like to go on a hike with me?" Sarah asked.

Question marks, periods, commas, and exclamation points should be placed *inside* quotation marks.

> The detective asked the witness several times,
> "Are you sure"?   ✗ INCORRECT

> The detective asked the witness several times,
> "Are you sure?"   ✓ CORRECT

Single quotation marks are used to denote a quotation within a quotation:

> Mrs. Juarez replied, "Sam said that he would 'need the car soon,'
> so don't keep it for too long."

It is not correct to use single quotation marks to show direct quotations. Double quotation marks should always be used for this purpose.

> The errand boy told his boss that he was
> 'just going out for a pizza run.'   ✗ INCORRECT

> The errand boy told his boss that he was
> "just going out for a pizza run."   ✓ CORRECT

Whenever quotation marks are used—either single or double—they should always precede and follow the quoted phrase. Both the beginning and ending quotation marks must be included.

> Everyone yelled, "Go team! and cheered the
> players to victory.   ✗ INCORRECT

> Everyone yelled, "Go team!" and cheered the
> players to victory.   ✓ CORRECT

In this example, the first sentence is missing the quotation marks after *team* that close the quoted phrase. The second example corrects this error by including the opening and closing quotation marks.

REVIEW QUESTIONS

1. Which of the following is an example of correctly punctuated direct dialogue in a sentence?

A) He explained, 'Rain gardens provide attractive landscaping that absorbs stormwater.'

B) He explained that "Rain gardens provide attractive landscaping that absorbs stormwater."

C) He explained, Rain gardens provide attractive landscaping that absorbs stormwater.

D) He explained, "Rain gardens provide attractive landscaping that absorbs stormwater."

2. Which of the following sentences correctly punctuates direct dialogue?

A) The conductor announced, "Our next selection is 'Spring' from Vivaldi's *Four Seasons*".

B) The conductor announced, "Our next selection is 'Spring' from Vivaldi's *Four Seasons*."

C) The conductor announced, "Our next selection is 'Spring' from Vivaldi's *Four Seasons*.'

D) The conductor announced, 'Our next selection is "Spring" from Vivaldi's *Four Seasons*.'

3. Which of the following sentences correctly applies the rules of punctuation?

A) In Hemingway's *The Sun Also Rises*, protagonist Jake Barnes explains, "You can't get away from yourself by moving from one place to another."

B) In Hemingway's *The Sun Also Rises*, protagonist Jake Barnes explains, 'You can't get away from yourself by moving from one place to another.'

C) In Hemingway's *The Sun Also Rises*, protagonist Jake Barnes explains, 'You can't get away from yourself by moving from one place to another'.

D) In Hemingway's *The Sun Also Rises*, protagonist Jake Barnes explains, "You can't get away from yourself by moving from one place to another".

4. In addition to perfect form, successful Olympic swimmers possess the following three qualities _____ strength, speed, and stamina.

In the blank above, write the punctuation mark that correctly completes the sentence. You can write either the symbol or the word.

5. Which of the following sentences correctly applies the rules of punctuation?

   A) Terence tested out of several first-year classes; therefore he will graduate one semester early.
   B) Terence tested out of several first-year classes; therefore, he will graduate one semester early.
   C) Terence tested out of several first-year classes, therefore, he will graduate one semester early.
   D) Terence tested out of several first-year classes; therefore; he will graduate one semester early.

6. Which of the following is an example of a correctly punctuated sentence?

   A) My friend asked "What are your travel plans this summer?"
   B) My friend asked "What are your travel plans this summer"?
   C) My friend asked, "What are your travel plans this summer"?
   D) My friend asked, "What are your travel plans this summer?"

7. Which of the following sentences is correctly punctuated?

   A) Because of the large number of runners expected at this year's marathon advanced registration is required.
   B) Because of the large number of runners expected at this year's marathon. Advanced registration is required.
   C) Because of the large number of runners expected at this year's marathon, advanced registration is required.
   D) Because of the large number of runners expected at this year's marathon; advanced registration is required.

8. Which of the following is an example of a correctly punctuated sentence?

   A) Anne owns a variety of cookbooks; however, she prefers to search for recipes online.
   B) Anne owns a variety of cookbooks, however, she prefers to search for recipes online.
   C) Anne owns a variety of cookbooks however, she prefers to search for recipes online.
   D) Anne owns a variety of cookbooks; however she prefers to search for recipes online.

9. Which of the following sentences contains the appropriate use of an apostrophe?

   A) The college held it's annual convocation last week.
   B) This season's harvest should be plentiful due to optimal weather.
   C) Students must complete they're capstone projects prior to graduation.
   D) We are joining the Anderson's for a barbecue next Saturday.

10. Circle the word below that is written correctly.

un-kind
re-adjust
all-inclusive
non-essential

11. Which of the following sentences is correctly punctuated?

A) After interviewing several candidates, the hiring committee made its recommendation.
B) After interviewing several candidates. The hiring committee made its recommendation.
C) After interviewing several candidates; the hiring committee made its recommendation.
D) After interviewing several candidates the hiring committee made its recommendation.

12. Which of the following sentences contains the appropriate use of an apostrophe?

A) Executive Council member's discussed the new initiative at their meeting last month.
B) Employment rates' in the region are starting to increase as the economy improves.
C) Signs directing patient's to the registration area are posted throughout the hospital.
D) Admissions counselors' schedules for next semester are posted in the office.

13. Which of the following sentences correctly applies the rules of punctuation?

A) Although it costs $11.50 to see the play, discounts are available for senior citizens.
B) Although it costs $11.50 to see the play. Discounts are available for senior citizens.
C) Although it costs $11.50 to see the play discounts are available for senior citizens.
D) Although it costs $11.50 to see the play; discounts are available for senior citizens.

14. Every summer, the Johnsons enjoy participating in the park's popular program, Happy Trails _____ 10 Short Hikes for Families and Children.

Which of the following punctuation marks correctly completes the sentence above?

A) ;
B) ,
C) :
D) -

15. Which of the following words is written correctly?

A) ex-chairperson
B) un-imaginative
C) re-apply
D) non-fiction

ANSWER KEY

1. D	**6.** D	**11.** A
2. B	**7.** C	**12.** D
3. A	**8.** A	**13.** A
4. : or colon	**9.** B	**14.** C
5. B	**10.** all-inclusive	**15.** A

ANSWERS AND EXPLANATIONS

1. (D) Choice D is an example of direct dialogue with proper use of quotation marks. In choice C, the quotation marks are incorrectly omitted, and choice A incorrectly uses single quotation marks. Choice B, an example of an indirect quote, does not need quotation marks.

2. (B) Choice B is correct because the song title is indicated by single quotation marks, and the entire quote is enclosed by double quotation marks. Choice A places the period at the conclusion of the sentence outside the quotation marks and is therefore incorrect.

3. (A) Choice A provides the only example of a sentence that is punctuated correctly. In this sentence, the direct quote from Jake Barnes is enclosed within double quotation marks, and the ending punctuation, a period, precedes the final quotation marks.

4. (: or colon) This sentence requires a colon after the word *qualities*. When a sentence includes a list, a colon should be used after the independent clause preceding the list.

5. (B) To punctuate this sentence properly, the conjunctive adverb *therefore* that connects the two independent clauses must be preceded by a semicolon and followed by a comma. Therefore, only choice B is correct.

6. (D) Choice D provides an example of a direct quote that is punctuated correctly. A comma is used following the introductory phrase to set off the direct quote, and double quotation marks enclose both the quoted material and the final punctuation (in this case, a question mark).

7. (C) The properly punctuated sentence, choice C, separates the dependent clause that begins the sentence from the independent clause in the latter part of the sentence with a comma. The other sentences are incorrect because choice A omits the comma, choice B creates a sentence fragment, and choice D uses a semicolon without two independent clauses.

8. (A) Choice A contains two independent clauses joined by a conjunctive adverb, so the placement of a semicolon before and a comma following the word *however* is correct. Since the other sentences do not follow this required punctuation, they are incorrect.

9. (B) Only choice B provides an example of an apostrophe used correctly, since *season's* shows possession and requires this mark of punctuation. Choices A and C are examples of contractions requiring apostrophes, but they are incorrectly used in place of the pronouns *its* and *their*. Choice D contains an unnecessary apostrophe since the plural form *Andersons* is needed.

10. (all-inclusive) A hyphen should be used following the prefixes *all*, *ex*, and *self*. The other choices do not require hyphenation and should be written as one word.

11. (A) Choice A is an example of a correctly punctuated sentence in which the dependent clause is separated from the independent clause by a comma. Choice B creates a sentence fragment, and choice D incorrectly omits the comma. A semicolon is not necessary in choice C, as the two clauses are not both independent.

12. (D) Only choice D provides an example of an apostrophe used correctly since *counselors'* shows plural possession. Choices A, B, and C are incorrect since these sentences have nouns that are plural, not possessive, and therefore do not require an apostrophe.

13. (A) Choice A is the only correctly punctuated sentence because a comma is needed to separate the dependent and independent clauses. Choice B incorrectly features a period after the dependent clause and a capital *D* to begin a new sentence, while choice C incorrectly has no punctuation after the dependent clause, and choice D has a semicolon after the dependent clause.

14. (C) Choice C is the correct answer since the title and subtitle of the program should be separated by a colon. Subtitles are not distinguished from titles with semicolons, commas, or hyphens, making the other choices incorrect.

15. (A) Since a hyphen should be used following the prefixes *all*, *ex*, and *self*, choice A is the correct answer. Choices B, C, and D incorrectly hyphenate compound nouns that should be written in closed form as one word.

CHAPTER 51

The Writing Process

For the TEAS, you will need to be familiar with the steps in the **writing process** and the resources and tools that writers use.

There are four basic steps in the writing process:

1. Prewriting
2. Drafting
3. Revising
4. Editing

Prewriting includes everything a writer does before composing the first draft. This may consist of brainstorming, researching, outlining, and so on.

Drafting occurs after the writer has an outline (either on paper or in his or her mind) of what he or she will write. Drafting is the process of actually writing the first draft of the text, either with pen and paper or on a computer.

Revising happens after the first draft is written. Revising consists of making large-scale changes to the text, such as changing the focus of the thesis, moving paragraphs around, deleting or adding blocks of text, and so on. The revision process may result in multiple subsequent drafts and continues until the writer is happy with the organization and content of the text.

Editing is the final step and consists of proofreading the draft and making minor changes to improve diction or correct errors. This is the step in which grammar, mechanics, and citation style (if citations are used) should be reviewed carefully. The editing process ends with a finished text.

PREWRITING TECHNIQUES

As mentioned above, prewriting includes everything a writer does before composing the first draft. Here are some common techniques a writer uses to gather ideas and organize them before writing the first draft of the text.

Brainstorming: Write down as much as you can think of about your topic. Don't worry about complete sentences or coherence. Just generate ideas.

Clustering or Mapping: This is a visual diagram made around your topic in the center. Branch off subtopics, and then add detail to each of them. Here is an example:

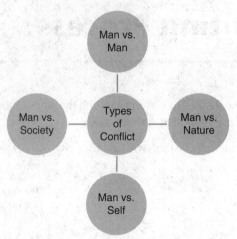

Interviewing: Ask other people questions about the topic. See what interests them about it and what more they would like to know.

Stream of Consciousness Writing: Just start writing about your topic and do not stop for a certain length of time (5–10 minutes minimum). It doesn't matter if you go off topic or write "I don't know what to write" 10 times. Just keep writing. Eventually you will generate ideas about your topic that can be useful to you.

Outlining: This should be done once you have at least some idea of what you will write about. An outline organizes your writing and creates a hierarchy that you can use to develop paragraphs or sections of your text. Begin by separating your topic into broad categories, and then develop those with subcategories. Here is an example:

Types of Conflicts in Literature

   I. Man vs. Nature
     a. *Moby Dick*
     b. *The Old Man and the Sea*
     c. *The Odyssey*
  II. Man vs. Man
     a. *Macbeth*
     b. *The Adventures of Tom Sawyer*
     c. *The Wonderful Wizard of Oz*
 III. Man vs. Self
     a. *Hamlet*
     b. *Requiem for a Dream*
 IV. Man vs. Society
     a. *To Kill a Mockingbird*
     b. *Romeo and Juliet*
     c. *The Handmaid's Tale*

PARAGRAPH ORGANIZATION

When drafting and revising a text, writers must pay attention to paragraph organization. Clear, effective writing is organized so that readers can understand the author's points. The TEAS may ask you about the order of sentences in a paragraph or what could be deleted or added to improve the flow and effectiveness of a paragraph.

A basic paragraph structure begins with a topic sentence that tells readers what the paragraph is about. The body of the paragraph will comprise details about that topic. The final sentence of the paragraph should summarize the information and tie it to the overall thesis of the text. Transitions should be used to move from one topic to the next, either at the end of one paragraph or at the beginning of the next.

CITATIONS

In researched writing, credit should be given to the words and ideas of others through citing the source for that material. There are several different citation styles (Chicago, APA, MLA, and so on) and you will not be tested on the format of any style. You will, however, be expected to know when material needs to include a citation. There are four basic rules for what material to cite:

1. **Quotations:** Anytime you use the exact words from another source, you must enclose the words in quotation marks and cite the source.
2. **Paraphrases:** Anytime you take language from another source and rephrase it in your own words, you must cite the source.
3. **Summary:** If you take an idea from another source and put a condensed version of it in your own words, you must cite the source.
4. **Data:** If you use facts, information, data, graphics, and so on from another source, you must cite that source. If you use an accepted, well-known fact that could be obtained from many different sources, such as a birthdate of a famous person or the date of a battle, then you do not need to cite a source for that information.

REVIEW QUESTIONS

1. Which of the following activities would be considered editing?

   A) Creating an outline
   B) Typing a first draft
   C) Interviewing subjects
   D) Correcting punctuation

Questions 2–4 refer to the following sentences.

> **(a)** I swam in a river with piranhas once and was not bitten.
> **(b)** There are only two situations in which a piranha is likely to bite a human.
> **(c)** In this case, they may attack anything that enters the pool.
> **(d)** The second situation is when too many piranhas are trapped in a pool with a low water level and become hungry and aggressive.
> **(e)** When confronted with a large animal, a piranha's instinct is to flee rather than to attack.
> **(f)** The first is when a piranha is lifted out of the water, usually by a fishing net, and the frightened fish may bite.
> **(g)** Although many people think of piranhas as man-eaters, they are rarely dangerous to humans.
> **(h)** For the most part, the man-eating piranha is a myth, just like the man-eating shark.
> **(i)** Piranhas mostly eat smaller fish and aquatic plants; they rarely feed on large animals.

2. If a writer constructs a paragraph with the sentences above, put the letters of the first four sentences that would compose the paragraph listed in the correct chronological order.

   _____ 1st sentence
   _____ 2nd sentence
   _____ 3rd sentence
   _____ 4th sentence

3. If a writer is constructing a paragraph with the sentences above, which of the following sentences should be omitted?

   A) *There are only two situations in which a piranha is likely to bite a human.*
   B) *I swam in a river with piranhas once and was not bitten.*
   C) *In this case, they may attack anything that enters the pool.*
   D) *Piranhas mostly eat smaller fish and aquatic plants; they rarely feed on large animals.*

4. Which of the following sentences is the best conclusion sentence for the paragraph?

   A) *Piranhas mostly eat smaller fish and aquatic plants; they rarely feed on large animals.*
   B) *There are only two situations in which a piranha is likely to bite a human.*
   C) *For the most part, the man-eating piranha is a myth, just like the man-eating shark.*
   D) *In this case, they may attack anything that enters the pool.*

5.

> **Parrots**
>
> I.   Behavior
>
>   a.
>
>   b.
>
> II.   Diet
>
>   a. In nature
>
>   b. In captivity
>
> III. Intelligence and Learning
>
>   a.
>
>   b.
>
> IV.   Breeding
>
>   a.
>
>   b.

Which of the following could be a subcategory under *Intelligence and Learning* in the outline above?

A) Sound imitation
B) Mating habits
C) Fresh produce
D) Conservation status

6. Which of the following phrases indicates a transition in a sequence?

A) by the same token
B) above all
C) to begin with
D) for example

7. Which of the following would require a citation?

A) A footnote in which the author includes a survey done by the American Medical Association.
B) The author gives her opinion on the popularity of a fad.
C) The author gives the value of Avogadro's number.
D) The author adds emphasis to a point he made earlier.

8. Which of the following could be a topic sentence for a paragraph?

A) That is why I prefer listening to music with stereo headphones.
B) A man with a body mass index, or BMI, of between 18.5 and 24.9 is considered normal.
C) Until we know more, the debate will continue.
D) The Battle of Waterloo in 1815 was a turning point for Napoleon.

9. Which of the following would NOT require a citation?

   A) The author summarizes the results of a research study published in a journal.
   B) The author composes an original poem as an example.
   C) The author puts an idea she read in a book into her own words.
   D) The author quotes her uncle.

10. Put the following steps of the writing process in order from first (1) to last (4).

   _____ Researching data to support an argument
   _____ Checking for spelling errors
   _____ Deleting an unnecessary paragraph
   _____ Choosing a topic for the essay

ANSWER KEY

1. D	**5.** A	**9.** B
2. g, i, e, b	**6.** C	**10.** 2, 4, 3, 1
3. B	**7.** A	
4. C	**8.** D	

ANSWERS AND EXPLANATIONS

1. (D) Correcting punctuation is part of the editing process. Interviewing and outlining are both prewriting activities, and writing a first draft is drafting.

2. (g, i, e, b) The best order is (g), (i), (e), (b). The topic sentence is: *Although many people think of piranhas as man-eaters, they are rarely dangerous to humans.* (i) and (e) expand on this idea: *Piranhas mostly eat smaller fish and aquatic plants; they rarely feed on large animals. When confronted with a large animal, a piranha's instinct is to flee rather than to attack.* (b) begins the discussion of the exceptions to the rule: *There are only two situations in which a piranha is likely to bite a human.*

3. (B) A sentence about the author's personal experience does not belong in this third-person paragraph.

4. (C) Choice C makes the best concluding sentence because it restates the topic sentence and provides a possible transition to a following paragraph about sharks.

5. (A) Sound imitation could be a subcategory under *Intelligence and Learning*. Mating habits and conservation status would fall under *Breeding*, and fresh produce would be part of one or both subcategories of *Diet*.

6. (C) The phrase *to begin with* indicates a step in sequence.

7. (A) Even in a footnote, material from an outside source must include a citation.

8. (D) The best choice is D. It introduces an idea that needs more explaining. Choices A and C are conclusions, while choice B is a supporting fact.

9. (B) Only choice B describes a situation in which no citation is needed. An original poem does not need a citation.

10. (2, 4, 3, 1) The first step would be to choose a topic, then do research. During revision, any unnecessary paragraphs would be removed. During editing, spelling would be checked.

CHAPTER 52

Vocabulary

Vocabulary questions on this part of the TEAS deal with figuring out the meaning of a word based on synonyms, context clues, tone, and your knowledge of roots, prefixes, and suffixes.

MEDICAL TERMS

SYNONYMS

Synonyms are two words with similar meanings. You may be asked to find a synonym for a certain word or to figure out the meaning of a word in a sentence that provides a synonym for the unknown word.

CONTEXT CLUES

These questions are similar to those in the reading section, but you may be given as little as a single sentence rather than a longer passage. You will need to use that limited context to figure out the meaning of a word. Look at the surrounding context for the word you are given. Figure out the setting in which the word is used. If the word is part of a series, the other words in the series can provide valuable clues. Review the section on homographs in the chapter on spelling. Questions in this section may use homographs to test whether you are paying attention to context. You should also consider the tone of the passage; it may give you a clue about the meaning of an unknown word.

WORD ORIGINS

You may also be asked questions about root words, prefixes, and suffixes. A **root word** is the base form of a word. **Affixes** are the parts we attach to modify the meaning of the root word. A **prefix** is attached before the root, and a **suffix** is attached after the root. You should spend some time becoming familiar with common affixes used in the medical profession. Here is a list of common roots to get you started:

- **abdomin:** abdomen
- **acous:** hearing
- **aden:** gland
- **adip:** fat
- **adrena:** adrenal
- **aero:** gas
- **andr:** male
- **angi:** vessel
- **anter:** front
- **aort:** aorta
- **arteri:** artery
- **arthr:** joint

- **audi:** hearing
- **bio:** life
- **bronch:** bronchus
- **carcin:** cancer
- **cardi:** heart
- **cerebr:** cerebrum
- **chol:** bile
- **chondr:** cartilage
- **col:** colon
- **cor:** pupil
- **crani:** cranium
- **cutane:** skin
- **cyst:** bladder
- **cyt:** cell
- **dactyl:** finger or toe
- **derma:** skin
- **dors:** back or posterior
- **encephal:** brain
- **enter:** intestine
- **esophag:** esophagus
- **esthesi:** sensation
- **faci:** face
- **fibr:** fiber
- **gastr:** stomach
- **gynec:** female
- **hemat/hemo:** blood
- **hepat:** liver
- **hist:** tissue
- **hyster/metr:** uterus
- **intestin:** intestine
- **kerat:** hard
- **lapar:** abdomen
- **laryng:** larynx
- **lipo:** fat
- **lymph:** lymph
- **mamm/mast:** breast
- **my:** muscle
- **myel:** spinal cord
- **nasal:** nose
- **necr:** death
- **nephr:** kidney
- **neur:** nerve
- **ocul/ophthalm:** eye
- **opt/optic:** seeing or sight
- **or:** mouth
- **orchid:** testicle or testis
- **oste:** bone
- **ot:** ear
- **ovari:** ovary
- **ox/oxy:** oxygen
- **pancreat:** pancreas
- **path:** disease
- **pector:** chest
- **ped/pod:** foot
- **pelv:** pelvis
- **pharmac/o:** drug
- **phleb:** vein
- **pneum:** air or lung
- **prostat:** prostate gland
- **pulmon:** lung
- **ren:** kidney
- **sept:** infection
- **somat:** body
- **stern:** breastbone, sternum
- **tendin:** tendon
- **test:** testicle or testis
- **thorac:** thorax/chest
- **thromb:** clot
- **thyr:** thyroid gland
- **vas:** duct/vessel
- **ven:** vein
- **ventr:** front of body
- **viscer:** viscera

Many medical terms are formed by combining one or more roots with a prefix and/or suffix, so you need to know the common affixes as well. Here is a list of common prefixes:

Prefix	Prefix Meaning	Example Term	Meaning
a / an / ar	not, without	amnesia	no memory
anti	against	antipsychotic	a mind-altering medication
dys	bad or difficult	dysentery	abnormal condition of intestines
endo	in, within	endoscopy	visual examination inside the body
epi	over, around	epidural	on or around the dura matter
exo / extra	outside	exoskeleton	external skeleton
hyper	beyond normal, high	hypertension	high blood pressure
hypo	low, under	hypoglycemia	low blood sugar
inter	between	interarticular	between joints
intra	within	intravenous	in a vein
macro	large, long	macroglossia	having an enlarged tongue
mal	bad	malaise	general sense of being unwell
micro	small	microscope	instrument for viewing small objects
neo	new	neoplasm	abnormal new growth of tissue
per	through	percutaneous	through the skin
peri	around, surrounding	pericardium	tissue surrounding the heart
poly	many, much	polydactyly	condition of too many fingers or toes
post	after	postmortem	after death
pre	before	prenatal	before birth
sub	below, under	subcutaneous	under the skin
super/supra	above	supraorbital	above the eye socket
tachy	rapid	tachycardia	fast heartbeat
trans	across, through	translucent	allowing light to shine through
un	not	unformed	not formed

Here is a list of common suffixes used in medical terminology:

Suffix	Suffix Meaning	Example Term	Meaning
ac/al/ar/ary	pertaining to	cardiac	pertaining to the heart
algia	pain	myalgia	muscle pain
ase	enzyme	lipase	enzyme that digests fats
asthenia	weakness	neurasthenia	weakness of nerves
crine	to secrete	endocrine	related to the glands
cyte	cell	leukocyte	white blood cell
dynia	pain	gastrodynia	stomach pain
ectomy/tomy	surgical removal	tonsillectomy	removal of tonsils
emia	blood	anemia	deficiency of red blood cells
gnosis	knowledge	prognosis	prediction for future
gram	picture or record	cardiogram	record of heart activity
ia/ism	state or condition	tachycardia	condition of a rapid heart rate
ic	pertaining to	therapeutic	pertaining to treatment
ist	one who specializes in	gynecologist	specialist in women's reproduction
itis	inflammation	sinusitis	inflammation of sinus tissues
lysis	breakdown, separate	paralysis	loss of ability to move or feel
lpsy	attack or seizure	epilepsy	neurological seizure disorder
ole/ule	small	molecule	smallest unit of a compound
ology	the study of	biology	the study of living things
oma	tumor	blastoma	cancer of precursor cells
osis	condition	ankylosis	abnormal joint stiffening
pathy	disease	neuropathy	relating to a nerve disorder
penia	deficiency	osteopenia	low bone mineral density
poiesis	formation	hematopoiesis	formation of blood cellular components
rrhage	excess fluid	hemorrhage	excessive bleeding
stasis	stopping, controlling	homeostasis	equilibrium

REVIEW QUESTIONS

1. Based on a review of the roots and affixes, which of the following is the surgical process of cutting into the chest wall?

   A) Thoracotomy
   B) Colectomy
   C) Thrombus
   D) Tracheotomy

Living alone seemed like more than she could bear.

2. Which of the following is the meaning of *bear* as it is used in the sentence?

   A) To carry
   B) To give birth to
   C) To turn and proceed in a direction
   D) To endure

3. Which of the following prefixes means *without*?

   A) mal
   B) an
   C) sub
   D) post

4. In which of the following sentences is *cool* used as an adjective meaning *having a lower temperature*?

   A) When you have a fever, a cool, wet cloth on your forehead can help.
   B) After you finish working on the roof, come inside and cool off.
   C) Sometimes teenagers only drink alcohol to appear cool to their friends.
   D) He played it cool when his mother noticed that the freshly baked cookies were missing.

After other treatment options had failed, the surgeon recommended a nephrectomy.

5. In the sentence, the root *nephr* indicates that the doctor will perform a removal of which body part? Write your answer in the blank:

   _____

6. Based on a review of the roots and affixes, which of the following is an abnormal thickening of the stratum corneum (the outer layer of the epidermis)?

A) Fibrosis
B) Hypotension
C) Hyperkeratosis
D) Gastritis

7. Which of the following words has a suffix that means *small*?

A) Gastronomy
B) Pustule
C) Paralytic
D) Neurocyte

The patient underwent a transesophageal echocardiogram test to get a detailed picture of her heart and its major blood vessels.

8. Based on your knowledge of roots and affixes, what does *transesophageal* mean?

A) Under the esophagus
B) Cutting across the esophagus
C) Outside the esophagus
D) Through the esophagus

The new kitchen cabinets and countertops are a perfect match.

9. Which of the following is the meaning of *match* as it is used in the sentence?

A) A contest or trial of skill
B) A marriage
C) A pair of items with mutually suitable characteristics
D) A stick of wood or paper with a tip coated with chemicals that ignite with friction

10. Which of the following prefixes would be added to *glycemia* to show that a person has a condition in which blood sugar is too high?

A) hyper
B) hypo
C) dia
D) trans

ANSWER KEY

1. A	5. kidney	9. C
2. D	6. C	10. A
3. B	7. B	
4. A	8. D	

ANSWERS AND EXPLANATIONS

1. (A) A *thoracotomy* would be the surgical process of cutting into the chest wall. The root *thorac* means *chest* and the suffix *tomy* means *surgical removal*.

2. (D) While each of the choices is a definition for *bear*, as it is used in the sentence it means *to endure*.

3. (B) The prefixes a, an, and ar mean *without*.

4. (A) Only in choice A is *cool* used as an adjective meaning *lower in temperature*. *Cool* describes the wet cloth, which is lower in temperature than a normal dry cloth.

5. (kidney) The root *nephr* means kidney.

6. (C) *Hyperkeratosis* is an abnormal thickening of the stratum corneum. The prefix *hyper* means *beyond normal*, the root *kerat* means *hard*, and the suffix *osis* means *condition*.

7. (B) The suffixes *ole* and *ule* mean *small*. A *pustule* is a small bump on the skin that contains pus.

8. (D) *Trans* means *across or through*, so *transesophageal* means *through the esophagus*.

9. (C) While each of the choices is a definition for *match*, as it is used in the sentence it means *a pair of items with mutually suitable characteristics*.

10. (A) *Hyper* means *abnormally high*. *Hypo* means *low*.

PART V

PRACTICE TEST

TEAS Practice Test: Answer Sheet

READING

1 1st 2nd 3rd 4th
2 (A) (B) (C) (D)
3 (A) (B) (C) (D)
4 (A) (B) (C) (D)
5 (A) (B) (C) (D)
6 (A) (B) (C) (D)
7 (A) (B) (C) (D)
8 (A) (B) (C) (D)
9 (A) (B) (C) (D)
10 (A) (B) (C) (D)
11 (A) (B) (C) (D)
12 1st 2nd 3rd 4th
13 (A) (B) (C) (D)
14 (A) (B) (C) (D)
15 (A) (B) (C) (D)

16 (A) (B) (C) (D)
17 (A) (B) (C) (D)
18 (A) (B) (C) (D)
19 _____
20 _ _ _ _ _ _
21 (A) (B) (C) (D)
22 (A) (B) (C) (D)
23 (A) (B) (C) (D)
24 (A) (B) (C) (D)
25 (A) (B) (C) (D)
26 (A) (B) (C) (D)
27 (A) (B) (C) (D)
28 (A) (B) (C) (D)
29 (A) (B) (C) (D)
30 (A) (B) (C) (D)

31 (A) (B) (C) (D)
32 (A) (B) (C) (D)
33 (A) (B) (C) (D)
34 _____
35 (A) (B) (C) (D)
36 (A) (B) (C) (D)
37 (A) (B) (C) (D)
38 (A) (B) (C) (D)
39 (A) (B) (C) (D)
40 (A) (B) (C) (D)
41 _____
42 (A) (B) (C) (D)
43 (A) (B) (C) (D)
44 (A) (B) (C) (D)
45 (A) (B) (C) (D)

MATHEMATICS

1 _____
2 (A) (B) (C) (D)
3 (A) (B) (C) (D)
4 (A) (B) (C) (D)
5 (A) (B) (C) (D)
6 (A) (B) (C) (D)
7 (A) (B) (C) (D)
8 (A) (B) (C) (D)
9 _ _ _ _ _
10 (A) (B) (C) (D)
11 (A) (B) (C) (D)
12 (A) (B) (C) (D)
13 _____

14 (A) (B) (C) (D)
15 _____
16 (A) (B) (C) (D)
17 (A) (B) (C) (D)
18 (A) (B) (C) (D)
19 (A) (B) (C) (D)
20 (A) (B) (C) (D)
21 (A) (B) (C) (D)
22 (A) (B) (C) (D)
23 (A) (B) (C) (D)
24 (A) (B) (C) (D)
25 (A) (B) (C) (D)
26 (A) (B) (C) (D)

27 (A) (B) (C) (D)
28 _____
29 (A) (B) (C) (D)
30 (A) (B) (C) (D)
31 (A) (B) (C) (D)
32 (A) (B) (C) (D)
33 (A) (B) (C) (D)
34 (A) (B) (C) (D)
35 (A) (B) (C) (D)
36 (A) (B) (C) (D)
37 (A) (B) (C) (D)
38 (A) (B) (C) (D) (E)

SCIENCE

1 Ⓐ Ⓑ Ⓒ Ⓓ
2 Ⓐ Ⓑ Ⓒ Ⓓ
3 _____
4 _____
5 Ⓐ Ⓑ Ⓒ Ⓓ
6 ___ ___ ___ ___
7 _____
8 Ⓐ Ⓑ Ⓒ Ⓓ
9 Ⓐ Ⓑ Ⓒ Ⓓ
10 Ⓐ Ⓑ Ⓒ Ⓓ
11 _____
12 Ⓐ Ⓑ Ⓒ Ⓓ
13 Ⓐ Ⓑ Ⓒ Ⓓ
14 _____
15 Ⓐ Ⓑ Ⓒ Ⓓ
16 Ⓐ Ⓑ Ⓒ Ⓓ
17 Ⓐ Ⓑ Ⓒ Ⓓ
18 Ⓐ Ⓑ Ⓒ Ⓓ

19 Ⓐ Ⓑ Ⓒ Ⓓ
20 Ⓐ Ⓑ Ⓒ Ⓓ
21 Ⓐ Ⓑ Ⓒ Ⓓ
22 Ⓐ Ⓑ Ⓒ Ⓓ
23 _____
24 Ⓐ Ⓑ Ⓒ Ⓓ
25 Ⓐ Ⓑ Ⓒ Ⓓ
26 Ⓐ Ⓑ Ⓒ Ⓓ
27 Ⓐ Ⓑ Ⓒ Ⓓ
28 _____
29 Ⓐ Ⓑ Ⓒ Ⓓ
30 Ⓐ Ⓑ Ⓒ Ⓓ
31 Ⓐ Ⓑ Ⓒ Ⓓ
32 ___ ___ ___ ___
33 Ⓐ Ⓑ Ⓒ Ⓓ
34 Ⓐ Ⓑ Ⓒ Ⓓ
35 Ⓐ Ⓑ Ⓒ Ⓓ
36 Ⓐ Ⓑ Ⓒ Ⓓ

37 Ⓐ Ⓑ Ⓒ Ⓓ
38 Ⓐ Ⓑ Ⓒ Ⓓ
39 Ⓐ Ⓑ Ⓒ Ⓓ
40 Ⓐ Ⓑ Ⓒ Ⓓ
41 Ⓐ Ⓑ Ⓒ Ⓓ
42 Ⓐ Ⓑ Ⓒ Ⓓ
43 Ⓐ Ⓑ Ⓒ Ⓓ
44 Ⓐ Ⓑ Ⓒ Ⓓ
45 Ⓐ Ⓑ Ⓒ Ⓓ
46 Ⓐ Ⓑ Ⓒ Ⓓ
47 Ⓐ Ⓑ Ⓒ Ⓓ
48 Ⓐ Ⓑ Ⓒ Ⓓ
49 Ⓐ Ⓑ Ⓒ Ⓓ
50 Ⓐ Ⓑ Ⓒ Ⓓ

ENGLISH AND LANGUAGE USAGE

1 Ⓐ Ⓑ Ⓒ Ⓓ
2 _____
3 Ⓐ Ⓑ Ⓒ Ⓓ
4 Ⓐ Ⓑ Ⓒ Ⓓ
5 Ⓐ Ⓑ Ⓒ Ⓓ
6 Ⓐ Ⓑ Ⓒ Ⓓ
7 Ⓐ Ⓑ Ⓒ Ⓓ
8 Ⓐ Ⓑ Ⓒ Ⓓ
9 Ⓐ Ⓑ Ⓒ Ⓓ
10 Ⓐ Ⓑ Ⓒ Ⓓ
11 Ⓐ Ⓑ Ⓒ Ⓓ
12 Ⓐ Ⓑ Ⓒ Ⓓ
13 Ⓐ Ⓑ Ⓒ Ⓓ

14 Ⓐ Ⓑ Ⓒ Ⓓ
15 _____
16 Ⓐ Ⓑ Ⓒ Ⓓ
17 Ⓐ Ⓑ Ⓒ Ⓓ
18 Ⓐ Ⓑ Ⓒ Ⓓ
19 Ⓐ Ⓑ Ⓒ Ⓓ
20 Ⓐ Ⓑ Ⓒ Ⓓ
21 Ⓐ Ⓑ Ⓒ Ⓓ
22 ___ ___ ___ ___
23 Ⓐ Ⓑ Ⓒ Ⓓ
24 Ⓐ Ⓑ Ⓒ Ⓓ
25 Ⓐ Ⓑ Ⓒ Ⓓ
26 Ⓐ Ⓑ Ⓒ Ⓓ

27 _____
28 Ⓐ Ⓑ Ⓒ Ⓓ
29 Ⓐ Ⓑ Ⓒ Ⓓ
30 Ⓐ Ⓑ Ⓒ Ⓓ
31 Ⓐ Ⓑ Ⓒ Ⓓ
32 Ⓐ Ⓑ Ⓒ Ⓓ
33 _____
34 Ⓐ Ⓑ Ⓒ Ⓓ
35 Ⓐ Ⓑ Ⓒ Ⓓ
36 Ⓐ Ⓑ Ⓒ Ⓓ
37 Ⓐ Ⓑ Ⓒ Ⓓ

Part I. Reading

45 questions / 55 minutes

1. Noah is buying a new car. He has decided that he wants a four-door sedan and has made a list of his top criteria:

   - Six-speed automatic transmission
   - At least 30 miles per gallon average fuel efficiency
   - Front wheel drive

   His maximum budget is $25,000. Circle the option below that would be an appropriate choice for Noah.

FUEL ECONOMY (CTY/HWY)	24/32 mpg
CAR TYPE	Sedan
TRANSMISSION	6-speed shiftable automatic
ENGINE TYPE	Gas
CYLINDERS	Inline 4
DRIVE TRAIN	Front Wheel Drive
MSRP (manufacturer's suggested retail price)	$23,995

FUEL ECONOMY (CTY/HWY)	25/35 mpg
CAR TYPE	Sedan
TRANSMISSION	8-speed automatic
ENGINE TYPE	Gas
CYLINDERS	Inline 4
DRIVE TRAIN	Front wheel drive
MSRP (manufacturer's suggested retail price)	$24,495

FUEL ECONOMY (CTY/HWY)	25/37 mpg
CAR TYPE	Sedan
TRANSMISSION	6-speed automatic
ENGINE TYPE	Gas
CYLINDERS	Inline 4
DRIVE TRAIN	Front wheel drive
MSRP (manufacturer's suggested retail price)	$26,050

FUEL ECONOMY (CTY/HWY)	26/36 mpg
CAR TYPE	Sedan
TRANSMISSION	6-speed shiftable automatic
ENGINE TYPE	Gas
CYLINDERS	Inline 4
DRIVE TRAIN	Front wheel drive
MSRP (manufacturer's suggested retail price)	$22,500

GO ON TO THE NEXT PAGE

Isabella wrote a paper on *Othello* for her English 1301 course. She went to the college's Student Writing Center for help with revising and editing her paper. As a result, she received a better grade than she had on the first paper she had written in that course.

2. The use of italics above signifies that the italicized word is

A) To be emphasized
B) A title
C) A foreign word
D) A word that is referenced in a footnote

Questions 3–8 refer to the following excerpt from *The Mound Builders* by George Bryce.

A mound of the kind found in our region is a very much flattened cone, or round-topped hillock of earth. It is built usually, if not invariably where the soil is soft and easily dug, and it is generally possible to trace in its neighborhood the depression whence the mound material has been taken. The mounds are as a rule found in the midst of a fertile section of country, and it is pretty certain from this that the mound builders were agriculturists, and chose their dwelling places with their occupation in view, where the mounds are found. The mounds are found accordingly on the banks of the Rainy River and Red River, and their affluents in the Northwest, in other words upon our best land stretches, but not so far as observed around the Lake of the Woods, or in barren regions. Near fishing grounds they greatly abound. What seem to have been strategic points upon the river were selected for their sites. The promontory giving a view and so commanding a considerable stretch of river, the point at the junction of two rivers, or the debouchure of a river into a lake or vice versa is a favorite spot. At the Long Sault on Rainy River there are three or four mounds grouped together along a ridge. Here some persons of strong imagination profess to see remains of an ancient fortification, but to my mind this is mere fancy. Mounds in our region vary from 6 to 50 feet in height, and from 60 to 130 feet in diameter. Some are circular at the base, others are elliptical.

The mounds have long been known as occurring in Central America, in Mexico, and along the whole extent of the Mississippi valley from the Gulf of Mexico to the great lakes. Our Northwest has, however, been neglected in the accounts of the mound-bearing region. Along our Red River I can count some six or eight mounds that have been noted in late years, and from the banks having been peopled and cultivated I have little doubt that others have been obliterated. One formerly stood on the site of

GO ON TO THE NEXT PAGE

the new unfinished Canadian Pacific Hotel in this city. The larger number of those known are in the neighborhood of the rapids, 16 or 18 miles below Winnipeg where the fishing is good. In 1879 the Historical Society opened one of these, and obtained a considerable quantity of remains. It is reported that there are mounds also on Nettley Creek, a tributary of the lower Red River, also on Lake Manitoba and some of its affluents. During the past summer it was my good fortune to visit the Rainy River, which lies some half way of the distance from Winnipeg to Lake Superior. In that delightful stretch of country, extending for 90 miles along the river there are no less than 21 mounds. These I identify with the mounds of Red River. The communication between Red and Rainy River is effected by ascending the Red Lake River, and coming by portage to a river running from the south into Rainy River. Both Red and Rainy River easily connect with the head waters of the Mississippi. Our region then may be regarded as a self-contained district including the most northerly settlements of the strange race who built the mounds. I shall try to connect them with other branches of the same stock, lying further to the east and south. For convenience I shall speak of the extinct people who inhabited our special region as the *Takawgamis*, or farthest north mound builders.

Source: Project Gutenberg

3. Which of the following is the best summary of the passage?

A) The author describes mounds and the types of places they are located. He identifies various locations of mounds within his part of the country and attempts to categorize them.

B) The author was out hiking when he discovered a native burial mound. This led him to explore other mounds in the region.

C) A scientist excavates several burial mounds to learn more about the people who built them and how they lived.

D) The author describes the ancient people who built mounds near his home. He then imagines what it must have been like for those people to travel from place to place.

4. Which of the following statements based on the passage is an opinion?

A) Both Red and Rainy River connect with the head waters of the Mississippi.

B) Rainy River lies some half way of the distance from Winnipeg to Lake Superior.

C) Our region then may be regarded as a self-contained district.

D) At the Long Sault on Rainy River there are three or four mounds grouped together along a ridge.

GO ON TO THE NEXT PAGE

5. In what part of North America does the author most likely live?

    A) A country in Central America
    B) Northwest Canada
    C) Southern Mexico
    D) The Gulf Coast region of the United States

6. What does the author most likely mean when he says, "The communication between Red and Rainy River is effected by ascending the Red Lake River"?

    A) The way to get from the Red River to the Rainy River is to go up the Red Lake River.
    B) It is difficult to reach the Rainy River from the Red River.
    C) In order to talk to someone in the Red River area, one must first call someone in the Red Lake area.
    D) One cannot get from the Red River to the Rainy River over land.

7. Why does the author believe that the mound builders were farming people?

    A) Mounds are located near rivers.
    B) Excavated mounds reveal farm tools.
    C) People in those areas today are farmers.
    D) Mounds are found in fertile parts of the country.

8. Which of the following best states the author's most likely purpose in writing this passage?

    A) The author seeks to educate readers about the mounds in his region since little has been published about them.
    B) The author argues that the mounds in his region were built by several different groups of people.
    C) The author wants readers to have instructions for how to build their own mounds.
    D) The author is trying to correct the misconception that the mounds were built by the *Takawgamis*.

All the students in Ms. Vinot's French class like ice cream. Some of them like chocolate, but others do not. Valerie is a student in Ms. Vinot's French class.

9. Which of the following can be concluded from the passage above?

    A) Valerie likes chocolate.
    B) Valerie does not like chocolate.
    C) Valerie likes ice cream.
    D) Valerie does not like ice cream.

GO ON TO THE NEXT PAGE

The next two questions are based on the following excerpt.

Women's Voices is a collection of eight essays examining select works of Finnish literature written by female authors and two short essays about feminist studies in other fields: art history and music. The editors each contribute one essay to the collection and aim to capture the diversity of female authorship and present a compact overview of Finnish feminist literary criticism. The essays are organized roughly by the time period of the literature being examined and progress from the mid-1800s to more contemporary writings in the 1990s. The first seven essays are classic literary criticism and the eighth is a marvelous essay on Sami women writers by Vuokko Hirvonen that blends literary criticism with history and anthropology. The book finishes with an essay on feminist art history by Tutta Palin and an essay on gender studies in music research by Taru Leppanen.

10. The passage above can be most properly categorized as a

    A) Paragraph from a book review
    B) Stanza of a poem
    C) Excerpt from a novel
    D) Newspaper article

11. As it is used in the passage above, the word *progress* means

    A) Improve
    B) Mature
    C) Move forward or develop
    D) Degenerate

How to Tie a Windsor Knot

First, cross the wide end of the tie over the thin end. Then continue up behind the thin end and wrap around to the front side. Cross the wide end in front, pull up and forward by the neck, and then down under itself. Pull the wide end to tighten the knot, then the thin end to make the finished tie snug against the neck.

12. In the instructions above, which sentence contains the second step in the process? Underline it.

Erlene needs to make a cake for her sister's birthday, so she went to the store to buy milk, eggs, sugar, and flour to make the cake. The sugar was on sale for $2.14 a bag, so she bought two bags. The store also had a sale on lemons, so she decided to buy a few lemons and make the cake lemon-flavored. After she made her purchases and went outside the store, she realized that she had forgotten to buy eggs.

GO ON TO THE NEXT PAGE

13. Which of the following is the best conclusion for the previous paragraph?

A) Erlene went back inside and returned the lemons.
B) Erlene made a chocolate cake for her sister.
C) Erlene went back inside and bought the eggs.
D) Erlene decided not to make her sister a cake.

The next three questions are based on the following information.

Students,

Your geography exam will be on Friday, the 22nd and will cover the five basic geography themes that we have reviewed in class. The exam will consist of 25 multiple-choice questions, ten short answer responses, and one essay question. The essay topic will be fairly narrow so that you will have time to adequately address the topic. Your essay should be at least one full page, however.

I have provided you with a summary below to help you study for the exam. The themes are shown on the left, and the types of ideas with which you should be familiar are in the middle. On the right, outlined in cloud shapes, are some examples of those ideas. The examples I have given are not the only examples of those ideas; feel free to come up with your own examples in your responses.

If you have any questions, you may see me during my regular office hours or schedule a time to meet with me.

—Ms. Babin

14. Based on the information in the diagram, how many types of characteristics of place will the students be tested on?

A) 2
B) 3
C) 4
D) 5

15. How many total questions will be on the exam?

A) 10
B) 25
C) 35
D) 36

16. What does the phrase "wear layers in ice" refer to in the diagram?

A) The movement of people from warmer climates to colder ones
B) People adapting to their environments
C) People behaving similarly across diverse regions
D) The human characteristics of a place

The next two questions are based on the following paragraph.

A recent study of working professionals found that people who are currently licensed as physicians had taken more biology classes as undergraduates than did people who work in other professions. The research concluded that people who take biology classes are more likely to become physicians.

17. Which of the following assumptions did the researchers make?

A) Taking more biology classes causes greater interest in becoming a physician.
B) Everyone takes a biology class in college.
C) No one becomes a physician without taking multiple biology classes in college.
D) People who want to become physicians need to take more biology classes.

GO ON TO THE NEXT PAGE

18. Which of the following, if true, would most weaken the conclusion drawn by the researchers?

A) Physicians are more likely than other students to take an anatomy class.

B) The physicians studied indicated that biology classes gave them important information about physical systems.

C) Many undergraduates who want to become physicians are advised to take biology classes.

D) Not all undergraduates who take biology classes become physicians.

19. The diagram shows an outdoor thermometer. What is the temperature shown in degrees Celsius? Write your answer in the blank:

_____

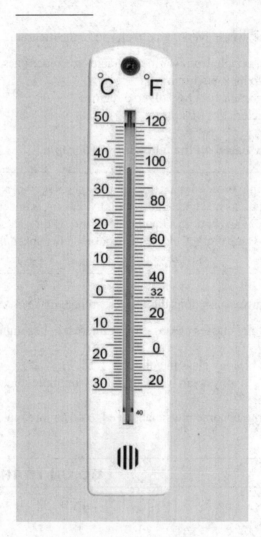

The next two questions refer to the following timeline.

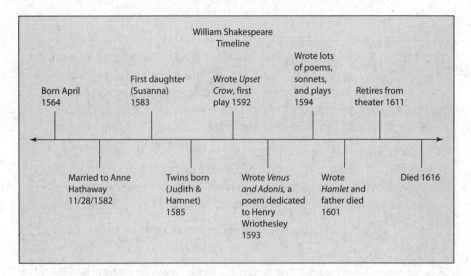

William Shakespeare Timeline

Born April 1564

Married to Anne Hathaway 11/28/1582

First daughter (Susanna) 1583

Twins born (Judith & Hamnet) 1585

Wrote *Upset Crow*, first play 1592

Wrote *Venus and Adonis*, a poem dedicated to Henry Wriothesley 1593

Wrote lots of poems, sonnets, and plays 1594

Wrote *Hamlet* and father died 1601

Retires from theater 1611

Died 1616

20. Put the following events in chronological order according to the timeline (1 = first / 5 = last).

_____ Wrote *Hamlet*

_____ Wrote *Upset Crow*

_____ Had twins

_____ Married Anne Hathaway

_____ Wrote *Venus and Adonis*

21. Which of the following events occurred in the same year that Shakespeare's father died?

A) Shakespeare wrote many sonnets.
B) Shakespeare himself died.
C) Shakespeare wrote *Hamlet*.
D) Anne Hathaway gave birth to Hamnet.

22. A research paper on the novel *The Sound and the Fury* quotes the novel itself, several different literary criticism essays, and a book review that was published in a newspaper just after the novel was released. The research paper also includes information gathered from maps of Mississippi. Which of those sources is a primary source?

A) The novel *The Sound and the Fury*
B) The newspaper's book review
C) The literary criticism essays
D) The maps of Mississippi

GO ON TO THE NEXT PAGE

Questions 23–28 refer to the excerpt above from *White Fang* by Jack London.

The day began auspiciously. They had lost no dogs during the night, and they swung out upon the trail and into the silence, the darkness, and the cold with spirits that were fairly light. Bill seemed to have forgotten his forebodings of the previous night, and even waxed facetious with the dogs when, at midday, they overturned the sled on a bad piece of trail.

It was an awkward mix-up. The sled was upside down and jammed between a tree-trunk and a huge rock, and they were forced to unharness the dogs in order to straighten out the tangle. The two men were bent over the sled and trying to right it, when Henry observed One Ear sidling away.

"Here, you, One Ear!" he cried, straightening up and turning around on the dog.

But One Ear broke into a run across the snow, his traces trailing behind him. And there, out in the snow of their back track, was the she-wolf waiting for him. As he neared her, he became suddenly cautious. He slowed down to an alert and mincing walk and then stopped. He regarded her carefully and dubiously, yet desirefully. She seemed to smile at him, showing her teeth in an ingratiating rather than a menacing way. She moved toward him a few steps, playfully, and then halted. One Ear drew near to her, still alert and cautious, his tail and ears in the air, his head held high.

He tried to sniff noses with her, but she retreated playfully and coyly. Every advance on his part was accompanied by a corresponding retreat on her part. Step by step she was luring him away from the security of his human companionship. Once, as though a warning had in vague ways flitted through his intelligence, he turned his head and looked back at the overturned sled, at his team-mates, and at the two men who were calling to him.

But whatever idea was forming in his mind, was dissipated by the she-wolf, who advanced upon him, sniffed noses with him for a fleeting instant, and then resumed her coy retreat before his renewed advances.

In the meantime, Bill had bethought himself of the rifle. But it was jammed beneath the overturned sled, and by the time Henry had helped him to right the load, One Ear and the she-wolf were too close together and the distance too great to risk a shot.

Too late One Ear learned his mistake. Before they saw the cause, the two men saw him turn and start to run back toward them. Then, approaching at right angles to the trail and cutting off his retreat they saw a dozen wolves, lean and grey, bounding across the snow. On the instant, the she-wolf's coyness and playfulness disappeared. With a snarl she sprang upon One Ear. He thrust her off with his shoulder, and, his retreat cut off and still

GO ON TO THE NEXT PAGE

intent on regaining the sled, he altered his course in an attempt to circle around to it. More wolves were appearing every moment and joining in the chase. The she-wolf was one leap behind One Ear and holding her own.

"Where are you goin'?" Henry suddenly demanded, laying his hand on his partner's arm.

Bill shook it off. "I won't stand it," he said. "They ain't a-goin' to get any more of our dogs if I can help it."

Gun in hand, he plunged into the underbrush that lined the side of the trail. His intention was apparent enough. Taking the sled as the centre of the circle that One Ear was making, Bill planned to tap that circle at a point in advance of the pursuit. With his rifle, in the broad daylight, it might be possible for him to awe the wolves and save the dog.

Source: Project Gutenberg

23. Which of the following best describes the primary mode of writing used in this passage?

   A) Expository
   B) Narrative
   C) Persuasive
   D) Descriptive

24. "They ain't a-goin' to get any more of our dogs if I can help it." This line from the passage is an example of

   A) Dialogue
   B) Exposition
   C) Summary
   D) Scene

25. What is Bill's most likely goal at the end of the passage?

   A) To kill all of the wolves
   B) To put down his injured dog
   C) To scare off the wolves
   D) To save himself from the she-wolf

26. Which of the following correctly describes the sequence of events in the passage?

   A) Bill goes after One Ear, and then the sled overturns.
   B) The sled overturns, and then the she-wolf lures One Ear away from the sled.
   C) One Ear meets the she-wolf, and she is joined by a dozen other wolves who lead One Ear away from the sled.
   D) One Ear follows the she-wolf away from the sled, and Bill overturns the sled attempting to catch them.

GO ON TO THE NEXT PAGE

27. Why does Bill not shoot the she-wolf as soon as she appears?

  A) He forgot to bring the rifle with them.
  B) Henry has the gun and is nearly out of bullets.
  C) He lost the gun in the sled accident.
  D) The rifle is trapped beneath the sled.

28. How does the author most likely feel about the wolves in this passage?

  A) They are clever and dangerous.
  B) They are dumb animals driven by instinct.
  C) They can be trained to help humans.
  D) They are beautiful creatures that should be protected.

Company	Price	Shipping
Toys for All	$12.59	$2.99
WINK, Inc.	$11.99	$1.99
Kim's Kritters	$14.99	Free shipping
Kid Stuff	$13.89	$1.49

29. Amee is buying a toy stuffed giraffe for her little brother. She does an online search and finds four companies that sell the giraffe she wants. In order to get the best price, from which company should she purchase the toy based on the information above?

  A) Toys for All
  B) WINK, Inc.
  C) Kim's Kritters
  D) Kid Stuff

The next two questions refer to the following letter.

Attn: Dr. Robert Meinhart
Dean of Humanities
Magnolia State College

Dear Dr. Meinhart:

I wish to seek a position in the Theater Department at Magnolia State College. Having spent a few years volunteering in the Theatre Department at Magnolia, I came to believe that Magnolia State is a college with a progressive reputation in a beautiful setting. I appreciate your mission statement encouraging "preparation for lifelong learning," a philosophy I've always held.

GO ON TO THE NEXT PAGE

My background includes a bachelor of fine arts in drama from Oklahoma State University and a master's in English from the University of Vermont. I have written several plays that have been performed for the community theater here in Oakland, and I have been invited to be a guest presenter at the Conference on Stagecraft in New Orleans in May 2017.

For the past six years I have been employed as the costume specialist for the Dance Department at Oakland College, and I teach the crew class. I have found that I especially enjoy teaching college-aged students. Prior to moving to Oakland, I taught English and speech classes at Jones High School in Burlington, Vermont for ten years.

I hope that my education, experience, and life practice will offer you a variety of assets and that you will welcome my application.

Sincerely yours,
Elena Furse

30. Which of the following lines from the letter expresses an opinion?

    A) I have been invited to be a guest presenter at the Conference on Stagecraft in New Orleans.
    B) I teach the crew class.
    C) Magnolia State is a college with a progressive reputation in a beautiful setting.
    D) I wish to seek a position in the Theater Department at Magnolia State College.

31. Which of the following best expresses the author's purpose?

    A) She is auditioning for a role in a Magnolia State College theater production.
    B) She is attempting to gain employment at Magnolia State College.
    C) She is looking for housing near Magnolia State College.
    D) She is describing her background for an article at the Conference on Stagecraft.

Matthew hoped that after the marathon there would be comfort and alleviation of his pain waiting for him.

32. Which of the following is the meaning of *alleviation* as used in the sentence above?

    A) Increasing
    B) Curing
    C) Raising
    D) Lessening

GO ON TO THE NEXT PAGE

The next two questions refer to the following information.

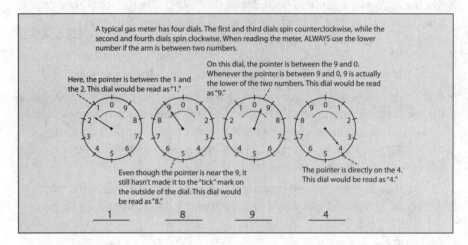

A typical gas meter has four dials. The first and third dials spin counterclockwise, while the second and fourth dials spin clockwise. When reading the meter, ALWAYS use the lower number if the arm is between two numbers.

Here, the pointer is between the 1 and the 2. This dial would be read as "1."

On this dial, the pointer is between the 9 and 0. Whenever the pointer is between 9 and 0, 9 is actually the lower of the two numbers. This dial would be read as "9."

Even though the pointer is near the 9, it still hasn't made it to the "tick" mark on the outside of the dial. This dial would be read as "8."

The pointer is directly on the 4. This dial would be read as "4."

<u>1</u>   <u>8</u>   <u>9</u>   <u>4</u>

33. If the second dial on the meter above had the arrow pointing between 9 and 0, what would the meter reading be?

A) 1994
B) 1894
C) 1094
D) 9894

34. What does the meter below read? Write your answer in the blank: _____

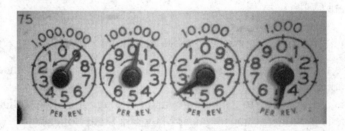

If Cheri spends any time in the intensive care unit, it's crowded and uncomfortable, and there's not really anywhere for parents to stay. Ronald McDonald House can save your sanity. It's on the 4th floor of the Abercrombie Building next to the orange elevators. They have sleep/nap rooms with private bathrooms, a living room, a fully stocked kitchen, and food, laundry, and a library with computer stations. Overnight stays (7:00 P.M.–11:00 A.M.) are assigned daily by the charge nurse of each unit, so ask her if you want to spend a night there. Nap rooms are open 1:00–5:00 P.M. and are first come, first served. The main area is open 9:00 A.M.–9:00 P.M.

GO ON TO THE NEXT PAGE

35. Who is the audience for the previous passage?

A) Tourists

B) Nurses

C) Hospital patients

D) Parents of hospital patients

36. Aaron is researching the annexation of Hawaii in 1898. He wants to find out what people in Hawaii thought about the annexation at the time it occurred. Which of the following would be his best source for this information?

A) A contemporary dictionary

B) An atlas published in 1899

C) A newspaper from Hawaii on the date Hawaii was annexed

D) A book about the formation of the United States

The next two questions refer to the following map.

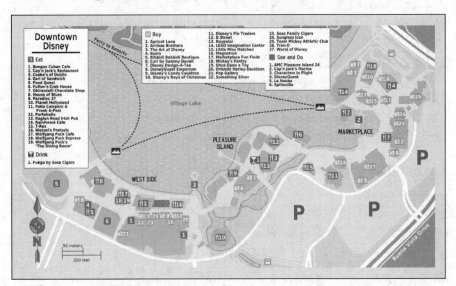

37. If a person playing games at DisneyQuest gets hungry, which restaurant is closest?

A) Food Quest

B) House of Blues

C) Bongos Cuban Café

D) Wetzel's Pretzels

38. Where is the Fuego bar located?

A) At the resorts

B) West Side

C) East Side

D) Pleasure Island

GO ON TO THE NEXT PAGE

The next two questions refer to the following passage.

Iridium is an extremely rare metal that is similar to platinum. Large concentrations of iridium are only found in meteorites (asteroids, meteors, or comets) that have crashed on earth or after large volcanic eruptions that thrust the iridium out from deep within the earth. Scientists concluded that a comet hit the earth and wiped out the dinosaurs because of the concentration of iridium found in rock stratum from 65 million years ago.

39. Which of the following, if true, most strongly supports the scientist's conclusion?

   A) Dinosaurs were not the only animals to die out 65 million years ago.
   B) A comet struck the earth approximately 28.5 million years ago, but no widespread extinction resulted from that collision.
   C) A volcano large enough to generate high concentrations of iridium is extremely rare.
   D) Most scientists agree that a comet impact wiped out the dinosaurs.

40. Which of the following methods of argument is used?

   A) Criticizing an opponent
   B) Examining evidence
   C) Making an analogy to a similar situation
   D) Appealing to readers' emotions

The next two questions refer to the following information.

1.	2.	3.	4.
5.	6. X	7.	8.
9.	10.	11.	12.
13.	14.	15.	16.

41. If the X in box 6 is moved up one space and then to the right two spaces, circle the number of the box it will now be in.

42. If the X in box 6 is moved left one space, then down two spaces, then right two spaces, which box will it be in?

   A) 1
   B) 7
   C) 11
   D) 15

GO ON TO THE NEXT PAGE

The next two questions refer to the following passage.

How to Start a Fire with an Artificial Flint Sparking Stick

First, you will need some tinder to start your fire. There are many things you can use for tinder, but it must be completely dry. You can use dry grass or leaves, tree bark or small sticks, paper, cloth, and so on. Use your knife to shred the tinder finely so that it will ignite from a spark. Once you have the tinder, put a bit of it into a small pile and place the sparking stick close to the tinder. Use the edged tool that comes attached to the sparking stick and draw it slowly downward over the sparking stick. If your flint does not have this tool, you can use your knife blade. Dragging the knife blade or edged tool across the surface of the sparking stick will produce hot sparks that will light the tinder if you have prepared it properly. Finally, when the fire is becoming established, you should gradually add more tinder, then thin sticks of wood. Larger pieces of wood should only be added once the fire is going well. Build your fire up gradually.

43. What step comes just after making a small pile of tinder?

A) Gathering dry leaves, small twigs, and grass
B) Adding larger pieces of wood
C) Using the sparking stick to produce sparks
D) Shredding the tinder with your knife

44. Vivian tried to make a fire using this method, but the sparks from her flint did not ignite the tinder. What might explain this? Select all that apply.

A) Her tinder was not shredded finely.
B) She used a knife blade to scrape the flint and produce the sparks.
C) Her tinder was not dry.
D) Her flint was purchased at a hardware store rather than at a camping store.

GO ON TO THE NEXT PAGE

Attn: Unit Four Employees,

The company picnic will be next Thursday from 11:00AM–1:00PM. The company will provide ham and fried chicken, as well as plates, napkins, and utensils. Employees are asked to bring one side dish or dessert to share and their own individual beverages. The picnic will be held in the common area outside near the fountain. We will have a number of outdoor activities for you to enjoy with your coworkers, such as bean bag toss, flying disc golf, sack races, and croquet. Dress code for Thursday is casual!

—Evelyn

45. Which of the following best states the author's purpose?

A) She wants to convince people to attend an event she is having.
B) She wants to give employees important information about the picnic.
C) She wants to make people feel guilty about not bringing food to the last picnic.
D) She wants to warn the employees to act professionally at social events.

STOP. THIS IS THE END OF PART I.

Part II. Mathematics

38 questions / 57 minutes

1. Put the following numbers in order from greatest (1) to least (4).

_____ −4.26

_____ $\dfrac{19}{5}$

_____ $-\dfrac{8}{3}$

_____ $\sqrt{3}$

2. A rug store adds 45% to the wholesale price it pays for each rug to set the selling price. What is the selling price of a rug that cost $90.00 wholesale?

A) $40.50
B) $90.45
C) $130.50
D) $135.00

3. Jim is making shortbread cookies. The recipe calls for 1 cup of butter, ½ cup sugar, and 2½ cups flour. Jim had already put in the 1 cup of butter and 2½ cups flour, but then he accidentally added 1 cup of sugar to the mixture. Which of the following shows how much butter and flour he must now add to achieve the proper proportion?

A) 1 cup of butter and 2½ cups flour
B) ½ cup of butter and 1 cup of flour
C) ¼ cup of butter and ½ cup of flour
D) 1 cup of butter and 1½ cups of flour

GO ON TO THE NEXT PAGE

4. Laura is recycling bottles to earn enough money to buy a new video game. Each bottle is worth 5 cents, and she has already collected 43 bottles. She wants to find out how many more bottles she would need to collect to earn a total of $40.00. Which of the following equations would give her the answer to her question?

A) $5(x + 43) = 40$
B) $.05(x + 43) = 40$
C) $.05(40) = x + 43$
D) $.05(x) = 40$

Test Score	Number of Students
100	1
95	2
90	1
85	3
80	4
75	3
70	1
65	1
60	0
55	1

5. Which of the following conclusions about the data shown in the chart above are true? Select all that apply.

A) The mode of the data set is greater than the median.
B) The mode of the data set is greater than the range.
C) The median of the data set is equal to the range.
D) The mode of the data set is equal to the median.

6. Which of the following describes values that are positively correlated?

A) A farmer noted that the older her chickens got, the fewer eggs they laid.
B) Nicholle filled up her car with gas each time the gas gauge showed that she had ¼ of a tank left because she did not ever want to run out of gas.
C) Kathy puts 5% of each paycheck into a retirement account. When she got a raise from $100 a week to $150 per week, the amount she put into the retirement account rose from $5 per week to $7.50 per week.
D) Zane missed 4 days of chemistry the first semester and got a B in the class. The second semester he missed 6 days and got a D in the class.

GO ON TO THE NEXT PAGE

7. Andy is building a ¼-scale model of his house, which means that ¼ inch equals 1 foot. The wall height of his actual living room is 14 feet, so the height of the living room walls in the model house is 3.5 inches. If the living room floor in his actual house measures 18 feet by 12 feet, how big should he make the model living room floor?

A) 18 inches by 12 inches
B) 9 inches by 6 inches
C) 6 inches by 4 inches
D) 4.5 inches by 3 inches

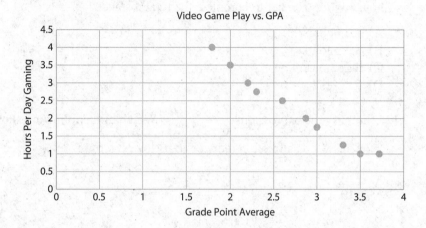

8. Which of the following conclusions is best supported by the data above?

A) In general, as the number of hours spent playing video games increases, GPA decreases.
B) It is not possible to achieve a 4.0 GPA if you play video games every day.
C) There is not a consistent relationship between the number of hours spent playing video games and GPA.
D) Video game play can benefit students by stimulating their creativity and teaching problem-solving skills.

9. Put the following values in order from least (1) to greatest (4).

_____ 0.3×320

_____ $\dfrac{3}{4} \times 75$

_____ 4^3

_____ 20% of 240

GO ON TO THE NEXT PAGE

10. Ryan's skateboard wheels have radii of 1.5 inches. How far does his skateboard travel in 4 complete revolutions of the wheels?

A) 3 inches
B) 3π inches
C) 12π inches
D) 48 inches

11. Vicki is running a 26.2-mile marathon. She has run ¼ of the distance in 75 minutes. If she keeps running at the same rate, how many more hours will it take her to complete the total distance?

A) 1.25 hours
B) 3.75 hours
C) 4.25 hours
D) 5 hours

12. Simplify the expression $\left(\dfrac{2}{6} \times \dfrac{3}{5}\right) + \dfrac{9}{11}$. Which of the following shows the answer as a fraction reduced to its lowest terms?

A) $\dfrac{112}{110}$

B) 1.02

C) $\dfrac{9}{55}$

D) $\dfrac{56}{55}$

13. Bruce received test scores of 83, 74, 92, 96, and 89. He has one more test this semester and would like to raise his test average. What would he need to score on the sixth test to raise his average to 90? Write your answer in the blank: _____

14. Simplify $5(4x^2 - 10)$.

A) $20x^2 - 10$
B) $20x^{10} - 10$
C) $20x^2 - 50$
D) $20x^{10} - 50$

GO ON TO THE NEXT PAGE

For questions 15–16, refer to the graph below.

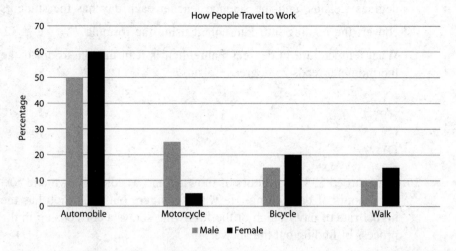

How People Travel to Work

■ Male ■ Female

15. In the chart above, circle the mode of transportation that is used the least overall.

16. If there were 540 women surveyed, how many of them said that they ride bicycles to work?

   A) 20
   B) 81
   C) 108
   D) 270

17. Which of the following is equal to 3.5% of 40?

   A) $\dfrac{35}{1,000} \times 40$

   B) $\dfrac{35}{1,000} \times 4$

   C) $\dfrac{35}{100} \times 40$

   D) 0.35×40

18. In the equation $6(x - 8) = -42$, what is the value of x?

   A) −1
   B) 1
   C) 6
   D) 7

GO ON TO THE NEXT PAGE

19. The science classroom temperature only measures temperature in degrees Celsius, and the science teacher each day has the students convert the reading into Fahrenheit using the formula $F = \frac{9}{5}C + 32$. What temperature in degrees Fahrenheit is it in the classroom if the thermometer reads 25 degrees Celsius?

A) 32
B) 57
C) 65
D) 77

20. John earned $58 for 4 hours of mowing and weeding a lawn and $73 for 6 hours of babysitting. He wants to figure out which job has the higher rate of pay. Which of the following shows a correct step in the process of finding out the answer?

A) $58 \div 6 = 9.7$
B) $73 \div 4 = 18.25$
C) $58 \div 4 = 14.5$
D) $58 + 73 \div 10 = 13.1$

21. The local baseball field is planning to build a 22-feet-long sidewalk from the gate to the concession stand. The architect's drawing of that sidewalk is 18 inches long. A section of the sidewalk that will be painted in the home team's colors measures 3 inches long on the drawing. How many feet long will that painted section be on the actual sidewalk?

A) 1.22
B) 2.45
C) 3.67
D) 4.28

22. Carolyn has two coupons she can use on a blanket she is buying. One coupon is for $10 off a purchase of $25 or more. The other is for 25% off any purchase. The blanket costs $75. Which of the following shows the discounted price (before tax) she would pay using the coupon with the greater discount?

A) $65.00
B) $56.25
C) $46.25
D) $18.75

GO ON TO THE NEXT PAGE

23. In a large orchestra, the ratio of woodwinds to horns to trumpets is 4:2:1. If the city of Lakeville is forming an 84-person orchestra, how many trumpet players will it need?

A) 12
B) 24
C) 36
D) 48

24. Solve the inequality $3x - 7 \geq 17$.

A) $x \leq 8$
B) $x \geq 8$
C) $x \geq 10$
D) $x \geq 24$

25. Preston charges $12 for a small carved box and $24 for a medium one. Which of the following expressions represents how much he will charge for an order of x small and y medium boxes?

A) $12 + 24$
B) $x + 2y$
C) $12y + 24x$
D) $12x + 24y$

26. Britt sold $9,000 worth of fish in July. That was an increase of 20% over his sales in June, but his June sales were 20% lower than his sales in May. Which of the following shows the amount he sold in May?

A) $7,500
B) $8,950
C) $9,000
D) $9,375

27. What is the value of y if $6x - 4y = -8$ and $7x + 4y = -18$?

A) -3
B) -2
C) -1
D) 1
E) 2

28. Nick has a 6-inch-tall drinking glass with a square base that has 4-inch sides. If he wants to fill the glass with water to exactly half of its volume, how many cubic inches of water will he need? Write your answer in the blank: _____

GO ON TO THE NEXT PAGE

29. Marisa is making curtains for two windows. Each window needs two panels that are 8 feet long. When Marisa gets to the fabric store, she sees that the fabric is measured by the yard. How many yards will she need to purchase to have enough for both windows?

A) $10\frac{2}{3}$

B) 8

C) $5\frac{1}{3}$

D) $2\frac{2}{3}$

30. Which of the following shows the best estimate of how many 6-foot shelves will be needed to hold 203 books with an average width of 1.4 inches?

A) 3 because 200×1 in. $= 200$ in., and $200 \div 12 \approx 16$ ft, so $16 \div 6 \approx 3$.

B) 3.95 because 203×1.4 in. $= 284.2$ in., and $284.2 \div 12 \approx 23.68$ ft, so $23.68 \div 6 \approx 3.95$.

C) 4 because 200×1.5 in. $= 300$ in., and $300 \div 12 = 25$ ft, so $25 \div 6 \approx 4.1$.

D) 5 because 200×1.5 in. $= 300$ in., and $300 \div 12 = 25$ ft, so $25 \div 6 \approx 4.1$ and $4.1 > 4$, so you need to round up to 5 shelves.

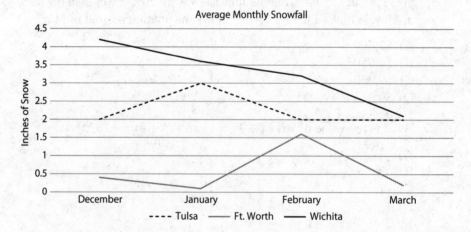

GO ON TO THE NEXT PAGE

31. Which of the following conclusions is supported by the graph on the previous page?

A) It is colder in Wichita than in Ft. Worth.
B) Ft. Worth has less snowfall between December and March than does either Tulsa or Wichita.
C) Tulsa's highest average monthly snowfall is higher than Wichita's highest average monthly snowfall.
D) Ft. Worth doesn't receive any snow before December.

32. Kalee normally walks the 1.5 miles from her home to her office at a pace of 3 miles per hour. Today she is late and has only 15 minutes to get to work. How fast does she need to walk to get there in 15 minutes?

A) 3 miles per hour
B) 5 miles per hour
C) 6 miles per hour
D) 9 miles per hour

33. Which of the following expresses 12.5% as a decimal?

A) 0.125
B) 1.25
C) 12.5
D) 125

34. A community center is recarpeting its music room. The room is a square with sides of 16 feet plus a semicircular performance area on one side as shown below. Which of the following shows the closest estimate of the number of square feet of carpet that will be needed to cover the total area?

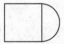

A) 450
B) 360
C) 250
D) 190

GO ON TO THE NEXT PAGE

35. Which of the following has the greatest value?

A) $\dfrac{8}{3}$

B) $\sqrt{2}$

C) 1.5

D) $\dfrac{5}{4}$

36. Solve $5x + 2(x - 9) = 4x + 6$ for the value of x.

A) −8
B) 0
C) 3
D) 8

37. Emma Lee is prescribed a new medication. She is to take 50 mg twice per day, and the prescription provides three refills. If there are 60 capsules in a full bottle and each capsule is 25 mg, how many doses does her new prescription provide, including the three refills?

A) 30
B) 60
C) 90
D) 120

38. If $3x \le x + 7$, which of the following are possible values for x? Select all that apply.

A) −1
B) 2
C) 3
D) 3.5
E) 4

STOP. THIS IS THE END OF PART II.

Part III. Science

50 questions / 60 minutes

1. Which of the following is one way the medulla oblongata controls respiration?

   A) It connects the larynx to the lungs.
   B) It secretes an aqueous surfactant.
   C) It moves oxygen to the blood.
   D) It monitors carbon dioxide levels.

2. Which of the following is a function of a lipid?

   A) To serve as a structural component of cell membranes
   B) To provide cells with short-term energy
   C) To store genetic information
   D) To speed up chemical reactions

3. Which type of muscle tissue makes up approximately 40% of your body mass? Write your answer in the blank: _____

4. These graphs show the same chemical reaction with and without using a catalyst. Circle the graph that shows the reaction *with* the catalyst.

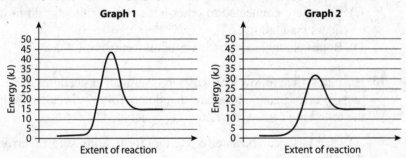

5. Which of the following tools would be most appropriate to measure the volume of a liquid substance?

   A) Electronic balance
   B) Microscope
   C) Graduated cylinder
   D) Measuring wheel

GO ON TO THE NEXT PAGE

6. The amount of energy in molecules of matter determines the state of matter. Put the following states of matter in order based on the amount of energy in their molecules. (1 = most energy / 4 = least energy)

_____ gas
_____ liquid
_____ plasma
_____ solid

7. Two identical copies of a chromosome formed during the cell cycle are called _____. Write your answer in the blank.

8. Which of the following do prokaryotic and eukaryotic cells have in common?

A) Nucleus
B) Circular DNA
C) Membrane-bound organelles
D) Cytoplasm

9. Which of the following describes a way in which the neuromuscular and skeletal systems work together?

A) Muscles in the lungs contract and relax to inhale and exhale.
B) Bones synthesize blood and immune cells and store minerals.
C) Bones are connected to other bones via ligaments and to muscle fibers via tendons.
D) Bones elongate and ossify as adolescents grow.

10. Hospitals that follow checklists for surgical procedures have lower rates of error than do hospitals that do not follow checklists. Which of the following can be most properly concluded?

A) Checklists can be an effective tool for fighting surgical errors.
B) All hospitals should use checklists for every step of patient care.
C) Doctors are more likely to make mistakes when they are not being watched.
D) Hospitals that care about their patients do not need to follow checklists.

11. There are _____ chromosomes in the typical human genome. Write the number in the blank.

GO ON TO THE NEXT PAGE

12. Which of the following describes the process of diffusion?

   A) A substance moves from an area of low concentration to an area of high concentration.
   B) A substance moves from an area of high concentration to areas of low concentration.
   C) A substance moves from the center toward two opposite poles.
   D) A liquid is turned into a gas through the application of heat.

13. Which of the following expresses the function of the glomerulus in a kidney?

   A) It carries urine from the kidney to the urinary bladder.
   B) It absorbs salt and water to produce urine.
   C) It carries blood from the kidney to the inferior vena cava.
   D) It filters waste products out of the blood.

14. In the image below, circle the dermis layer of the skin.

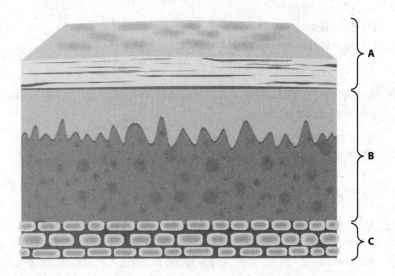

15. Which plane of reference divides the human body into left and right sides?

   A) Median
   B) Coronal
   C) Transverse
   D) Frontal

GO ON TO THE NEXT PAGE

16. Which of the following are types of macromolecules? Select all that apply.

    A) Carbohydrate
    B) Amino acid
    C) Nucleic acid
    D) Oxygen

17. What is the result when a person's pancreas stops releasing insulin?

    A) Proteins in food cannot be properly digested, leading to malnutrition.
    B) Sugar will not enter cells, causing high blood sugar levels and diabetes.
    C) Too much thyroid hormone will be produced, leading to Graves' disease.
    D) It will lead to low levels of progesterone, which can cause infertility.

18. Blood plasma contains which of the following? Select all that apply.

    A) Hormones
    B) Nutrients
    C) Hemoglobin
    D) Antibodies

19. Which of the following shows the correctly balanced chemical equation for photosynthesis?

    A) $CO_2 + H_2O \rightarrow C_6H_{12}O_6 + O_2$
    B) $3CO_2 + 6H_2O \rightarrow C_6H_{12}O_6 + 6O_2$
    C) $3CO_2 + 3H_2O \rightarrow C_6H_{12}O_6 + 6O_2$
    D) $6CO_2 + 6H_2O \rightarrow C_6H_{12}O_6 + 6O_2$

20. A student wants to determine whether mold grows faster on bread at a higher temperature. He sets up several groups of bread slices from the same loaf to test at different temperatures. Which of the following would be the most accurate way to measure the amount of mold that grows on the bread?

    A) Count how many pieces of bread have mold and how many do not. The amount of mold can be expressed as the ratio of molded pieces to nonmolded pieces.
    B) Designate three levels of mold: light, medium, and heavy. These labels can be used to describe the mold growth at various temperatures.
    C) Use a transparent grid overlay to measure the surface area of the bread and the size of the mold spots. The amount of mold can be expressed as a percentage of the total bread surface area.
    D) Weigh the bread before the experiment. When mold appears, tear out the moldy parts and then weigh the bread again. Divide the original weight by the new weight.

GO ON TO THE NEXT PAGE

21. Which of the following substances has a neutral pH?

A) Lemon juice with a pH of 2
B) Water with a pH of 7
C) Soapy water with a pH of 12
D) Milk with a pH of 6

22. Which of the following describes an ionic bond?

A) Two atoms of the same element share a pair of electrons in the middle of the two atoms.
B) One metallic and one nonmetallic atom bond by attracting oppositely charged ions.
C) Two metallic atoms bond through the electrostatic attractive force between conduction electrons and positively charged metal ions.
D) Two nonmetallic atoms bond by sharing their electrons.

Questions 23–25 refer to the following information and chart.

A new weight-loss medication has entered clinical trials. Six subjects in a study were given two pills each day and told not to make any changes in their diet or exercise levels. Six more subjects were given the same instructions, but the pills were placebos that did not contain any of the drug being tested. Weight was measured at the start of the trial, after six months on the medication, and after two years on the medication. The control group saw no significant long-term effects on weight. The group given the medication saw significant changes in weight. Their results are shown below.

Subject	Starting Weight	Weight After 6 Months	Weight After 2 Years
A: male	230 lb	200 lb	180 lb
B: female	200 lb	170 lb	120 lb
C: female	180 lb	160 lb	110 lb
D: male	285 lb	225 lb	195 lb
E: male	305 lb	250 lb	220 lb
F: female	220 lb	180 lb	125 lb

23. In the chart, circle the subject who had the greatest amount of weight lost after two years.

24. Which of the following conclusions can be drawn from the information in the chart above?

A) Males lost more weight than did females initially, but females lost more weight overall.
B) At the end of the two-year study, males lost more weight than did females.
C) The weight-loss regimen is effective for short-term weight loss but not for long term.
D) No clear pattern of weight loss can be determined from the data.

GO ON TO THE NEXT PAGE

25. Which of the following best describes the instruction to make no changes in diet or exercise?

A) It forms the control group, in which subjects were given placebos.
B) It establishes a controlled setting, in which only one variable is changed.
C) It establishes two separate groups for men and women.
D) It eliminates the possibility of unintentional bias in the study.

26. Identify the cell structure marked below.

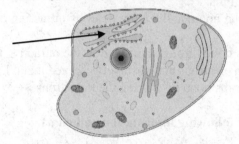

A) Smooth endoplasmic reticulum
B) Golgi apparatus
C) Mitochondria
D) Rough endoplasmic reticulum

27. Which of the following most accurately describes the role of the pancreas in digestion?

A) It produces sugar and growth-regulating biochemicals that empty directly into the bloodstream.
B) It absorbs water and nutrients from digesting food before the food enters the large intestine.
C) It produces hormones and digestive juices and secretes them into the duodenum.
D) It produces mucus to lubricate the food that is being digested in the stomach.

28. The chart below shows the names of various nitrogenous bases. Circle the nitrogenous base that is unique to DNA.

adenine
cytosine
guanine
thymine
uracil

GO ON TO THE NEXT PAGE

29. Which of the following hormones causes the uterine lining to thicken during ovulation?

A) Luteinizing hormone
B) Testosterone
C) Melatonin
D) Estrogen

30. Which of the following are type of white blood cells? Select all that apply.

A) Monocyte
B) Lymphocyte
C) Granulocyte
D) Erythrocyte

31. Which of the following is a membrane around the lungs?

A) Surfactant
B) Pleura
C) Alveoli
D) Bronchioles

32. A pathogen spreads to a susceptible host through a chain of infection. Put the following steps of that chain in order (1 = first; 5 = last).

_____ Portal of exit from reservoir
_____ Reservoir
_____ Portal of entry into host
_____ Mode of transmission

33. In Mendelian inheritance, what is the ratio of dominant to recessive traits in a dihybrid cross?

A) 9:3:3:1
B) 9:6:3:1
C) 6:2:1
D) 3:1

34. Which of the following responses can the body use to regulate its temperature on a hot day?

A) The pancreas releases insulin to signal the cells to uptake sugar.
B) The thyroid gland releases hormones to regulate metabolic rate.
C) Adrenal glands produce hormones to regulate blood pressure.
D) Sebaceous glands produce sweat to cool the surface of the skin.

GO ON TO THE NEXT PAGE

35. Which is the most appropriate unit to measure the mass of a paper clip?

A) Kilograms
B) Grams
C) Meters
D) Liters

36. In order to multiply, a virus must _____.

A) invade a host cell
B) combine with another virus
C) produce antigens
D) generate its own energy

37. Which of the following would be an effective surgical treatment for severe gastroesophageal reflux disease (GERD)?

A) A fundoplication to wrap the top part of the stomach around the lower part of the esophagus and tighten it
B) An appendectomy to remove the infected appendix and alleviate the severe abdominal pain
C) An esophagectomy to remove cancerous tumors from the esophagus
D) A tonsillectomy to remove the tonsils in the throat that cause repeated infections

38. Pulmonary respiration is the exchange of gases between the blood in the capillaries and the _____ of the lungs.

A) pharynx
B) alveoli
C) bronchi
D) bronchioles

39. Which type of reasoning moves from specific observations to more general theories?

A) Deductive
B) Operational
C) Inductive
D) Descriptive

40. Which of the following organs is used by both the reproductive and genitourinary systems in males?

A) Uterus
B) Kidney
C) Testes
D) Urethra

GO ON TO THE NEXT PAGE

41. Which of the following describes diastole?

   A) A contraction of the heart muscle
   B) A relaxation of the heart muscle
   C) The filtration of interstitial fluid
   D) The production of red blood cells

42. Which property of water allows water to stick to the sides of a straw?

   A) Solubility
   B) Surface tension
   C) Adhesion
   D) Cohesion

43. Laura wants to test her hypothesis that adding plant food to tomato plants will help them grow more tomatoes. Which of the following is the dependent variable?

   A) Type of soil used
   B) Number of tomatoes produced
   C) Amount of water used
   D) Addition of plant food

44. Which of the following types of motion do the molecules of a liquid exhibit?

   A) Lateral and translational
   B) Translational only
   C) Vibrational and translational
   D) Vibrational only

45. Which of the following are functions of the kidneys? Select all that apply.

   A) Produce white blood cells
   B) Remove waste products from the body
   C) Balance the body's fluids
   D) Release hormones that regulate blood pressure

46. Which equation shows the synthesis of water?

   A) $2Na + Cl_2 \rightarrow 2NaCl$
   B) $2H_2 + O_2 \rightarrow 2H_2O$
   C) $NaOH \rightarrow Na + OH$
   D) $4Fe + 3O_2 \rightarrow 2Fe_2O_3$

GO ON TO THE NEXT PAGE

47. In an experiment to test whether more time spent studying for a test will increase test scores, which of the following is the independent variable?

A) The subject matter of the test the students are given
B) The number of questions on the test
C) The scores the students receive on the test
D) The amount of time each student spends studying

48. How do the respiratory and circulatory systems work together?

A) The circulatory system carries blood to and from the lungs for gas exchange.
B) Blood is carried throughout the body by blood vessels.
C) The lungs exhale carbon dioxide out of the body and into the atmosphere.
D) The diaphragm and intercostal muscles contract and relax to allow air in and push air out of the lungs.

49. Which of the following is a name for a short, branched extension of a nerve cell that receives impulses from other cells?

A) Axon
B) Myofibrils
C) Dendrite
D) Synapse

50. Which of the following bones articulate at a hinge joint?

A) Humerus and scapula
B) L1 and L2 vertebrae
C) Radius and ulna
D) Femur and tibia

STOP. THIS IS THE END OF PART III.

Part IV. English and Language Usage

37 questions / 37 minutes

1. Which of the following sentences is punctuated correctly?

A) Lori told Sergio, "Hurry up! Were going to be late."
B) Lori told Sergio, "Hurry up! We're going to be late."
C) Lori told Sergio, "Hurry up! We're going to be late".
D) Lori told Sergio "Hurry up! We're going to be late."

> The rate of illegitimacy in both countries has risen dramatically, indicating a general acceptence of the practice among the populations.

2. Circle the word that is misspelled in the sentence above.

3. The use of the prefix *hyper* in the word *hypertension* indicates that a patient has which of the following?

A) High blood pressure
B) Low blood pressure
C) Fluctuating blood pressure
D) Irregular blood pressure

4. Which of the following are complete sentences? Select all that apply.

A) Word meanings can shift over time.
B) Some words acquire additional meanings, some words lose meanings.
C) Many words evolve entirely new meanings, and this is known as semantic change.
D) Why the changes occur is more difficult to determine.

> After the storm, Amee found a shivering puppy huddled under a tree branch.

5. Which of the following is the closest synonym to *huddled* as it is used in the sentence above?

A) Sleeping
B) Panting
C) Hiding
D) Curled up

GO ON TO THE NEXT PAGE

6. Which of the following uses correct capitalization?

    A) I invited my Uncle.
    B) Turn South on Bumguardner Street.
    C) Talk to Ms. Elba about your grade.
    D) Were you born in houston, Texas?

7. Which of the following is a simple sentence?

    A) I called my friend Dean to pick me up from the bus station.
    B) I told him to pick me up at noon, but the bus was late.
    C) While he has waiting, he read an entire magazine!
    D) Because he had nearly fallen asleep by the time I arrived.

The easy fit of the dress allows and emphasizes motion.

---

8. Which of the following shows the complete predicate from the sentence above?

    A) allows
    B) the easy fit of the dress
    C) emphasizes
    D) allows and emphasizes

9. For which of the following sentences would a citation be needed?

    A) Dr. Michael E. DeBakey was born on September 7, 1908.
    B) The patient's husband said, "Without this procedure, she would not have survived."
    C) It is important to provide continuous blood flow during operations.
    D) I believe that students should be required to take more science courses in high school.

10. Which of the following would be the best topic sentence for a paragraph about how the character Betty Crocker was created?

    A) Betty was a common female name in the early 1920s.
    B) Crocker was the name of the company's late secretary and director.
    C) Betty Crocker was not a real person, but a persona created by the advertising department.
    D) The Washburn-Crosby Company manufactured Gold Medal flour.

GO ON TO THE NEXT PAGE

11. Which of the following words is spelled correctly?

A) definite
B) seperate
C) infintave
D) recieve

12. Based on your knowledge of root words and affixes, which of the following means "the creation of bone"?

A) pathogenesis
B) osteogenesis
C) osteoarthritis
D) carcinogenesis

The teacher felt that the study session went well.

13. Which part of speech is *well*, as it is used in the sentence above?

A) adjective
B) verb
C) noun
D) adverb

I was just trying to ask the lady for the time, but she went bananas and started yelling.

14. Which of the following words from the sentence above is considered a colloquialism?

A) lady
B) time
C) bananas
D) yelling

She could not answer his question _____ she was too distracted by the ringing phone.

15. Write the correct punctuation mark in the blank above.

GO ON TO THE NEXT PAGE

Some of the old warehouses near the river have been torn down.

Some of them have been remodeled and converted to studio apartments.

16. Which of the following shows the best way to combine the two sentences above into one sentence that preserves the same meaning?

A) Some of the old warehouses near the river have been torn down and remodeled and converted to studio apartments.
B) Some of the old warehouses near the river have been torn down, but then they have been remodeled and converted to studio apartments.
C) Some of the old warehouses near the river have been torn down, remodeled, or converted to studio apartments.
D) Some of the old warehouses near the river have been torn down, while others have been remodeled and converted to studio apartments.

17. Which of the following suffixes means "examination or inspection"?

A) ology
B) opsy
C) osis
D) oid

The company is bankrupt due to the maladroit way in which the president handled purchases.

18. Which of the following best states the meaning of the word *maladroit* as it is used above?

A) Inept
B) Stupid
C) Greedy
D) Rude

19. Which of the following words is shown in its correct plural form?

A) Stratum
B) Syllabuses
C) Diagnoses
D) Axises

GO ON TO THE NEXT PAGE

> In the novel, we see the prewar ideals of chaste female and protective male that are implicit in imperial power being overthrown by the destabilizing and destructive force of the war.

20. The sentence above most likely came from which of the following sources?

    A) An advertisement
    B) A research paper
    C) A personal letter
    D) A company memo

21. Which of the following sentences shows correct subject-verb agreement?

    A) Each of the men bring a lunch to work.
    B) Twenty percent of the class like field trips.
    C) The girl and her mother quickly runs back home.
    D) Riding horses is my favorite activity.

22. Put the following steps of the writing process in the correct order from first (1) to last (4).

    _____ Proofread for spelling errors
    _____ Write a rough draft
    _____ Brainstorm ideas for examples
    _____ Revise the order of the paragraphs

23. Which of the following shows the verb *to follow* in singular past perfect tense?

    A) followed
    B) has followed
    C) following
    D) had followed

> She had intense cravings for salty foods, to the point that it interfered with her work.

24. Which of the following is the best synonym for *intense* as it is used in the sentence above?

    A) Mean
    B) Strong
    C) Hard
    D) Upsetting

GO ON TO THE NEXT PAGE

The cheetah ran very swiftly after the fleeing gazelle.

25. Which of the following words is used as an adjective in the previous sentence?

    A) cheetah
    B) ran
    C) very
    D) swiftly

26. Which of the following sentences shows correct word choice?

    A) I had to stay up late last night to write a paper for my biology class.
    B) I had to stay up late last night to wright a paper for my biology class.
    C) I had to stay up late last night to rite a paper for my biology class.
    D) I had to stay up late last night to right a paper for my biology class.

Questions 27–28 refer to the following paragraph.

(1) Making shortbread cookies is very simple and requires only three ingredients: butter, flour, and sugar. (2) I made them once for my mother and she loved them. (3) First, preheat the oven to 300°. (4) Then use an electric mixer to cream 1 cup butter and ½ cup sugar together. (5) Slowly mix in 2½ cups of flour. (6) Press the dough into an ungreased 9-by-13-inch pan, prick the dough all over with a fork, and sprinkle the top with more sugar. (7) Bake the dough for about 40 minutes until the edges are golden brown. (8) Let the pan cool for about 10 minutes and then cut the cookies into squares.

27. Circle the number of the sentence that should be removed from the paragraph.

28. Which of the following sentences would best conclude the paragraph?

    A) You can also cut them into other shapes before you bake them.
    B) Be sure to use the best quality butter you can find to make the cookies rich.
    C) If you don't have an electric mixer, just stir the butter and sugar together until you don't see granules of sugar anymore.
    D) Let the cookies cool completely before removing them from the pan or they may crumble.

GO ON TO THE NEXT PAGE

29. Which sentence below is punctuated correctly?

A) Anna Belle decided to go to the party since she had finished her homework.
B) Anna Belle decided to go to the party; since she had finished her homework.
C) Anna Belle decided to go to the party, since she had finished her homework.
D) Anna Belle decided to go, to the party, since she had finished her homework.

30. Which of the following is a run-on sentence?

A) William walked slowly back to the car after he had an exhausting day at the water park.
B) Slowly walking back to the car after William had an exhausting day at the water park.
C) William walked slowly back to the car; he had an exhausting day at the water park.
D) William walked slowly back to the car, he had an exhausting day at the water park.

31. At which stage of the writing process would the writer check for grammatical errors?

A) Prewriting
B) Drafting
C) Revising
D) Editing

32. In which of the following sentences does *set* mean *decide on*?

A) Cassie wanted to set the date for the dinner party.
B) Randy said he would cook the dinner if Cassie set the table.
C) That night, Cassie forgot to put the salt and pepper shaker set on the table.
D) After having cocktails, the dinner guests set their empty glasses on a tray.

Carson took a very long walk around the wooded area behind the baseball fields.

33. Circle the word in the sentence above that is an adverb.

GO ON TO THE NEXT PAGE

The next two questions refer to the following sentence.

> The patient exhibited hyposensitivity to pain, and his mother said he did not react when he burned his hand on the stove.

34. What type of sentence structure is used in the sentence above?

    A) Simple
    B) Compound
    C) Complex
    D) Compound-complex

35. In the sentence above, what is the meaning of the prefix *hypo*?

    A) Under
    B) Extreme
    C) Painful
    D) Large

The next two questions refer to the following sentence.

> There are three things Trisha loves spending time with her family, working as a welder, and roller skating with total abandon.

36. What punctuation mark should go after the word *loves* in the sentence above?

    A) Comma
    A) Semicolon
    B) Colon
    C) Quotation mark

37. What is the best synonym for *abandon* as it is used in the sentence above?

    A) Freedom
    B) Leave
    C) Renounce
    D) Recklessness

STOP. THIS IS THE END OF PART IV.

TEAS Practice Test: Answer Key

PART I: READING

1.	Fourth chart	19.	38	37.	A
2.	B	20.	5, 3, 2, 1, 4	38.	D
3.	A	21.	C	39.	C
4.	C	22.	A	40.	B
5.	B	23.	B	41.	Box 4
6.	A	24.	A	42.	D
7.	D	25.	C	43.	C
8.	A	26.	B	44.	A and C
9.	C	27.	D	45.	B
10.	A	28.	A		
11.	C	29.	B		
12.	Second sentence	30.	C		
13.	C	31.	B		
14.	A	32.	D		
15.	D	33.	A		
16.	B	34.	9035		
17.	A	35.	D		
18.	C	36.	C		

PART II: MATHEMATICS

1.	4, 1, 3, 2	14.	C	27.	C
2.	C	15.	Walk	28.	48
3.	A	16.	C	29.	A
4.	B	17.	A	30.	C
5.	B and D	18.	B	31.	B
6.	C	19.	D	32.	C
7.	D	20.	C	33.	A
8.	A	21.	C	34.	B
9.	4, 2, 3, 1	22.	B	35.	A
10.	C	23.	A	36.	D
11.	B	24.	B	37.	D
12.	D	25.	D	38.	A, B, C, and D
13.	106	26.	D		

PART III: SCIENCE

1. D
2. A
3. skeletal
4. Graph 2
5. C
6. 3, 2, 1, 4
7. chromatids
8. D
9. C
10. A
11. 46
12. B
13. D
14. B
15. A
16. A and C
17. B
18. A, B, and D
19. D
20. C
21. B
22. B
23. Subject F
24. A
25. B
26. D
27. C
28. thymine
29. D
30. A, B, and C
31. B
32. 2, 1, 4, 3
33. A
34. D
35. B
36. A
37. A
38. B
39. C
40. D
41. B
42. C
43. B
44. C
45. B, C, and D
46. B
47. D
48. A
49. C
50. D

PART IV: ENGLISH AND LANGUAGE USAGE

1. B
2. acceptence
3. A
4. A, C, and D
5. D
6. C
7. A
8. D
9. B
10. C
11. A
12. B
13. D
14. C
15. ;
16. D
17. B
18. A
19. C
20. B
21. D
22. 4, 2, 1, 3
23. D
24. B
25. C
26. A
27. 2
28. C
29. A
30. D
31. D
32. A
33. very
34. D
35. A
36. C
37. A

TEAS Practice Test: Explanatory Answers

Part I: Reading

1. Fourth chart. The first chart has an average fuel efficiency of only 28 miles per hour. The second chart has an eight-speed transmission rather than a six-speed. The third chart is over his maximum budget. The fourth chart is the only one that meets all the criteria.

2. B. *Othello* is italicized because it is the title of a play.

3. A. The first paragraph describes how mounds are formed and the types of places they are generally located. The second paragraph discusses the specific regions near the author in which mounds are found. Choice A is the best summary of the passage.

4. C. This statement is a conclusion drawn by the author, not a statement of proven fact.

5. B. The author most likely lives in northwest Canada. In the second paragraph, he refers to the area as *our Northwest* and mentions the *Canadian Pacific Hotel*.

6. A. When the author says *communication*, he means the way to travel from one river to another. *Ascending* means going up, so the sentence as a whole means that the way to travel from the Red River to the Rainy River is to go up the Red Lake River.

7. D. The first paragraph of the passage says, "The mounds are as a rule found in the midst of a fertile section of country, and it is pretty certain from this that the mound builders were agriculturists."

8. A. The passage is mostly a description of the mounds, and the second paragraph of the passage says, "Our Northwest has, however, been neglected in the accounts of the mound-bearing region." Therefore, the author's purpose is most likely to provide an account of the mounds to contribute to scholarship about them. The best answer is A.

9. C. Since all the students in Ms. Vinot's French class like ice cream and Valerie is a student in Ms. Vinot's French class, she must like ice cream.

10. A. This paragraph is most likely from a book review since it discusses the structure of a book of essays.

11. C. Since the paragraph is describing the development and layout of the book, the word *progress* means "to develop or move forward."

12. Second sentence. The first step is to cross the wide end over the thin end. The second step is to continue up behind the thin end and wrap around to the front side.

13. C. Since she needs eggs to make the cake, the most logical thing for her to do is go back inside and buy the eggs.

14. A. The diagram shows two characteristics of place: physical characteristics and human characteristics.

15. D. There are 25 multiple-choice questions, 10 short-answer, and one essay question. That is a total of 36 questions.

16. B. "Wear layers in ice" is shown as an example in the category of "Interaction of People with Environment" in the area of Relationships. The best answer is B.

17. A. The study showed a correlation between having taken more biology classes in college and being a licensed physician. It concludes that taking biology classes makes a person more likely to become a physician. The assumption made is that taking the classes *caused* the person to want to be a physician.

18. C. The conclusion is faulty because it states that taking biology classes makes a person more likely to become a physician. The causality of that statement is not proven by the argument. If a person already wanted to become a physician and therefore took more biology classes in order to achieve that goal, then taking the classes did not cause the person to want to become a physician. Choice D may seem as if weakens the argument, but it does not actually affect the conclusion.

19. 38. The thermometer reads 38 degrees Celsius.

20. 5, 3, 2, 1, 4. According to the timeline, Shakespeare married Anne Hathaway in 1582, had twins in 1585, wrote *Upset Crow* in 1592, wrote *Venus and Adonis* in 1593, and wrote *Hamlet* in 1601.

21. C. Shakespeare wrote *Hamlet* in 1601, the same year his father died.

22. A. The novel itself is the primary source.

23. B. The excerpt is primarily a narrative, though description is used.

24. A. The line shown is dialogue between Bill and Henry.

25. C. At the end of the passage, Bill goes into the brush with his gun. The passage says "it might be possible for him to awe the wolves and save the dog," which implies that he will shoot at the wolves to scare them away.

26. B. First, the sled overturns. Then the she-wolf lures One Ear away before she is joined by other wolves. Finally, Bill follows One Ear into the brush.

27. D. The passage says that the rifle "was jammed beneath the overturned sled, and by the time Henry had helped him to right the load, One Ear and the she-wolf were too close together and the distance too great to risk a shot." The best answer is D.

28. A. The description of how the she-wolf lures One Ear away from the sled provides a picture of her cleverness. Once the wolf pack appears, their danger is evident.

29. B. Add the shipping price to the purchase price. The best total price is from WINK, Inc.

30. C. Choice C expresses her opinion about the college. The other three statements are facts.

31. B. The letter is a job application.

32. D. To alleviate is to make something easier to endure or to lessen the effects of something.

33. A. If the second dial on the meter had the arrow pointing between 9 and 0, then that dial would be read as a 9, and the meter would read 1994.

34. 9035. This meter reads 9035 because the first dial is exactly on the 9, the second dial is between 0 and 1, the third dial is between 3 and 4, and the fourth dial is exactly on the 5.

35. D. The intended audience is a parent of a child who is staying in the intensive care unit of a hospital.

36. C. Since he wants the views of Hawaiians at the time the annexation occurred, the best source would be a newspaper from Hawaii on the date Hawaii was annexed.

37. A. DisneyQuest is #4 on the West Side, and the closest restaurant is Food Quest at #5.

38. D. Fuego is the only bar, #1 with the drink symbol, and is located in Pleasure Island.

39. C. If high levels of iridium are only caused by volcanic eruption or by meteorites, and volcanic eruptions of that magnitude are rare, then the likelihood of the iridium being deposited by a meteorite increases. Choice C best strengthens the scientists' argument.

40. B. The scientists examined physical evidence and drew a logical conclusion from that evidence.

41. Box 4. The X is moved up one space to box 2 and then right two spaces to box 4.

42. D. The X is moved left one space to box 5, then down two spaces to box 13, then right two spaces to box 15.

43. C. After making a pile of tinder, you make sparks with the sparking stick to light the tinder.

44. A and C. The directions emphasize that the tinder must be shredded finely and that the tinder must be dry.

45. B. The author is giving people helpful information about the company picnic.

Part II: Mathematics

1. 4, 1, 3, 2. Estimate the values of the fractions and the root. $\sqrt{3} \approx \sqrt{4} \approx 2$. $-\dfrac{8}{3} \approx -\dfrac{8}{4} \approx -2$. $\dfrac{19}{5} \approx \dfrac{20}{5} \approx 4$. The values from greatest to least would be: $\dfrac{19}{5}, \sqrt{3}, -\dfrac{8}{3}, -4.26$.

2. C. If the rug costs \$90.00 wholesale, first find the 45% increase: $90 \times \dfrac{45}{100} = \dfrac{4050}{100} = 40.5$. Now add that to the original \$90.00: $90 + 40.5 = 130.50$.

3. A. Since the amount of sugar he used was twice the original amount, he must also double the butter and flour. He should add 1 cup of butter and 2½ cups flour.

4. B. Each bottle is worth 5 cents, but she should use this number expressed in dollars (\$.05) since she is trying to get to \$40.00. This would let her write the equation .05 $(x) = 40$. Since she already has 43 bottles, though, the equation should be modified to .05 $(x + 43) = 40$.

5. B and D. Check each answer choice to see whether it is true. The mode of the data set is 80 since 4 students scored an 80. The median is found by adding up the number of values and identifying the middle value: there are 17 students, so the middle value will be number 9. That score is an 80. Choice A is not true. Choice B asks about the range. $100 - 55 = 45$, so choice B is true. Choice C is not true since the median and range are not equal. Choice D is true since the median and mode are both 80.

6. C. Since the percent of Kathy's salary that she puts into her retirement plan remains constant, the amount she puts in goes up when her salary goes up. Those values are positively correlated. Choices A and D show negative correlations.

7. D. Divide each measurement by 4: $\dfrac{18}{4} = 4.5$ and $\dfrac{12}{4} = 3$, so the model living room should measure 4.5 inches by 3 inches.

8. A. The data points show that GPA generally decreases with more time spent playing video games.

9. 4, 2, 3, 1. Calculate the values. Choice A: $0.3 \times 320 = 96$. Choice B: $\dfrac{3}{4} \times 75 = 56.25$. Choice C: $4^3 = 64$. Choice D: 20% of $240 = 48$. Now put them in order from least to greatest.

10. C. If the wheel radius is 1.5 inches, then the diameter is 3 inches. Use the circumference formula to find the distance around the wheel in 1 revolution. $c = \pi d$, so $c = 3\pi$. Since the question asks the distance travelled in 4 revolutions, multiply the circumference by 4: $3\pi \times 4 = 12\pi$.

11. B. Since she has run ¼ the distance in 75 minutes, she has ¾ of the distance left. At the same rate, she will run that in $75 \times 3 = 225$ minutes. The question asks for the answer in hours, so divide 225 by 60 to get the answer in hours. $225 \div 60 = 3.75$ hours.

12. D. First multiply the fractions in parentheses: $\dfrac{2}{6} \times \dfrac{3}{5} = \dfrac{6}{30} = \dfrac{1}{5}$. Then add the final fraction. $\dfrac{1}{5} + \dfrac{9}{11} = \dfrac{11}{55} + \dfrac{45}{55} = \dfrac{56}{55}$. This is already reduced to its lowest terms.

13. 106. To find an average, add up the total number of points and divide by the number of terms you added up. For example, you could find his current average: $83 + 74 + 92 + 96 + 89 = 434$. Divide by 5 scores to find the average. $434 \div 5 = 86.8$. If he wants an average of 90, then he will need a total of 540 points since $6 \times 90 = 540$. Find the difference. $540 - 434 = 106$ points.

14. C. Distribute the 5 across the parentheses. $5(4x^2 - 10) = 20x^2 - 50$.

15. Walk. Average the percentage for men and women for each mode of transportation. Combined, about 55% use an automobile, 15% use a motorcycle, 17.5% use a bicycle, and 12.5% walk.

16. C. According to the chart, 20% of the women surveyed ride bicycles. If 540 women were surveyed, then $540 \times .2 = 108$ women ride bicycles.

17. A. Since 3.5% is the same as $\dfrac{35}{1,000}$, choice A shows 3.5% of 40: $\dfrac{35}{1,000} \times 40$.

18. B. First, distribute the 6 across the parentheses:

$$6(x - 8) = -42$$
$$6x - 48 = -42$$

Now add 48 to both sides. $\qquad 6x = 6$
Divide both sides by 6. $\qquad\quad x = 1$

19. D. Use the formula $F = \dfrac{9}{5}C + 32$. Since the Celsius temperature is 25 degrees, plug that into the formula for C. $F = \dfrac{9}{5} \times 25 + 32$. Now solve for F.

$$F = \frac{9}{5} \times 25 + 32$$
$$F = 45 + 32$$
$$F = 77$$

20. C. To find the rate for each job, she would need to divide her pay by the number of hours worked. For the first job, that would be $58 \div 4 = 14.5$, which is choice C.

21. C. Set up a proportion with actual feet on top and inches on the drawing on the bottom. $\frac{22}{18} = \frac{x}{3}$. Now solve for x.

$$22 \times 3 = 18x$$
$$66 = 18x$$
$$x = \frac{66}{18} = 3.67$$

22. B. If she uses the $10-off coupon, the price will be $65. If she uses the 25%-off coupon, then the discount will be $75 \times .25 = 18.75$. $75 - 18.75 = 56.25$. That would be the lowest price, so the answer is B.

23. A. If the ratio is 4 parts woodwinds to 2 parts horns to 1 part trumpet, then there are 7 total parts. Since the total number of people is 84, divide that by the 7 total parts to get a multiplier of 12. For the trumpets, then, there will be 1 part times the multiplier of 12. $1 \times 12 = 12$.

24. B. The inequality is: $3x - 7 \geq 17$. Add 7 to both sides to get $3x \geq 24$. Divide both sides by 3 to get $x \geq 8$.

25. D. If x is the number of small boxes at $12 each and y is the number of medium boxes at $24 each, then the expression will be $12x + 24y$.

26. D. You know the July sales, so start there. July is $9,000 and that is 120% of June's sales. Let June $= x$. $9,000 = 1.2x$. $x = 7,500$. Now you know June's sales. Let May $= y$. June $= 80\%$ of May, so $7,500 = .8y$, and then $y = 9,375$.

27. C. Line up the two equations so that you can add them.

$$\begin{array}{r} 6x - 4y = -8 \\ +7x + 4y = -18 \\ \hline 13x = -26 \\ x = -2 \end{array}$$

Since the question asks for the value of y, plug $x = -2$ into one of the equations to solve for y.

$$6x - 4y = -8$$
$$6(-2) - 4y = -8$$
$$-12 - 4y = -8$$
$$-4y = 4$$
$$y = -1$$

28. 48. To find the volume of a rectangle, you need the area of the base times the height: $V = lwh$. Since the base is 4 inches square and the height is 6, $V = 4 \times 4 \times 6 = 96$. We only need half the volume, so $V = 48$.

29. A. She needs two 8-foot panels for each of two windows, so that is 32 feet total. Since the fabric is measured in yards, you must convert 32 feet to yards. Set up a proportion: $\frac{32\,\text{feet}}{x\,\text{yards}} = \frac{3\,\text{feet}}{1\,\text{yard}}$. $32 \times 1 = 3 \times x$.

$x = \frac{32}{3} = 10.67$ or $10\frac{2}{3}$.

30. C. Choice C provides the best estimate by rounding the number of books down slightly to 200 and their average width up slightly to 1.5. Choice B shows the actual calculations, which is not an estimate.

31. B. On the graph, Ft. Worth's entire line lies beneath those of Tulsa and Wichita. It can be concluded that Ft. Worth has less snowfall between December and March than does either Tulsa or Wichita.

32. C. Use the formula $d = r \times t$. The distance is 1.5 miles and she needs to cover that distance in 15 minutes. You are looking for her rate in miles per hour, so make sure you use the formula with t expressed in hours rather than in minutes. 15 minutes $= \dfrac{1}{4}$ hour.

$$1.5 \text{ miles} = r \times \frac{1}{4}$$

Divide both sides by $\dfrac{1}{4}$ to find the rate: $\dfrac{1.5}{4} = r$, so $r = 6$ mph.

33. A. 12.5% can be written as $\dfrac{12.5}{100}$ or 0.125.

34. B. The area of the square is $16 \times 16 = 256$. The area of the semicircle is $\dfrac{1}{2}\pi r^2 = \dfrac{1}{2}\pi 8^2 = 32\pi$. You can estimate $\pi = 3$. That gives you an area of $32 \times 3 = 96$ for the semicircle. $256 + 96 = 352$. Since you rounded down a bit to estimate π, the actual amount will be a bit bigger than 352. The best estimate shown is 360.

35. A. Estimate the values: $\dfrac{8}{3} > 2$, $\sqrt{2} \approx 1.7$; $\dfrac{5}{4} = 1.25$. The greatest is $\dfrac{8}{3}$.

36. D. Solve for x.

$5x + 2(x - 9) = 4x + 6$	Distribute the 2 across the parentheses.
$5x + 2x - 18 = 4x + 6$	Combine $5x + 2x$.
$7x - 18 = 4x + 6$	Add 18 to both sides.
$7x = 4x + 24$	Subtract $4x$ from both sides.
$3x = 24$	Divide both sides by 3.
$x = 8$	

37. D. $60 \times 25 = 1{,}500$; $1{,}500 \times 4$ bottles $= 6{,}000$; $6{,}000 \div 50 \dfrac{\text{mg}}{\text{dose}} = 120$.

38. A, B, C, and D. $3x \leq x + 7$. Subtract x from both sides: $2x \leq 7$; divide both sides by 2: $x \leq 3.5$.

Part III: Science

1. D. The medulla oblongata controls respiration by monitoring carbon dioxide levels and detecting blood pH.

2. A. Lipids serve as structural components of cell membranes, store energy, provide long-term energy, and have some important signaling functions.

3. Skeletal. Skeletal muscle tissue makes up approximately 40% of a person's body mass.

4. Graph 2. A catalyst increases the rate of a reaction, which reduces the amount of activation energy needed for the reaction.

5. C. Of the options given, only a graduated cylinder measures volume.

6. 3, 2, 1, 4. The molecules in plasma have the most energy, while the molecules in a solid have the least.

7. Chromatids. Chromatids are two identical copies of a chromosome formed during the cell cycle.

8. D. Both prokaryotic and eukaryotic cells have cytoplasm. Only eukaryotic cells have a nucleus and membrane-bound organelles, while only prokaryotic cells have circular DNA.

9. C. Bones physically join with the neuromuscular system via connective tissues such as ligaments and tendons.

10. A. The scenario presented suggests a causal relationship between checklists for surgical procedures and rate of errors. This means that checklists can be an effective tool for fighting surgical errors. Choice B draws a further conclusion and is too extreme.

11. 46. Humans typically have 23 pairs of chromosomes for a total of 46 chromosomes.

12. B. In the process of diffusion, a substance moves from an area of high concentration to areas of low concentration.

13. D. The function of the glomerulus is to bring blood (and the waste products it carries) to the nephron. Glomeruli carry out the primary filtering action of the kidney.

14. B. The skin can be divided into three layers: epidermis, dermis, and hypodermis. The dermis is the middle layer.

15. A. The median plane divides the human body vertically into left and right sides.

16. A and C. The four types of macromolecules are carbohydrates, lipids, proteins, and nucleic acids.

17. B. If the pancreas stops releasing insulin, then sugar will not enter cells. This will cause high blood sugar levels and diabetes.

18. A, B, and D. Blood plasma contains nutrients, hormones, antibodies, and other immune proteins. Hemoglobin is contained in red blood cells.

19. D. This equation shows a total of six carbon atoms, 18 oxygen atoms, and 12 hydrogen atoms on each side of the equation.

20. C. The most accurate way shown to measure the amount of mold growth would be choice C: to measure the surface area with a ruler and express the mold growth as a percent of the total area.

21. B. Neutral pH measures 7 on the pH scale.

22. B. An ionic bond is usually between a metal and a nonmetal. They bond by attracting oppositely charged ions.

23. Subject F. Calculate the weight loss for each subject by subtracting the weight after two years from the starting weight. The subject who had the greatest amount of weight lost after two years is Subject F, with a weight loss of 95 lb.

24. A. Choice A is true. The three males lost 145 pounds combined at the six-month mark, while the females had only lost 90 pounds combined. However, at the end of two years, the females had lost 245 pounds combined, and the men had lost 225 pounds combined.

25. B. The instructions not to change diet or exercise constitute a controlled setting, with only one variable: the medication.

26. D. The structure identified is the rough endoplasmic reticulum.

27. C. The pancreas produces hormones and digestive juices and secretes them into the duodenum.

28. Thymine. DNA and RNA both have adenine, cytosine, and guanine. DNA also has thymine, while RNA has uracil.

29. D. Estrogen causes the uterine lining to thicken during ovulation.

30. A, B, and C. Monocytes, lymphocytes, and granulocytes are types of white blood cells, while erythrocytes are red blood cells.

31. B. The pleura is a membrane around the lungs.

32. 2, 1, 4, 3. An infectious agent moves from its normal location (reservoir) through some portal of exit. The mode of transmission is how the pathogen comes into contact with a potential host. If that host has a portal of entry, the pathogen can then move into the host.

33. A. In Mendelian inheritance, the ratio of dominant to recessive traits in a dihybrid cross is 9:3:3:1.

34. D. When the body gets too hot, the sebaceous glands produce sweat to cool the surface of the skin.

35. B. The best unit of measure for the mass of a paper clip would be in grams. Kilograms also measure mass, but would be more appropriate units to use for larger items.

36. A. Viruses must invade a host cell in order to use energy from that cell to multiply. Viruses do not produce their own energy.

37. A. Gastroesophageal reflux disease (GERD) is a condition in which acidic stomach contents come back up into the esophagus. One surgical treatment for GERD is a fundoplication to wrap the top part of the stomach around the lower part of the esophagus and tighten it so that the acid does not splash out.

38. B. Pulmonary respiration is the exchange of gases between the blood in the capillaries and the alveoli of the lungs.

39. C. Inductive reasoning involves forming a generalization based on specific observations or experiments.

40. D. The urethra is used by both the reproductive and genitourinary systems.

41. B. Diastole is the phase of the heartbeat in which the heart muscle relaxes and allows the chamber to fill with blood.

42. C. Adhesion is the attraction between water and other molecules. Water exhibits adhesion when its attraction to another substance is greater than the water's attraction to itself (cohesion).

43. B. The number of tomatoes grown is the dependent variable, while the addition of plant food is the independent variable.

44. C. The molecules of a liquid exhibit both vibrational and translational motion.

45. B, C, and D. The kidneys remove waste products from the body, balance the body's fluids, release hormones that regulate blood pressure, produce a hormone that stimulates red blood cell production, and produce an active form of vitamin D. They do not produce white blood cells.

46. B. Synthesis of water is shown by combining two hydrogen and one oxygen atoms: $2H_2 + O_2 \rightarrow 2H_2O$

47. D. The independent variable is the thing that is changed in the experiment. In this case, that would be the amount of time each student spends studying. The dependent variable is the scores the students receive on the test. The subject matter of the test and the number of questions on the test are controls since they would be the same for everyone.

48. A. The respiratory and circulatory systems work together in exchanging oxygen and carbon dioxide. The circulatory system carries deoxygenated blood to the lungs, which exhale carbon dioxide and oxygenate the blood that is returned to the body.

49. C. Dendrites are short, branched extensions of nerve cells that receive impulses from other cells.

50. D. The femur and tibia are articulated with a hinge joint at the knee.

Part IV: English and Language Usage

1. B. Choice A omits the apostrophe in the contraction *we're*. Choice C has the period outside the quotation marks. Choice D does not use a comma to introduce the quote.

2. Acceptence. The correct spelling is *acceptance*.

3. A. The prefix *hyper* means *too much* or *a lot*, so a person with hypertension has high blood pressure.

4. A, C, and D. Choice B has two independent clauses joined together improperly with a comma.

5. D. *Huddled* means *curled up* or *nestled*.

6. C. Choice A should not use a capital for *Uncle* unless it also uses the person's name, such as *Uncle Jack*. Choice B should not capitalize *South*. Choice D should capitalize both the city and state.

7. A. Choice A is a simple sentence with one independent clause.

8. D. This sentence has a compound predicate: *allows and emphasizes*.

9. B. Direct quotations always require a citation. Choice A does not require a citation because it is a fact that can be easily verified from many sources.

10. C. This sentence introduces the idea of Betty Crocker as a character. The other choices provide details about the name and background on the company.

11. A. *Definite* is spelled correctly.

12. B. Osteogenesis is the formation of bone. The prefix *osteo* means *relating to* bone and the root *genesis* means *creation*.

13. D. *Well* is used as an adverb to describe how the study session was going.

14. C. *Bananas* is a colloquialism meaning *crazy*.

15. ;. The phrases shown are both related independent clauses, so they can be joined by a semicolon. They could also be joined by a period, but the second phrase would need to begin with a capital letter to start the new sentence.

16. D. Since the original sentences show two different outcomes for the old warehouses, the new sentence needs to preserve that meaning. Choice D does that best.

17. B. The suffix *opsy* means *examination* or *inspection*.

18. A. *Maladroit*, in this context, means *inept*.

19. C. The correct plural word is *diagnoses*.

20. B. This sentence is most likely from a research paper. It does not appear to promote anything, it is too formal for a personal letter, and it uses academic rather than professional language.

21. D. Choice D uses correct subject-verb agreement. Choice A incorrectly uses the plural verb *bring* with the singular subject *each*. Choice B incorrectly uses the plural verb *like* with the singular *class*. Choice C has a compound subject *the girl and her mother* but uses the singular verb *runs*.

22. 4, 2, 1, 3. The first of these steps would be brainstorming, followed by drafting, revising, and proofreading.

23. D. The past perfect of *to follow* is *had followed*.

24. B. The best synonym for *intense* is *strong*.

25. C. *Very* is an adjective modifying the adverb *swiftly*.

26. A. The correct word choice for this situation is *write*.

27. B. The personal note does not need to be a part of the recipe.

28. C. Choice C adds an important final step to the instructions.

29. A. Choice A is correct. No punctuation is needed before *since*.

30. D. Choice D is a run-on sentence. Two independent clauses cannot be joined by just a comma.

31. D. The writer should check for grammatical errors during the final editing phase of the writing process.

32. A. In choice A, *set the date* means to decide on a date for the party.

33. Very. The word *very* is an adverb that modifies the adjective *long. Baseball* and *wooded* are also adjectives.

34. D. This is a compound-complex sentence because it has two independent clauses joined by a comma and coordinating conjunction, plus the dependent clause *when he burned his hand on the stove.*

35. A. *Hypo* means less than normal, or under. The patient showed a less than normal response to pain.

36. C. There should be a colon after *loves* because the rest of the sentence is a list of the three things.

37. A. As used in the sentence, *abandon* means she is completely uninhibited. The best synonym is *freedom.*

NOTES

NOTES

NOTES

NOTES

NOTES

NOTES

NOTES

NOTES

NOTES

NOTES